Zang Fu
PATTERN IDENTIFICATION
Study Guide

Zang Fu
PATTERN IDENTIFICATION
Study Guide

Qiao Yi
with Julie Liu

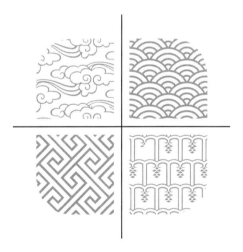

EASTLAND PRESS · SEATTLE

Copyright 2021 by Qiao Yi

Published by Eastland Press, Inc.
P.O. Box 99749
Seattle, WA 98139, USA
www.eastlandpress.com

All rights reserved. No part of this book may be reproduced or transmitted in any form or by any means, electronic or mechanical, including photocopying, recording, or by any information storage and retrieval system, without the prior written permission of the publisher, except where permitted by law.

Library of Congress Control Number: 2020938294
ISBN: 978-0-939616-96-1
Printed in the United States of America

2   4   6   8   10   9   7   5   3   1

Book design by Gary Niemeier

Table of Contents

ACKNOWLEDGEMENTS, xiii

INTRODUCTION, xv

▣ PART 1: ZANG ORGANS 1

Chapter 1: **Heart Disease Patterns** 2

    Physiological characteristics and functions of the Heart 2

    Pathological changes and major clinical manifestations of Heart disease 4

    Common etiological factors in Heart patterns 4

    Common patterns in Heart disease 9

      1. **Heart Qi Deficiency Pattern** | 心氣虛証 | 10

      2. **Heart Yang Deficiency Pattern** | 心陽虛証 | 11

      3. **Heart Yang Collapse Pattern** | 心陽暴脱証 | 12

        Comparison: Heart Qi Deficiency vs. Heart Yang Deficiency vs. Heart Yang Collapse 13

      4. **Heart Blood Deficiency Pattern** | 心血虛証 | 14

      5. **Heart Yin Deficiency Pattern** | 心陰虛証 | 15

        Comparison: Heart Blood Deficiency vs. Heart Yin Deficiency 16

      6. **Heart Fire Blazing Pattern** | 心火上炎証 | 17

      7. **Phlegm-Fire Harassing the Heart Pattern** | 痰火擾心証 | 18

        Comparison: Heart Fire Blazing vs. Phlegm-Fire Harassing the Heart 20

      8. **Phlegm Misting the Heart Pattern** | 痰謎心竅証 | 20

        Comparison: Phlegm Misting the Heart vs. Phlegm-Fire Harrassing the Heart 22

      9. **Heart Vessels Obstruction Pattern** | 心脈瘀阻 | 22

    Summary of Heart Disease Patterns 25

Chapter 2: **Lung Disease Patterns** 26

    Physiological characteristics and functions of the Lung 26

    Common etiological factors in Lung patterns 28

    Pathological changes and major clinical manifestations of Lung disease 29

    Common patterns in Lung disease 33

1. **Lung Qi Deficiency Pattern** | 肺氣虛証 | 34
2. **Lung Yin Deficiency Pattern** | 肺陰虛証 | 35
3. **Wind-Cold Invading the Lung Pattern** | 風寒犯肺 | 36
   Comparison: Wind-Cold Invading the Lung vs. Exterior Wind-Cold   37
4. **Wind-Heat Invading the Lung Pattern** | 風熱犯肺 | 38
   Comparison: Wind-Cold Invading the Lung vs. Wind-Heat Invading the Lung   39
   Comparison: Wind-Heat Invading the Lung vs. Exterior Wind-Heat   40
5. **Dryness Invading the Lung Pattern** | 燥邪犯肺 | 41
   Comparison: Dryness Invading the Lung vs. Exterior Dryness   43
   Comparison: Dryness Invading the Lung vs. Lung Yin Deficiency   43
   Comparison: Exopathogenic Factors Invading the Lung   44
6. **Wind-Water Invading the Lung Pattern** | 風水犯肺 | 46
7. **Cold Invading the Lung Pattern** | 寒邪客肺 | 47
8. **Turbid Phlegm Obstructing the Lung Pattern** | 痰濁阻肺 | 48
   Comparison: Wind-Cold Invading the Lung vs. Cold Invading the Lung vs. Cold-Phlegm Obstructing the Lung   50
9. **Heat Congesting the Lung Pattern** | 熱邪壅肺 | 51
   Comparison: Wind-Heat Invading the Lung vs. Heat Congesting the Lung vs. Heat-Phlegm Obstructing the Lung   52
10. **Cold-Water Shooting into the Lung Pattern** | 寒水射肺 | 53
    Comparison: Cold-Phlegm Obstructing the Lung vs. Cold-Water Shooting into the Lung   55

Summary of Lung Disease Patterns   56

Chapter 3: **Spleen Disease Patterns**   57

Physiological characteristics and functions of the Spleen   57
Common etiological factors in Spleen patterns   58
Pathological changes and major clinical manifestations of Spleen disease   59
Common patterns in Spleen disease   62

1. **Spleen Qi Deficiency Pattern** | 脾氣虛証 | 63
2. **Spleen Qi Sinking Pattern** | 脾氣下陷 | 64
3. **Spleen Not Controlling Blood Pattern** | 脾不統血 | 66
4. **Spleen Yang Deficiency Pattern** | 脾陽虛証 | 67
   Comparison: Spleen Qi Deficiency vs. Spleen Qi Sinking vs. Spleen Not Controlling Blood vs. Spleen Yang Deficiency   68
5. **Spleen Yin Deficiency Pattern** | 脾陰虛証 | 70

6. **Cold-dampness Encumbering the Spleen Pattern** | 寒濕睏脾 | **71**

   Comparison: Cold-Dampness Encumbering the Spleen vs. Spleen Yang Deficiency with Cold-Dampness   72

   Comparison: Cold-Dampness Encumbering the Spleen vs. Water-Dampness Immersion   73

7. **Damp-Heat Encumbering the Spleen Pattern** | 濕熱睏脾 | **74**

   Comparison: Damp-heat Encumbering the Spleen vs. Cold-dampness Encumbering the Spleen   76

Summary of Spleen Disease Patterns   77

Chapter 4: Liver Disease Patterns   78

Physiological characteristics and functions of the Liver   78

Common etiological factors in Liver patterns   80

Pathological changes and major clinical manifestations of the Liver   81

Common patterns in Liver disease   85

1. **Liver Blood Deficiency Pattern** | 肝血虛証 | **87**
2. **Liver Yin Deficiency Pattern** | 肝陰虛証 | **88**

   Comparison: Liver Yin Deficiency vs. Liver Blood Deficiency   90

3. **Liver Qi Stagnation Pattern** | 肝鬱氣滯証 | **90**
4. **Liver Fire Blazing Pattern** | 肝火上炎証 | **92**

   Comparison: Liver Fire Blazing vs. Heart Fire Blazing   93

5. **Liver Yang Rising Pattern** | 肝陽上亢証 | **94**

   Comparison: Liver Fire Blazing vs. Liver Yang Rising   95

   Comparison: Liver Yin Deficiency vs. Liver Yang Rising   96

6. **Liver Wind Stirring Internally Pattern** | 肝風內動 | **97**

6.1. **Liver Yang Transforming into Wind Pattern** | 肝陽化風 | **97**

6.2. **Extreme Heat Generating Wind Pattern** | 熱極生風 | **99**

6.3. **Blood Deficiency Generating Wind Pattern** | 血虛生風 | **100**

6.4. **Yin Deficiency Generating Wind Pattern** | 陰虛生風 | **101**

   Comparison: Liver Yang Rising vs. Liver Yang Transforming into Wind   102

   Comparison: Liver Yang Transforming into Wind vs. Wind-Phlegm Disturbing Upward   103

7. **Cold Stagnation in Liver Channel Pattern** | 寒滯肝脈 | **104**
8. **Liver Blood Stagnation Pattern** | 肝血瘀滯 | **105**

Liver disease patterns relationship and development   106

Summary of Liver Disease Patterns   107

Chapter 5: **Kidney Disease Patterns**   108

Physiological characteristics and functions of the Kidney   108
Common etiological factors in Kidney disease   112
Pathological changes and major clinical manifestations of the Kidney   112
Common patterns in Kidney disease   115

1. **Kidney Qi Deficiency Pattern** | 腎氣虛証 | 117
2. **Kidney Qi Failing to Secure Pattern** | 腎氣不固 | 118
   Comparison: Kidney Qi Failing to Secure vs. Spleen Qi Sinking   120
3. **Kidney Failing to Grasp Qi Pattern** | 腎不納氣 | 120
   Comparison: Kidney Failing to Grasp Qi vs. Lung Qi Deficiency   122
4. **Kidney Yang Deficiency Pattern** | 腎陽虛証 | 122
   Comparison: Kidney Qi Failing to Secure vs. Kidney Yang Deficiency   124
   Comparison: Kidney Qi Deficiency vs. Kidney Yang Deficiency vs. Kidney Qi Failing to Secure vs. Kidney Failing to Grasp Qi   125
5. **Kidney Yang Deficiency with Water Effusion** | 腎虛水泛 | 126
   Comparison: Kidney Yang Deficiency with Water Effusion vs. Cold-Water Shooting into the Lung vs. Water Qi Encroaching on the Heart   128
6. **Kidney Yin Deficiency Pattern** | 腎陰虛証 | 129
7. **Kidney Essence Deficiency Pattern** | 腎精不足 | 131
   Comparison: Kidney Yin Deficiency vs. Kidney Essence Deficiency   132

Kidney disease patterns relationship and development   133
Summary of Kidney Disease Patterns   134

PART 2: FU ORGANS ········ 135

Chapter 6: **Stomach Disease Patterns**   136

Physiological characteristics and functions of the Stomach   136
Common etiological factors in Stomach patterns   137
Pathological changes and major clinical manifestations of the Stomach   137
Common patterns in Stomach disease   141

1. **Stomach Yin Deficiency Pattern** | 胃陰虛 | 142
   Comparison: Stomach Yin Deficiency vs. Spleen Yin Deficiency   143
   Comparison: Stomach Yin Deficiency vs. Large Intestine Dryness   144
2. **Stomach Deficiency Cold Pattern** | 胃中虛寒 | 145
   Comparison: Stomach Deficiency Cold vs. Spleen Yang Deficiency   146
3. **Stomach Fire Pattern** | 胃熱熾盛 | 147
   Comparison: Stomach Fire vs. Stomach Yin Deficiency   148

4. **Cold Invading the Stomach Pattern** | 寒邪犯胃 | **149**

   Comparison: Cold Invading the Stomach vs. Stomach Deficiency Cold   151

   Comparison: Cold Invading the Stomach vs. Cold-Dampness Encumbering the Spleen   152

5. **Food Stagnation Pattern** | 食滯腸胃 | **153**

6. **Blood Stagnation in the Stomach Pattern** | 血瘀胃脘 | **154**

Summary of Stomach Disease Patterns   155

Chapter 7: **Small Intestine Disease Patterns**   156

Physiological characteristics and functions of the Small Intestine   156

Pathological changes and major clinical manifestations of Small Intestine disease   157

Common etiological factors in Small Intestine patterns   157

Common patterns in Small Intestine disease   160

1. **Small Intestine Deficiency Cold Pattern** | 小腸虛寒 | **160**

2. **Small Intestine Excess Fire Pattern** | 小腸實火 | **162**

3. **Small Intestine Qi Stagnation Pattern** | 小腸氣滯 | **163**

Summary of Small Intestine Disease Patterns   164

Chapter 8: **Large Intestine Disease Patterns**   165

Physiological characteristics and functions of the Large Intestine   165

Common etiological factors in Large Intestine patterns   166

Pathological changes and major clinical manifestations of Large Intestine disease   166

Common patterns in Large Intestine disease   168

1. **Large Intestine Deficiency Cold Pattern** | 大腸虛寒 | **169**

   Comparison: Large Intestine Deficiency Cold vs. Spleen Yang Deficiency vs. Kidney Yang Deficiency   170

   Comparison: Large Intestine Deficiency Cold vs. Small Intestine Deficiency Cold   171

2. **Large Intestine Dryness Pattern** | 大腸液虧 | **172**

3. **Large Intestine Cold-Dampness Pattern** | 大腸寒濕 | **173**

   Comparison: Large Intestine Cold-Dampness vs. Large Intestine Deficiency Cold   174

4. **Large Intestine Damp-Heat Pattern** | 大腸濕熱 | **175**

   Comparison: Large Intestine Damp-Heat vs. Large Intestine Cold-Dampness   176

   Comparison: Large Intestine Damp-Heat vs. Damp-Heat Encumbering the Spleen   177

5. **Large Intestine Heat Accumulation Pattern** | 大腸熱結 | **178**

   Comparison: Large Intestine Heat Accumulation vs. Large Intestine Dryness   180

   Comparison: Large Intestine Heat Accumulation vs. Large Intestine Damp-Heat   181

Summary of Large Intestine Disease Patterns   182

Chapter 9: **Gallbladder Disease Patterns**   **183**

Physiological characteristics and functions of the Gallbladder   183
Common etiological factors in Gallbladder patterns   184
Pathological changes and major clinical manifestations of the Gallbladder   184
Common patterns in Gallbladder disease   186

    1. **Gallbladder Qi Deficiency Pattern** | 膽氣虛証 | **187**

    2. **Gallbladder Heat Pattern** | 膽熱証 | **188**
        Comparison: Gallbladder Heat vs. Liver Fire Blazing   189

    3. **Gallbladder Stagnation with Phlegm Disturbance** | 膽鬱痰擾証 | **191**
        Comparison: Gallbladder Stagnation with Phlegm Disturbance vs. Gallbladder Heat   192
        Comparison: Gallbladder Stagnation with Phlegm Disturbance vs.
         Heart Fire Blazing   193
        Comparison: Gallbladder Stagnation with Phlegm Disturbance vs. Phlegm-Fire
         Harassing the Heart   194

Summary of Gallbladder Disease Patterns   195

Chapter 10: **Urinary Bladder Disease Patterns**   **196**

Physiological characteristics and functions of the Urinary Bladder   196
Common etiological factors in Urinary Bladder patterns   197
Pathological changes and major clinical manifestations of the Urinary Bladder   197
Common patterns in Urinary Bladder disease   198

    1. **Urinary Bladder Deficiency Cold Pattern** | 膀胱虛寒 | **199**
        Comparison: Urinary Bladder Deficiency Cold vs. Kidney Yang Deficiency   200
        Comparison: Urinary Bladder Deficiency Cold vs. Small Intestine Deficiency Cold   201

    2. **Urinary Bladder Damp-Heat Pattern** | 膀胱濕熱証 | **202**
        Comparison: Urinary Bladder Damp-Heat vs. Small Intestine Excess Fire   203

Summary of Urinary Bladder Disease Patterns   205

▌ PART 3: COMPOUND PATTERNS ········ 207

Methods to identify compound *zàng fǔ* patterns   208
Common compound *zàng fǔ* patterns   209

Chapter 11: **Heart and Lung**   **210**

Pathophysiological relationship between the Heart and Lung   210

    1. **Heart and Lung Qi Deficiency Pattern** | 心肺氣虛証 | **210**

Chapter 12: **Heart and Spleen** 212

Pathophysiological relationship between the Heart and Spleen 212

    1. **Heart and Spleen Deficiency Pattern** | 心脾兩虛証 | 213

Chapter 13: **Heart and Liver** 215

Pathophysiological relationship between the Heart and Liver 215

    1. **Heart and Liver Blood Deficiency Pattern** | 心肝血虛証 | 217

Chapter 14: **Heart and Kidney** 218

Pathophysiological relationship between the Heart and Kidney 218

    1. **Heart and Kidney Yang Deficiency Pattern** | 心腎陽虛 | 220

    2. **Heart and Kidney Disharmony Pattern** | 心腎不交 | 222

        Comparison: Heart and Kidney Disharmony vs. Heart Fire Blazing 223

Chapter 15: **Heart and Small Intestine** 224

Pathophysiological relationship between the Heart and Small Intestine 224

    1. **Heart Fire Transmits to the Small Intestine Pattern** | 心火下移小腸証 | 225

        Comparison: Heart Fire Transmits to the Small Intestine vs. Small Intestine Excess Fire 226

Chapter 16: **Spleen and Lung** 227

Pathophysiological relationship between the Spleen and Lung 227

    1. **Spleen and Lung Qi Deficiency Pattern** | 脾肺氣虛証 | 229

Chapter 17: **Spleen and Kidney** 230

Pathophysiological relationship between the Spleen and Kidney 230

    1. **Spleen and Kidney Yang Deficiency Pattern** | 脾腎陽虛証 | 231

Chapter 18: **Spleen and Stomach** 233

Pathophysiological relationship between the Spleen and Stomach 233

    1. **Spleen and Stomach Disharmony Pattern** | 脾胃不和証 | 235

Chapter 19: **Lung and Kidney** 236

Pathophysiological relationship between the Lung and Kidney 236

    1. **Lung and Kidney Yin Deficiency Pattern** | 肺腎陰虛 | 238

Chapter 20: **Liver and Kidney** 240

Pathophysiological relationship between the Liver and Kidney 240

1. **Liver and Kidney Yin Deficiency Pattern** | 肺腎陰虛 | 241

Comparison: Liver and Kidney Yin Deficiency vs. Liver Yang Rising 242

Chapter 21: **Liver and Spleen/Stomach** 244

Pathophysiological relationship between the Liver and Spleen/Stomach 244

1. **Liver and Spleen Disharmony Pattern** | 肝脾不和証 | 245
2. **Liver and Stomach Disharmony Pattern** | 肝胃不和証 | 246

Comparison: Liver and Spleen Disharmony vs. Liver and Stomach Disharmony 248

Chapter 22: **Liver and Lung** 249

Pathophysiological relationship between the Liver and Lung 249

1. **Liver Fire Invading the Lung Pattern** | 肝火犯肺証 | 250

Comparison: Liver Fire Invading the Lung vs. Heat Congesting the Lung 251

Chapter 23: **Liver and Gallbladder** 252

Pathophysiological relationship between the Liver and Gallbladder 252

1. **Liver and Gallbladder Damp-Heat Pattern** | 肝膽濕熱証 | 253

Comparison: Liver and Gallbladder Damp-Heat vs. Gallbladder Heat 255

■ PART 4: QUESTIONS & ANSWERS FOR DEEPER INSIGHT ········ 257

The Questions in Summary 258

Chapter 24: **The Questions and Answers** 260

■ PART 5: COMPREHENSIVE EXAMINATION ········ 341

Chapter 25: **Exam Questions and Answer Key** 342

Answer Key 404

BIBLIOGRAPHY, 407
GENERAL INDEX, 411

Acknowledgements

This book originated from my classroom handouts for *zàng fǔ* courses that I taught 15 years ago at Emperor's College. After many years of rewriting, editing, and translating, this book has finally come into being. In this long and complicated process, there are many people who gave me encouragement, support, and advice for which I express my heartfelt gratitude.

I would like to thank my late colleague and dear friend, Dr. Al Stone. We co-authored two books before this one, but unfortunately, he passed away due to illness just as we were preparing to write this book together. His spirit, friendship, sense of humor, knowledge, enthusiasm, and dedication to traditional Chinese medicine will always remain in my heart. My thanks also to Julie Liu, L.Ac, my coauthor on this book, for her hard work and incredible job.

Most of all, I would like to thank all my students in the *zàng fǔ* classes for their challenges and criticisms. Special thanks go to Richard Vigorelli, L.Ac., Bruce Gustafson, L.Ac., DOM, and Olivia McMullen Fields, L.Ac., for helping me edit the class handouts. Your help is deeply appreciated.

Finally, I wish to express my thanks and deep appreciation to my family. Their patience and support were the foundation upon which I was able to complete this book.

Introduction

Zàng fǔ pattern identification (臟腑辯證 *zàng fǔ biàn zhèng*) is a method used to analyze signs and symptoms of disease according to the physiological functions and pathological characteristics of the *zàng fǔ* organs. It is used to infer the etiopathology, location, and nature of a disease. It also reveals the condition of the body's antipathogenic qi and its ability to battle pathogenic qi.

All physiological functions and pathological changes are associated with the *zàng fǔ* organs. Most often, the occurrence and development of disease is the result of *zàng fǔ* organ dysfunction. *Zàng fǔ* pattern identification is one of the core diagnosis methods in traditional Chinese medicine and is the foundation for clinical analysis and differentiation of every disease, particularly for interior and chronic conditions.

Relationship with other pattern identification methods

Qi, blood, and body fluids are the fundamental materials in the composition of the human body as well as the motive force for maintaining the body's physiological activities. The production and proper use of qi, blood, and body fluids depends on the proper functioning of the *zàng fǔ* organs.

When there is abnormal function of the *zàng fǔ* organs, there must also be a pathological change in qi, blood, and body fluids; likewise a dysfunction of qi, blood, and body fluids must in turn cause abnormalities in the function of the *zàng fǔ* organs. They coexist and are codependent, mutually affecting each other physiologically and pathologically. Therefore, it is common in the clinic to combine *zàng fǔ* pattern identification (臟腑辯證 *zàng fǔ biàn zhèng*) with qi, blood, and body fluids pattern identification (氣血津液辨證 *qì xǔe jīn yè biàn zhèng*).

Eight principles pattern identification (八網辨證 *bā gāng biàn zhèng*) organizes clinical manifestations of disease into the general categories of yin and yang. A disease location can be classified as exterior or interior, the thermal nature of the pathogen can be divided into either cold or heat, and the strength of the antipathogenic qi against the pathogenic qi can be characterized as either excessive or deficient. *Zàng fǔ* pattern identification is an application of the eight principles pattern identification to the particular disharmony of a specific *zàng fǔ* organ.

The signs and symptoms of any disease reflect the pathological reactions of the body to certain pathogenic factors. Pathogenic factors invade and lodge in the *zàng fǔ* organs, disrupting the state of relative balance, leading to dysfunction and the development of disease. Therefore, *zàng fǔ* pattern identification should be integrated with etiology pattern identification (病因辨證 *bìng yīn biàn zhèng*) in order to establish proper treatment strategies for eliminating the pathogens.

Eight principles pattern identification; etiology pattern identification; qi, blood, and body fluids pattern identification; and *zàng fǔ* pattern identification are systems for analyzing pathological change, but do so from different perspectives. Each method has its special emphasis, characteristics, and focus, but they are related and supplemental to each other. The first three methods are the basis for *zàng fǔ* pattern identification, while *zàng fǔ* pattern identification is also the basis for all other pattern identification methods. Qing dynasty physician Tang Rong-Chuan (唐容川, 1846-1897) notably stated: "If a doctor doesn't know *zàng fǔ* pattern identification, then he cannot identify the location and cause of the disease nor establish the proper treatment principle."

Method and procedure

In *zàng fǔ* pattern identification, the diseased *zàng fǔ* organs should be identified first on the basis of their physiological functions and pathological characteristics and then on the nature of the disease, such as heat or cold, deficiency or excess, as distinguished according to the eight principles.

After identifying the location and nature of a condition, if a pattern is characterized as excessive, then further analysis should be combined with etiology pattern identification to find the causative factors such as wind, cold, heat, blood stasis, or phlegm. If the condition is considered a deficiency pattern, then further analysis should use the qi, blood, and body fluids pattern identification method.

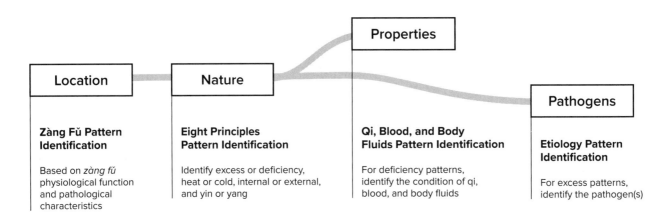

Chart 1 Method and Procedure of *Zàng Fǔ* Pattern Identification

Signs and symptoms reflect the physiological and pathological changes of the *zàng fǔ* organs. Each *zàng fǔ* organ has its unique physiological functions, and therefore has its unique set of associated diseases and patterns. It is the theoretical foundation of *zàng fǔ* pattern identification to diagnose a pattern on the basis of differing physiology and pathology of the *zàng fǔ* organs. When identifying a pattern, the following aspects should be taken into consideration:

(1) Nature, character, and pathological changes of the *zàng fǔ* organ and its related channel.
For example, the Heart governs the blood and houses the *shén*; if blood deficiency results

in a failure to nourish the Heart, then *shén* is disrupted. The Heart is a yang organ, is associated with the fire phase, and governs yang qi. Thus when pathogens invade the Heart they tend to be transformed into heat or fire, which then disturbs the *shén*. Therefore, *shén* disorders are always related to the Heart.

(2) The relationship with other organs and tissues. For example, the Heart opens into the tongue. If Heart fire flares up, it can cause a red tongue or canker sores.

(3) The relationship with other *zàng fǔ* organs. For example, the Heart and Small Intestine are related as an internal-external pair; Heart fire can transmit to the Small Intestine, resulting in burning and painful urination.

Through the three aspects above, we can identify pathological changes in the *zàng fǔ* organs to provide evidence for pattern identification.

Part 1

ZANG ORGANS

Zàng (臟) organs include the Heart, Lung, Spleen, Liver, and Kidney. These yin organs produce, transform, regulate, and store fundamental substances such as qi, blood, essence, and body fluids. They are solid organs that do not have empty cavities. Based on the physiological function and anatomical structure of *zàng* organs, their pathological changes are mostly due to an insufficiency in producing and storing, which more often results in deficiency patterns.

CONTENTS

CHAPTER 1: HEART DISEASE PATTERNS, 2

CHAPTER 2: LUNG DISEASE PATTERNS, 26

CHAPTER 3: SPLEEN DISEASE PATTERNS, 57

CHAPTER 4: LIVER DISEASE PATTERNS, 78

CHAPTER 5: KIDNEY DISEASE PATTERNS, 108

Chapter 1
Heart Disease Patterns

Physiological characteristics and functions of the Heart

The Heart is located in the middle of the chest, where it is protected by the Pericardium. The Heart channel emerges from the axilla and continues through the medial side of the arm into the palm. It is internally-externally connected with the Small Intestine, opens into the tongue, and manifests on the face. The fluid of the Heart is sweat and its related emotion is joy.

The Heart is called the sovereign organ (君主之官 *jūn zhú zhī guān*) and the root of life (生命之本 *shēng mìng zhī běn*), and is in charge of spirit and vitality. It is the sun within the yang organs, responsible for the blood circulation of the entire body as well as for mental activities. The Heart is a fire organ, the storage place for sovereign fire (君火 *jūn huǒ*), and governs yang qi. It is associated with the summer season.

The nature of the Heart is inward and conservative, favoring calm and quiet while disfavoring heat. So, when pathogenic heat attacks the body, it tends to cause Heart dysfunction.

Heart	Relationship
Spirit	Consciousness, the mind/spirit (神 *shén*)
Internal-external connection	Small Intestine
Open orifice	Tongue
Controls	Blood
External manifestation	Face
Fluid	Sweat
Fire	Sovereign fire
Emotion	Joy
Season	Summer
Five phase	Fire
Six climate factor	Fire

Table 1.1 Heart and its related properties

1 | Governs blood and controls blood vessels

The Heart is responsible for:
(1) Promoting blood circulation. Heart qi is the motive force that keeps blood circulating inside vessels continuously.
(2) Generating blood. Heart fire transforms body fluids into blood and sends it into the vessels.
(3) Keeping blood vessels elastic and smooth.

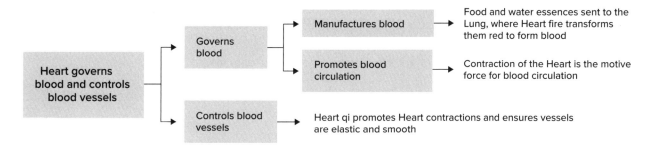

Chart 1.1 Heart governs blood and vessels

2 | Houses the *shén*

The Heart is the center for consciousness and vitality, influencing both mental and physical activities.
(1) The Heart governs blood, which nourishes *shén*; blood is the fundamental material for physical and mental activities.
(2) The Heart accepts external stimuli and has correct response capabilities. *Spiritual Pivot*, Chapter 8 (靈樞, 本神 *líng shū, běn shén*) states:

> The Heart is responsible for all kinds of mental activities, which are caused by external stimuli. When the Heart has memory and retains information, it is called thought or intention (意 *yì*). When thought or intention exists, then willpower and determination (志 *zhì*) develops.

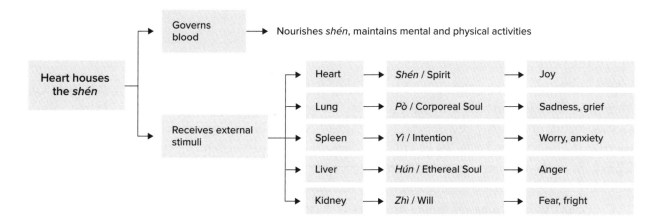

Chart 1.2 Heart houses the *shén*

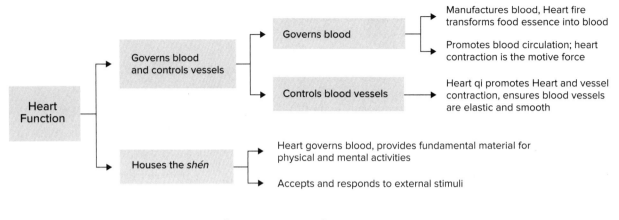

Chart 1.3 Heart function summary

Common etiological factors in Heart patterns

Heart patterns are mainly caused by endopathogenic factors, but exopathogens can also attack the Heart directly. The following are common etiological factors for Heart disease patterns:

(1) Congenital weakness
(2) Chronic illness with improper care leading to internal *zàng fǔ* organs deficiency
(3) Emotional stress: excessive anxiety and worry damaging Heart and Spleen
(4) Exopathogenic heat or cold directly attacking the Heart
(5) Improper diet creating phlegm or malnutrition leading to qi and blood deficiency or stagnation

Pathological changes and major clinical manifestations of Heart disease

Pathological changes of the Heart are mostly due to its failure to govern blood, control blood vessels, and house the *shén*. There are four major clinical manifestations of Heart dysfunction: palpitations, sleep disorder, mental disorder, and chest distress or pain.

1 | Palpitations

Definition: Refers to a sensation of the heart beating that is felt in the chest by the patient. It is caused by either an increase in heart rate, an increase in heart contraction, or by irregular heartbeats. It is often present in various kinds of coronary heart disease, cardioneurosis, anemia, and hyperthyroidism. Palpitations can also arise in a healthy person during periods of exercise or emotional excitement. Depending on its severity, palpitations can be divided into the following categories:

- **Fright palpitations** (驚悸 *jīng jì*): refers to heart palpitations that occur when there is fright. It is usually due to some external cause. They come and go quickly and are of short duration. This condition is mild and patients do not usually seek treatment for fright palpitations.

- **Continuous palpitations** (怔忡 *zhēng chōng*): refers to severe throbbing of the heart, which is often felt from the chest down to the umbilicus. It is a progression of fright palpitations, usually due to internal causes, and is induced or aggravated by exertion. Prolonged duration of this condition is severe and may require medical attention.

Etiology and pathomechanisms: Palpitations appear in all Heart patterns and are directly related to the condition of the Heart. Under normal conditions, the motive force of the Heart keeps the organ pumping regularly, ensuring smooth blood circulation. The *shén* resides in the Heart and is nourished by blood, qi, essence, and body fluids.

When the Heart is attacked by pathogenic factors, emotional stress, or trauma resulting in phlegm or blood stasis, or when the Heart is deprived of nourishment due to a deficiency of qi, blood, yin, or yang from improper diet, chronic illness, or a weak constitution, then the motive force becomes insufficient and the Heart cannot keep blood circulation smooth. The *shén* will be disturbed and restless, causing fright palpitations.

Continuous palpitations represent an exacerbation of fright palpitations and is viewed as damage to the Heart organ rather than a functional pathology. Thus the lack of the Heart's motive force and *shén* disturbance are the pathomechanisms of palpitations.

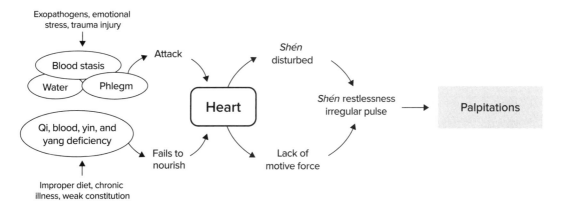

Chart 1.4 Etiology and pathomechanism of palpitations

2 | Insomnia

Definition: A sleep disorder that may involve a lack of sleep, sleepiness, oversleeping or sleeping at inappropriate times. Insomnia describes a variety of symptoms associated with sleep disturbance, which include:
- difficulty falling asleep after retiring to bed
- early awakening
- intermittent waking through the period of attempted sleep
- inability to sleep through the night, restlessness at night
- dream-disturbed sleep

Etiology and pathomechanisms: The Heart is the major organ directly related to sleep. The Heart houses the *shén*, which is responsible for both the body's external manifestation of vitality as well as the internal conscious and subconscious mental activity. During the daytime, the yang qi is abundant and the *shén* is active towards the outside of the body. When yang qi increases in the mornings, one will therefore awaken and become active.

The yin governs the nighttime when the *shén* that was active on the outside during the day moves inwards to be stored in the Heart. If Heart and *shén* remain peaceful and calm, there will be sleep. Heart qi and yang promote the activities of the *shén*, while Heart blood and yin are the substances that nourish the *shén*. Thus changes to the Heart qi, blood, yin, and yang will affect the Heart *shén*.

The two pathomechanisms of insomnia are: pathogenic factors (especially heat) disturbing the *shén* and a loss of nourishment to the Heart. Pathogenic heat can cause the *shén* to lose its anchor in the Heart at night and become restless. This can be the heat of an exopathogenic factor or heat that arises from an endopathogenic factor such as stagnation or deficiency of vital substances. These patterns are often found in old age, chronic illness, or the later stages of a febrile disease.

Loss of nourishment may be attributed to either excess or deficiency. In the case of excess, the stagnation of qi, blood, phlegm, or food can block the flow of qi and blood to the Heart, leading to a shortage of the vital substances necessary for the nourishment of the *shén*. Such stagnation can occur because of emotional stress, traumatic injury, or improper diet. As for deficiency, the lack of qi, blood, yin, or essence cannot sufficiently nourish the Heart, and therefore cannot anchor the *shén*.

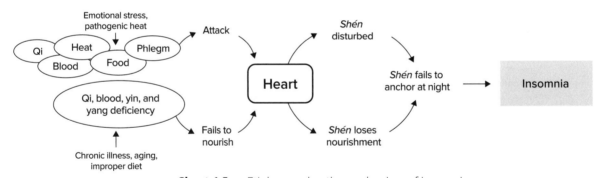

Chart 1.5 Etiology and pathomechanism of insomnia

3 | *Shén* disturbance

Definition: *Shén* disturbance means that consciousness is obscured or lost, manifesting with abnormal mental behaviors. This condition is usually found in one of the following patterns, each caused by unique etiologies and pathogenesis:
- irritability and restlessness (煩躁 *fán zào*)
- restless organ disorder (臟躁 *zàng zào*)
- hysteria (百合病 *bǎi hé bìng*)
- yin madness (癲 *diān*)
- yang madness (狂 *kuáng*)
- epilepsy (癇 *xián*)

Etiology and pathomechanisms: Under normal circumstances, *shén* is housed in the Heart and nourished by the blood. At nighttime, *shén* anchors in the Heart and the person falls asleep. In the daytime, when a person wakes up, the *shén* will move out of the Heart through the Heart orifice and perform all conscious and subconscious activities, such as thinking, memory, behavior, and speech.

There are two major reasons for *shén* disturbance. One is due to the attack by pathogenic factors, especially heat and phlegm. Pathogenic heat disturbs the *shén*, causes it to be unsettled and leads to restlessness, irritability, vexation, incoherent speech, or manic behaviors. When pathogenic heat pushes *shén* out of the Heart, coma and unconsciousness may result. Phlegm can also obstruct the Heart orifice, inhibiting the *shén* from performing mental activities, resulting in chronic depression, madness, laughing or crying inappropriately, or even loss of consciousness and delirium.

Pathogenic heat is usually caused by external heat attack, febrile disease, or emotional stress, but can also result from a disorder of the internal organs. Phlegm can be generated by improper diet, long-term emotional stress, and a disorder of the internal organs.

The second reason for *shén* disturbance is qi, blood, yin, yang, and essence insufficiency. The *shén* requires these nutritional substances to maintain normal function. When nutritional substances are insufficient due to chronic illness, aging, or improper diet the *shén* will not be able to function, resulting in mental depression, possible hallucinations, disorientation, frequent attacks of melancholy, soliloquies (獨語 *dú yǔ*), paraphasia (錯語 *cuò yǔ*), and poor memory.

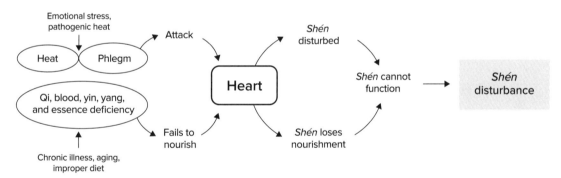

Chart 1.6 Etiology and pathomechanism of *shén* disturbance

4 | Chest distress or pain

Definition: A sensation of pain, oppression, discomfort, and stifling in the chest.

Etiology and pathomechanisms: Stagnation in the chest can cause chest distress or pain, such as when pathogenic cold attacks the Heart, leading to an obstruction of vessels. *Zàng fǔ* organ dysfunction caused by emotional stress, improper diet, or trauma injury can also lead to phlegm, blood stasis, or qi stagnation. Improper diet, chronic illness, or a weak constitution can lead to qi deficiency. When qi is deficient, there is not enough power to circulate the qi and blood, resulting in stagnation.

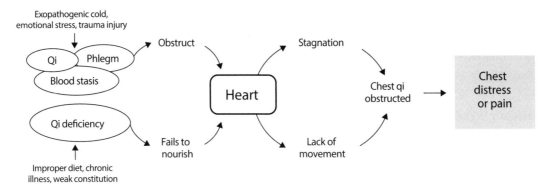

Chart 1.7 Etiology and pathomechanism of chest distress or pain

5 | Other signs and symptoms related with the Heart

The following signs and symptoms can also appear in Heart patterns: canker sores, pale or dark facial complexion, poor memory, tongue ulcers, knotted, abrupt, or intermittent pulse, excessive sweating, red tongue tip or crimson tongue, and yellow urine with burning and painful sensation.

Physiological Function	Pathological Change	Clinical Manifestation
Governs blood and controls the blood vessels	Qi and blood circulation obstruction	Fright or continuous palpitations, shortness of breath, chest tightness and pain, irregular pulse
	Pathogenic heat disturbs blood	Vomiting blood, nosebleed, blood in the urine, bruising
	Blood deficiency, unable to nourish the Heart	Palpitations, dizziness
Houses the *shén*	Blood deficiency, unable to nourish the *shén*	Insomnia, dream-disturbed sleep, poor memory, depression
	Heat disturbs the *shén*	Irritability, mania, delirium, coma
Opens to the tongue	Excess heat	Red prickles on tongue tip or ulcers
	Blood stagnation	Purple or dusky (pale purple) tongue or dark spots on tongue
	Pathogens obstructing tongue channels and collaterals	Stiffness of tongue, flaccid tongue, difficult speech, or inability to speak
Manifests in the complexion	Qi, blood, or yang deficiency	Pale face
	Blood stagnation	Dark or purple complexion
Related to the Small Intestine	Heart fire transmits to the Small Intestine	Frequent, scanty, and dark yellow urine with painful and burning sensation

Table 1.2 Physiological functions, pathological changes, and clinical manifestations of the Heart

Common patterns in Heart disease

There are nine different Heart patterns commonly seen in the clinic and they can be divided into two categories:

(1) Deficiency patterns: Heart qi deficiency, Heart yang deficiency, which can develop into Heart yang collapse, Heart blood deficiency, and Heart yin deficiency

(2) Excess patterns: Phlegm misting the Heart, phlegm-fire harassing the Heart, Heart fire blazing, and Heart vessels obstruction, which, depending on the etiology and pathogenesis, can be subdivided into phlegm obstruction of the Heart vessels, qi stagnation in the Heart vessels, blood stasis obstruction of the Heart vessels, and excess cold obstruction of the Heart vessels.

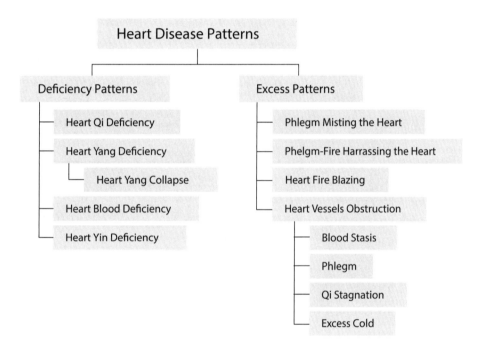

Chart 1.8 Common Heart disease patterns

	Etiology	Patterns
Deficiency	Emotional stress, over-worrying and -thinking, congenital insufficiency, or chronic illness impairs *zàng fǔ* organs	Heart Blood Deficiency, Heart Yin Deficiency, Heart Qi Deficiency, Heart Yang Deficiency, Heart Yang Collapse
Excess	Improper diet, emotional stress, chronic illness, pathogenic heat or cold attacking	Phlegm-Fire Harassing the Heart, Phlegm Misting the Heart, Heart Fire Blazing, Heart Vessels Obstruction

Table 1.3 Classification of common Heart patterns

1 Heart Qi Deficiency Pattern 心氣虛証

Definition: A group of signs and symptoms caused by a weakness of motive force, which slows blood circulation, resulting in the Heart losing nourishment.

Clinical manifestations: Fright or continuous palpitations, chest tightness, shortness of breath that worsens with exertion, fatigue, pale face, spontaneous sweating, pale tongue with white coating, weak pulse, rapid pulse without strength, knotted pulse, or abrupt pulse.

Key points: Fright or continuous palpitations, chest distress, plus qi deficiency signs and symptoms.

Etiology and pathogenesis: This pattern is most closely related to chronic illness, improper diet leading to malnutrition, congenital weakness, or aging. Qi deficiency can be caused by impaired body fluids or blood deficiency. It also can develop from long-term severe emotional stress such as overthinking and worrying.

The Heart qi provides the motive force for blood circulation, which involves proper heart muscle contractions for propelling the blood to flow smoothly through the vessels, thereby maintaining the normal physiological activities of all *zàng fǔ* organs and tissues. Thus when Heart qi is insufficient it cannot push blood to flow smoothly inside the vessels, resulting in palpitations and irregular pulses.

Weakness of the Heart's motive force makes it difficult for the blood to flow upward and outward, causing a pale complexion, pale tongue, or weak pulse. The deficient qi is unable to flow adequately, so there can be shortness of breath along with chest tightness and distress. Sweat is the fluid of the Heart, and thus when deficient Heart qi fails to secure the body's surface, the interstitial spaces (腠理 *còu lǐ*) loosen and leak body fluids, resulting in spontaneous sweating.

Physical activity consumes qi, therefore, in deficiency patterns, all of the above signs and symptoms are aggravated by exertion.

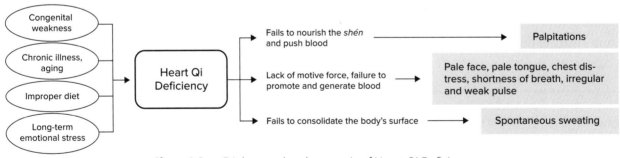

Chart 1.9 Etiology and pathogenesis of Heart Qi Deficiency

TCM Disease	Western Disease	Herbal Formulas		Acupuncture	
Palpitations (心悸)	Anemia, angina, coronary artery disease, arrhythmia, menopause syndrome, panic attack, anxiety	Yang Xin Tang	Si Jun Zi Tang, Huang Qi	HT-5, PC-6, BL-15, CV-6, CV-17, ST-36	HT-6, HT-7, HT-8, CV-14, BL-19
Insomnia (失眠)	Neurosis, menopause syndrome, depression, anxiety		Bao Yuan Tang Gui Pi Tang		HT-7, SP-6, Anmian
Chest painful obstruction (胸痹)	MI, angina, CAD, cor pulmonale, myocarditis, pericarditis, pulmonary embolism		Sheng Mai San, Shen Fu Tang		HT-7, BL-44, CV-4, GV-20
Fatigue (虛勞)	Anemia, CHF, valvular heart disease, COPD, arrhythmia, Lyme disease, hypothyroidism, depression		Shen Mai San Si Jun Zi Tang		CV-3, CV-4, CV-5, CV-6, CV-12, BL-20, BL-23, GV-4
Forgetfulness (健忘)	Dementia, Alzheimer's, sleep apnea, depression, hypothyroidism, ADD/ADHD		Gui Pi Tang		BL-20, BL-23, KI-7, Sishengcong

Table 1.4 Diseases and treatments related to Heart Qi Deficiency

2 Heart Yang Deficiency Pattern |心陽虛証|

Definition: A group of signs and symptoms that are a result of Heart qi deficiency and weakness of motive force with internal pathogenic cold.

Clinical manifestations: Fright or continuous palpitations, chest distress with tightness or pain, intolerance to cold, cold limbs, shortness of breath, fatigue, spontaneous sweating, a pale face, a pale flabby tongue with moist white coating, and a pulse that is weak, minute, knotted, or deep without strength.

Key points: Fright or continuous palpitations, chest pain or distress, irregular pulse, plus yang deficiency signs and symptoms.

Etiology and pathogenesis: This pattern usually develops from Heart qi deficiency. When a patient suffers from Heart qi deficiency and does not receive proper treatment, Heart function continues to be impaired and eventually develops into yang deficiency.

When yang fails to warm and push the blood, the channels and vessels in the Heart become obstructed causing stagnation and chest distress with tightness or pain. In yang deficiency, the yang is unable to perform its warming function, causing cold limbs and intolerance of cold (畏寒 wèi hán). A slow pulse with a pale, flabby, and moist tongue are also the signs of yang deficiency.

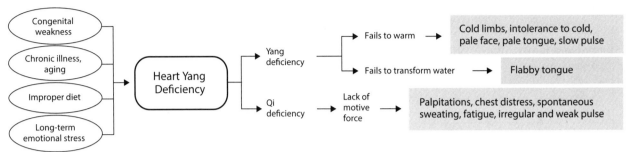

Chart 1.10 Etiology and pathogenesis of Heart Yang Deficiency

TCM Disease	Western Disease	Herbal Formulas		Acupuncture	
Palpitations (心悸)	Anemia, angina, coronary artery disease, arrhythmia, menopause syndrome, panic attack, anxiety	Shen Fu Tang, Bao Yuan Tang	Si Jun Zi Tang + Huang Qi	HT-5, PC-6, BL-15, CV-6, CV-17, GV-14	HT-6, HT-7, HT-8, CV-14, BL-19
Chest painful obstruction (胸痹)	MI, angina, CAD, cor-pulmonale, myocarditis, pericarditis, pulmonary embolism		Sheng Mai San + Shen Fu Tang		HT-7, BL-44, CV-4, GV-20
Fatigue (虛勞)	Anemia, CHF, valvular heart disease, COPD, arrhythmia, Lyme disease, hypothyroidism, depression		Sheng Mai San + Si Jun Zi Tang		CV-3, CV-4, CV-5, CV-6, CV-12, BL-20, BL-23, GV-4

Table 1.5 Diseases and treatments related to Heart Yang Deficiency

3 Heart Yang Collapse Pattern 心陽暴脫証

Definition: A critical clinical condition due to extreme Heart yang deficiency, leading to the sudden collapse of Heart yang.

Clinical manifestations: Sudden start of severe palpitations; profuse cold, oily, pearl-like sweat; severely cold limbs; pale complexion; feeble breath; severe chest pain; cyanosis of the lips; minute, faint, or irregular pulse; or even a loss of consciousness and coma.

Key points: Sudden severe palpitations, profuse cold, oily, pearl-like sweat, plus Heart yang deficiency and yang collapse signs and symptoms.

Etiology and pathogenesis: This pattern usually develops from Heart yang deficiency, but can also be caused by excessive pathogenic cold damaging Heart yang or phlegm obstructing the Heart orifice.

When yang fails to secure the body's surface, body fluids leak out, producing sweat that is oily, profuse, and cold. When yang fails to perform its warming function, the body and limbs become severely cold.

Gathering qi (宗氣 zōng qì) is in charge of breathing and is motivated by chest yang (胸陽 xiōng yáng). When yang fails, gathering qi leaks out and cannot assist the Lung, resulting in feeble breath. When Heart yang collapses, the *shén* housed in the Heart loses support and nourishment, becoming disturbed and unsettled. This can lead to stupor or even coma. In yang failure there is a loss of motive force, and hence the pulse is faint, minute, or irregular.

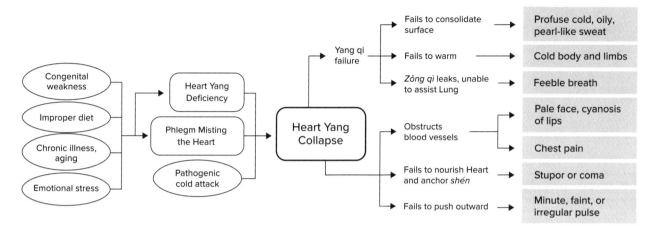

Chart 1.11 Etiology and pathogenesis of Heart Yang Collapse

TCM Disease	Western Disease	Herbal Formulas	Acupuncture
Palpitations (心悸)	Anemia, angina, coronary artery disease, arrhythmia, menopause syndrome, panic attack, anxiety	Shen Fu Tang, Du Shen Tang, Sheng Mai San	CV-4, CV-6, CV-8, GV-4, GV-14, GV-20, ST-36, PC-6, BL-15, BL-20, BL-23
Collapse syndrome (脱证)	Obstructive cardiac diseases, or cardiac arrhythmias, heart failure, hypoglycemia, dehydration		
Chest painful obstruction (胸痹)	MI, angina, CAD, COPD, myocarditis, pericarditis		
Wind-stroke (中風)	CVA		
Sweating syndrome (汗証)	Anemia, MI, heart failure, hypoglycemia, ectopic pregnancy, dehydration		

Table 1.6 Diseases and treatments related to Heart Yang Collapse

Comparison: Heart Qi Deficiency vs. Heart Yang Deficiency vs. Heart Yang Collapse

Heart qi deficiency (心氣虛 *xīn qì xū*), Heart yang deficiency (心陽虛 *xīn yáng xū*), and Heart yang collapse (心陽暴脫 *xīn yáng bào tuō*) are Heart hypofunction patterns that differ in degree of severity. The major pathogenesis for all three patterns is the failure of Heart qi to nourish and promote. Thus, they present with palpitations, shortness of breath, chest distress and tightness, become worse with exertion, and an irregular pulse.

Heart qi deficiency is the first pattern to appear when Heart qi becomes insufficient due to chronic illness, improper diet, aging, or congenital weakness. Without proper treatment, Heart qi deficiency can develop into Heart yang deficiency, which will present with signs and symptoms caused by deficiency cold, such as cold limbs, intolerance of cold, chest pain, and pale facial complexion in addition to the signs and symptoms of qi deficiency. Heart yang collapse develops from chronic and severe Heart yang deficiency and is the late and critical stage of the illness. At this point, yin and yang separate, yang fails to hold yin, and there is a sudden collapse with profuse cold, oily sweat.

The key points to distinguish these three patterns are as follows:
1) Severity
2) Coldness and cold, oily sweat

Pattern		Heart Qi Deficiency	Heart Yang Deficiency	Heart Yang Collapse
Pathogenesis		Heart qi insufficiency leads to Heart hypofunction	Heart yang fails to promote and warm	Yang collapse, fails to warm, promote, consolidate, and nourish
Symptoms	Common	Palpitations, shortness of breath, chest distress or tightness, worse with exertion, irregular pulse		
	Different		Chest pain, cold limbs, intolerance to cold, dark lips, pale complexion, thin and faint pulse	Sudden severe palpitations and chest pain with cold, oily sweating, stupor, or coma
Severity		Mild	Severe	Critical
Tongue & pulse		Pale tongue with white coating; weak pulse, rapid pulse without strength, knotted pulse, or abrupt pulse	Pale flabby tongue with moist white coating; weak, minute, knotted, or deep pulse without strength	Bluish-purple lips; faint, minute pulse
Treatment strategy		Nourish the Heart, calm *shén*	Tonify qi, warm yang	Restore yang, tonify yuan qi, rescue qi from collapse
Herbal formulas		Yang Xin Tang	Shen Fu Tang, Bao Yuan Tang	Shen Fu Tang, Du Shen Tang, Sheng Mai San

Table 1.7 Comparison of Heart Qi Deficiency, Heart Yang Deficiency, and Heart Yang Collapse

4 Heart Blood Deficiency Pattern 心血虛証

Definition: A group of signs and symptoms caused by blood deficiency that leads to the Heart losing nourishment.

Clinical manifestations: Fright or continuous palpitations, insomnia, dream-disturbed sleep, dizziness, poor memory and concentration, pale or sallow complexion, pale lips, pale nails and tongue, a thin and weak pulse.

Key points: Palpitations, insomnia, poor memory, plus blood deficiency signs and symptoms.

Etiology and pathogenesis: This pattern is usually caused by chronic illness, which impairs blood; or Spleen and Stomach function disorder, which weakens the production of blood; or improper diet; or chronic bleeding; or long-term emotional stress (overthinking, worry), which consumes blood.

The Heart governs blood and houses the *shén*. When blood is insufficient and unable to nourish the *shén*, the *shén* becomes unsettled, leading to poor memory and concentration, insomnia, and dream-disturbed sleep. Heart blood deficiency also leads to the weakening of motive force, causing symptoms of fright or continuous palpitations. When blood is insufficient and unable to nourish and fill the body, symptoms include a pale and sallow complexion along with pale nails, lips, and tongue. This insufficiency means that blood cannot properly fill the vessels, resulting in a thin and deficient pulse.

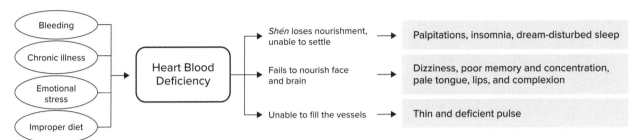

Chart 1.12 Etiology and pathogenesis of Heart Blood Deficiency

TCM Disease	Western Disease	Herbal Formulas		Acupuncture	
Palpitations (心悸)	Anemia, coronary artery disease, arrhythmia, anxiety or panic attack	Dan Shen Si Wu Tang, Gui Pi Tang, Zhi Gan Cao Tang	Shen Qi Si Wu Tang	PC-6, CV-14, CV-17	HT-7, BL-15, BL-17, BL-20, ST-36, CV-4, CV-6, CV-14, SP-6
Fatigue (虛勞)	Anemia, CHF, valvular heart disease, COPD	Si Wu Tang		CV-4, CV-6, CV-12, BL-23	
Insomnia (失眠)	Neurasthenia, menopause syndrome, depression or anxiety	Suan Zao Ren Tang, Gui Pi Tang		HT-5, HT-6, Anmian	
Forgetfulness (健忘)	Dementia, Alzheimer's, sleep apnea, depression, ADD/ADHD, hypothyroidism	Gui Pi Tang		Sishencong, BL-23, KI-6	
Dizziness (眩暈)	Anemia, hypotension, hypothyroidism, hypoglycemia	Huang Qi Si Wu Tang		GV-20, GB-20	
Restless organ disorder (臟躁)	Anxiety, depression, postpartum depression, hysteria, neurosis, menopause syndrome, PTSD	Gan Mai Da Zao Tang		PC-5, HT-9, GV-20, LR-3	

Table 1.8 Diseases and treatments related to Heart Blood Deficiency

5 Heart Yin Deficiency Pattern | 心陰虛証 |

Definition: A group of signs and symptoms that are caused by yin deficiency heat that affects the Heart.

Clinical manifestations: Palpitations, insomnia, dream-disturbed sleep, low-grade fever in the afternoon or evening, five-center heat, night sweats, a red tongue with scanty coating, and a thin rapid pulse.

Key points: Palpitations, insomnia, plus yin deficiency heat signs and symptoms.

Etiology and pathogenesis: This pattern can develop from febrile diseases because high fevers can severely impair yin; from excess long-term overthinking and worrying, which gradually consumes blood and yin fluid; or from chronic illness, which impairs the generation of yin. Additionally, Heart yin deficiency can develop from chronic illness related to Liver and Kidney yin deficiency or aging.

When Heart yin is deficient, it fails to nourish the *shén*, which becomes unstable and causes palpitations. Yin deficiency leads to yang excess, making it difficult for the *shén* to be anchored with yin at night, resulting in insomnia. When deficiency heat flares up at night, it disturbs the *shén*, causing excessive dreaming and vexation.

As a person falls asleep, this heat combines with protective qi at night and evaporates the body fluids, leading to night sweats. There are also heat sensations in the five centers, a red tongue with a scanty coating, and a thin rapid pulse.

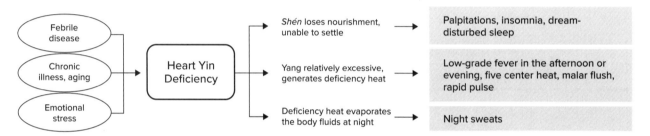

Chart 1.13 Etiology and pathogenesis of Heart Yin Deficiency

TCM Disease	Western Disease	Herbal Formulas		Acupuncture	
Palpitations (心悸)	Anemia, arrhythmia, hyperthyroidism, CAD, neurasthenia, anxiety	Huang Lian E Jiao Tang	Tian Wang Bu Xin Dan	HT-6, HT-7, CV-14, BL-15, GV-14, SP-6, KI-6, KI-7	PC-6, CV-17
Insomnia (失眠)	Hyperthyroidism, menopause syndrome, neurasthenia, anxiety, ADD/ADHD				Anmian
Fatigue (虛勞)	Anemia, valvular heart disease, COPD, CHF, hyperthyroidism		Sheng Mai San		ST-36, CV-4, CV-6

Table 1.9 Diseases and treatments related to Heart Yin Deficiency

Comparison: Heart Blood Deficiency vs. Heart Yin Deficiency

Heart blood deficiency (心血虛 *xīn xuè xū*) and Heart yin deficiency (心陰虛 *xīn yīn xū*) both present with palpitations, insomnia, dream-disturbed sleep, and a thin pulse. However, the etiology and pathogenesis are different, so there are different clinical manifestations and treatments.

Heart blood deficiency is mostly caused by bleeding, chronic illness, malnutrition, or long-term emotional stress that all consume or lead to an inadequate generation of blood. Insufficient blood to nourish the Heart and *shén* manifests with dizziness, poor memory and concentration, low spirits, depression, pale complexion, and pale tongue. Heart yin deficiency is mostly due to febrile disease, chronic illness, or long-term emotional stess that consumes yin and gives rise to yin deficiency, which is unable to anchor yang, leading to a relative excess of yang. Therefore, Heart yin deficiency manifests more as yin deficiency heat, such as low-grade fever in the afternoon or evening, five-center heat, and night sweats. Deficiency heat flaring upward may cause irritability, anxiety, moodiness, malar flush, a red cracked tongue, and a rapid pulse.

The key points to distinguish these two patterns are as follows:
1) Facial and tongue color: pale color vs. red color
2) Heat signs and symptoms vs. no heat signs and symptoms
3) *Shén*: fails to be nourished vs. disturbed by heat

Pattern		Heart Blood Deficiency	Heart Yin Deficiency
Etiology		Chronic illness, long-term emotional stress, aging	
		Bleeding	Febrile disease
Pathogenesis		Heart fails to be nourished	
		Blood deficiency, Heart loses nourishment	Heart yin deficiency fails to nourish, generates internal deficiency heat
Symptoms	Common	Palpitations, insomnia, dream-disturbed sleep, thin pulse	
	Different	Blood deficiency: dizziness, pale complexion, lips, tongue, and nails	Yin deficiency heat: low-grade fever in the afternoon or evening, five center heat, night sweats, red tongue, rapid pulse
	Shén	Depression, low spirits, poor memory and concentration	Irritable, moody, anxious
Tongue & pulse		Pale tongue with thin coating; weak thin pulse	Red tongue with scanty or no tongue coating; thin rapid pulse
Treatment strategy		Nourish and tonify Heart blood	Nourish and tonify Heart yin
Herbal formulas		Shen Qi Si Wu Tang	Huang Lian E Jiao Tang, Bu Xin Tang

Table 1.10 Comparison of Heart Blood Deficiency and Heart Yin Deficiency

6 Heart Fire Blazing Pattern 心火上炎証

Definition: A group of signs and symptoms caused by internal excess heat that flares up and disturbs Heart *shén*. It is also called excess Heart fire (心火亢盛 *xīn huǒ kàng shèng*).

Clinical manifestations: Red face and lips, irritability, anxiety, vexation, insomnia, bitter taste, thirst, canker sores or sores on lips or tongue. A red tongue tip, or deep red tongue with yellow coating, and a rapid pulse. In some cases there are manic behaviors, delirium, nosebleed, vomiting blood, or skin sores or boils. There could also be burning and painful urination.

Key points: Insomnia, irritability, anxiety, a red tongue tip, canker sores, plus internal excess heat signs and symptoms.

Etiology and pathogenesis: This pattern can be caused by improper diet, such as overeating hot, spicy, greasy foods and overconsumption of alcohol or heat-generating herbs and products. Another factor is emotional stress, which can transform qi stagnation into heat. Other disorders of the internal organs can also generate internal heat.

When pathogenic heat flares upward it disturbs the *shén*, preventing it from anchoring or settling, leading to insomnia, anxiety, manic behavior, irritability, or delirium. When heat following the Heart channel flames upward, there is a red tongue tip and canker sores. If the heat damages the channels and collaterals, nosebleed or vomiting of blood may result. Heat toxicity can accumulate in the channels and collaterals, causing local qi and blood to stagnate, leading to skin sores or boils. Red face, thirst, constipation, and yellow urine are all symptoms of excess internal heat.

Since the Heart and Small Intestine are internally and externally related, pathogenic heat may transform from the Heart into the Small Intestine, leading to painful and burning urination. If pathogenic heat impairs the vessels, this could cause blood in the urine.

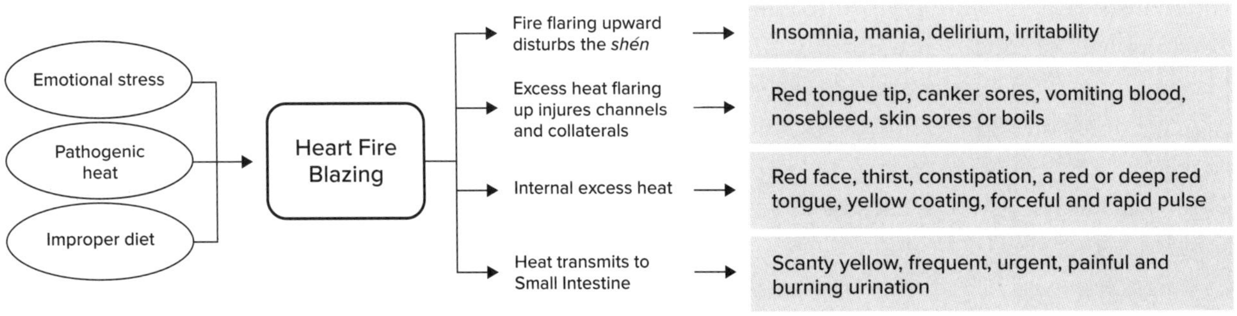

Chart 1.14 Etiology and pathogenesis of Heart Fire Blazing

<table>
<tr><th>TCM Disease</th><th>Western Disease</th><th colspan="2">Herbal Formulas</th><th colspan="2">Acupuncture</th></tr>
<tr><td>Palpitations (心悸)</td><td>Panic attack, anxiety, hyperthyroidism, SVT, VT, arrhythmia</td><td rowspan="5">Xie Xin Tang, Dao Chi San</td><td>Huang Lian Wen Dan Tang, Chai Hu Jia Long Gu Mu Li Tang</td><td rowspan="5">HT-7, HT-8, HT-9, CV-15, SP-6, LI-11, GV-19, GV-24</td><td>BL-15, CV-14, CV-17, PC-6</td></tr>
<tr><td>Bloody painful urinary dribbling (血淋)</td><td>UTI, kidney infections, bladder infections, kidney stones</td><td>Xiao Ji Yin Zi</td><td>BL-28, CV-3, SP-9, SP-10</td></tr>
<tr><td>Insomnia (失眠)</td><td>Menopause syndrome, anxiety, neurosis, ADD/ADHD</td><td>Zhu Sha An Shen Wan</td><td>Anmian, KI-6, PC-6</td></tr>
<tr><td>Tongue ulcer (舌瘡)</td><td>Tongue ulcer</td><td rowspan="2">Jia Wei Dao Chi San</td><td rowspan="2">PC-8, LI-4, ST-6, ST-36, CV-23</td></tr>
<tr><td>Canker sores (口瘡)</td><td>Canker sores</td></tr>
</table>

Table 1.11 Diseases and treatments related to Heart Fire Blazing

7 Phlegm-Fire Harassing the Heart Pattern | 痰火擾心証

Definition: A group of signs and symptoms caused by Heart fire combining with phlegm that harasses the Heart *shén* and manifests with various kinds of *shén*-disturbed conditions. This can occur in exogenous febrile disease as well as in endogenous disease.

Clinical manifestations: Fever, irritability, red face and eyes, thirst, heavy breathing, bitter taste in the mouth, manic agitation, incoherent speech, mental confusion, rash and violent behavior, uncontrolled laughter or crying, shouting, muttering to oneself, or even coma and delirium, a red tongue with yellow greasy coating, and a slippery and rapid pulse.

Key points: Exogenous: acute, short course, high fever, profuse phlegm, and coma or delirium. Endogenous: chronic or recurrent. Manic behavior plus heat-phlegm signs and symptoms.

Etiology and pathogenesis: Exogenous febrile disease due to exopathogenic factors attacking and excessive emotional stress are the two major etiological factors leading to this pattern. Exopathogenic factors invasion can cause heat to scorch inside, leading to yang excess. Long-term or excessive emotional stress can cause qi stagnation that can transform into fire, also known as 'five emotions transform into fire' (五志化火 wǔ zhì huà huǒ).

Internal excess heat scorches the fluids and engenders phlegm. This accumulation of heat and phlegm then rises and harasses the Heart, disturbs the *shén*, and leads to insomnia, dream-disturbed sleep, irritability, and agitation. Other symptoms can include coma and delirium, manic behavior, rash and violent behavior, mental confusion, incoherent speech, and uncontrolled laughter or crying.

Heat tends to rise upward, causing a red face, eyes, and tongue. When it impairs body fluids it then leads to thirst. Other signs of heat include heavy breathing, bitter taste in the mouth, yellow urine, yellow tongue coating, constipation, and a rapid pulse. When phlegm accumulates in the throat area, it can cause a rattling sound, a thick greasy tongue coating, and a slippery pulse.

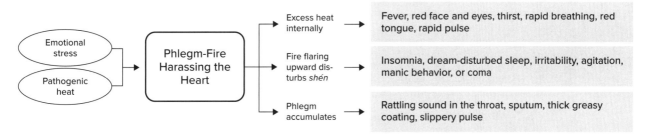

Chart 1.15 Etiology and pathogenesis of Phlegm-Fire Harassing the Heart

TCM Disease	Western Disease	Herbal Formulas	Acupuncture
Yang mania (陽狂)	Schizophrenia, hysteria, neurosis, psychosis OCD, anxiety, ADD/ADHD	Meng Shi Gun Tan Wan, Sheng Tie Luo Yin	GV-14, GV-16, GV-26, PC-6, ST-40
Wind-stroke (中風)	CVA	An Gong Niu Huang Wan, Zhi Bao Dan	GV-20, GV-26, ST-40, LR-3, KI-1, jing-well points on hands
Insomnia (失眠)	Menopausal syndrome, neurosis, anxiety, ADD/ADHD	Wen Dan Tang	HT-7, HT-9, SP-6, Anmian, ST-40

(Huang Lian Wen Dan Tang spans all three rows of Herbal Formulas column)

Table 1.12 Diseases and treatments related to Phlegm-Fire Harassing the Heart

Comparison: Heart Fire Blazing vs. Phlegm-Fire Harassing the Heart

Heart fire blazing (心火上炎 *xīn huǒ shàng yán*) and phlegm-fire harassing the Heart (痰火擾心 *tán huǒ rǎo xīn*) both involve excess heat invading the Heart. Thus they share many signs and symptoms such as irritability, red face, restlessness, agitation, fidgeting, vexation, fever, insomnia, yellow urine, constipation, red tongue with yellow coating, and a rapid pulse.

However, in addition to the excess heat disturbance seen in the pattern of Heart fire blazing, phlegm-fire harassing the Heart also exhibits signs of phlegm obstruction such as abnormal manic behavior, shouting, uncontrollable laughing or crying, slurred speech, incoherent speech, rattling sounds in the throat, yellow sputum, a thick, yellow, greasy tongue coating, and a slippery pulse.

The key points to distinguish these two patterns are as follows:
1) *Shén* disturbance: normal behavior vs. abnormal manic behavior. Both patterns present with signs and symptoms caused by heat disturbing the *shén* such as irritability, restlessness, agitation, or fidgeting. However, in phlegm-fire harassing the Heart, patients show more extreme abnormal manic behavior such as shouting and improper laughing and crying.
2) Tongue and pulse.

Pattern		Heart Fire Blazing	Phlegm-Fire Harassing the Heart
Pathogenesis		Heart fire blazes upward, disturbing the shen	Heat and phlegm accumulation rises and harasses the Heart, disturbing the shen
Symptoms	Common	Irritability, flushed face, restlessness, agitation, fidgeting, vexation, bitter taste, fever, insomnia, yellow urine, constipation, thirst, red tongue with yellow coating, rapid pulse	
	Mental Condition	In severe cases: delirium, coma	Slurred speech, incoherent speech, uncontrollable laughing or crying, shouting, manic behavior
		Mild, acute	Severe, sub-acute or chronic
	Other	Canker sores, tongue ulcers, nose bleeding, vomiting with blood	Rattling sound in the throat, yellow sputum
Tongue & pulse		Red body or red tip, yellow tongue coating; rapid pulse	Red body, thick, yellow, greasy tongue coating; rapid and slippery pulse
Treatment strategy		Drain fire from the Heart	Clear heat from the Heart, transform phlegm, open orifices
Herbal formulas		Xie Xin Tang, Dao Chi San	Huang Lian Wen Dan Tang, Meng Shi Gun Tan Wan

Table 1.13 Comparison of Heart Fire Blazing and Phlegm-Fire Harassing the Heart

8 Phlegm Misting the Heart Pattern 痰謎心竅証

Definition: A group of signs and symptoms caused by phlegm obstructing the Heart orifice, presenting with abnormal mental behavior.

Clinical manifestations: Mental fatigue, somnolence or stupor, abnormal behavior accompanied by cough with phlegm or breathing with phlegm sounds in the throat, a thick greasy tongue coating, and a slippery pulse. This pattern can be subdivided into yin manic psychosis (癲 *diān*), epilepsy (癇 *xián*), and phlegm collapse (痰厥 *tán júe*).

Diseases	Common Symptoms	Different Symptoms
Yin mania (癲)	Abnormal behavior, cough with phlegm or breathing with rattling sound, a thick greasy tongue coating, and a slippery pulse	Chronic depression, aversion to speaking or mumbling to oneself, laughing, or crying inappropriately
Epilepsy (癇)		Sudden syncope with drooling saliva and spasms of the limbs; a short blackout or period of confused memory, odd changes in the way things look, sound, smell or feel; after the symptoms pass, the patient manifests no abnormality
Phlegm collapse (痰厥)		Dim complexion, sense of fuzziness, ambiguous speech, breathing with phlegm sound, syncope, loss of consciousness

Table 1.14 Clinical manifestation of Phlegm Misting the Heart

Key points: Abnormal mental behavior combined with phlegm signs and symptoms.

Etiology and pathogenesis: This pattern is mostly caused by dampness invasion obstructing qi circulation or emotional stress leading to qi stagnation. Dampness invasion may be due to the external environment or weather; improper diet such as overconsumption of sweet, greasy, raw, and cold foods; or overconsumption of alcohol. When qi fails to move and distribute body fluids, there will be fluid accumulation, which engenders phlegm. Chronic illness with Lung, Spleen, or Kidney deficiency or a weak constitution may also cause water metabolism dysfunction that generates phlegm.

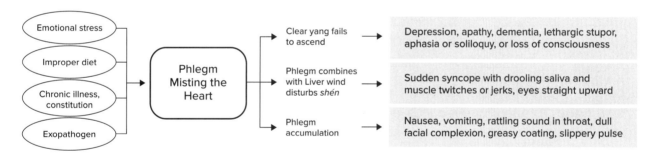

Chart 1.16 Etiology and pathogenesis of Phlegm Misting the Heart

TCM Disease	Western Disease	Herbal Formulas		Acupuncture	
Constraint presentations (鬱証)	Depression, neurosis, menopause syndrome, ADD/ADHD, autism	Dao Tan Tang, Gun Tan Wan, Di Tan Tang	Yue Ju Wan	PC-5, HT-9, BL-15, BL-20, ST-40, GV-14, GV-26, CV-12	BL-15, BL-18, BL-20, HT-7
Seizure presentations (癇証)	Epilepsy		Shun Qi Dao Tan Wan		GV-20, CV-15, SI-3, LR-3, BL-62
Yin mania (陰狂)	Schizophrenia, hysteria, neurosis, OCD, PTSD, ADD/ADHD		Ding Xian Wan		GV-20, PC-6, HT-7

Table 1.15 Diseases and treatments related to Phlegm Misting the Heart

Comparison: Phlegm Misting the Heart vs. Phlegm-Fire Harrassing the Heart

Phlegm misting the Heart (痰謎心竅 *tán mí xīn qiào*) and phlegm-fire harassing the Heart (痰火擾心 *tán huǒ rǎo xīn*) both display signs and symptoms of phlegm obstruction, including abnormal behavior, a thick greasy tongue coating, and a slippery pulse.

However, phlegm-fire harassing the Heart, regarded as 'yang madness,' involves excess heat and violent behavior, exhibiting irritability, restlessness, slurred or incoherent speech, shouting, and uncontrollable laughing or crying. In contrast, phlegm misting the Heart, regarded as 'yin madness,' does not involve heat signs but exhibits depressive behavior such as stupor, mental confusion, depression, muttering, aphasia, and lethargy.

The key points to distinguish these two patterns are as follows:
1) Excitement and irritability vs. depression and stupor
2) Excess heat signs vs. no obvious heat signs

Pattern		Phlegm Misting the Heart	Phlegm-Fire Harassing the Heart
Pathogenesis		Phlegm obstructs the Heart orifice, clear yang fails to ascend to nourish the brain, phlegm may combine with Liver wind and disturb the *shén*	Heat and phlegm accumulation rises and harasses the Heart, disturbs the shen
Symptoms	Common	Abnormal behaviors, with phlegm obstruction signs and symptoms, such as rattling sounds in the throat, a thick greasy tongue coating, and a slippery pulse	
	Mental condition	Mental fatigue, somnolence, stupor, depression, autism, epilepsy, loss of consciousness	Slurred speech, incoherent speech, uncontrollable laughing or crying, muttering, shouting, violent behavior
		Yin	Yang
Tongue & pulse		Thick greasy tongue coating; slippery pulse	Red body, thick, yellow, greasy tongue coating; slippery and rapid pulse
Treatment strategy		Transform phlegm, open orifices	Clear heat from Heart, transform phlegm, open orifices
Herbal formulas		Dao Tan Tang, Gun Tan Wan, Di Tan Tang	Huang Lian Wen Dan Tang, Meng Shi Gun Tan Wan

Table 1.16 Comparison of Phlegm Misting the Heart and Phlegm-Fire Harassing the Heart

9 Heart Vessels Obstruction Pattern | 心脈瘀阻 |

Definition: A group of signs and symptoms caused by pathogenic factors such as blood stasis, turbid phlegm, excess cold, or qi stagnation obstructing heart vessels, resulting in palpitations, pain, and oppression in the chest.

Clinical manifestations: The common signs and symptoms include fright or continuous palpitations, tight sensation or distress in the chest, intermittent chest pain attacks, and pain radiating to the shoulders and arms. The following table indicates signs and symptoms caused by different pathogenic factors.

Common Symptoms	Pathogenesis	Symptoms and Signs
Continuous or fright palpitations, chest tightness and distress, chest pain intermittent attack and pain radiates to shoulder and arm	Blood stasis	Sharp pain which is like a needle prick, purple tongue or purple spots on the tongue, a thready and choppy pulse
	Phlegm	Heavy and tightness pain, obesity, heavy sensation of the body, tiredness, white greasy tongue coating, deep and slippery pulse
	Excess cold	Sudden onset, severe pain, relieved by warmth, cold limbs, pale tongue with white coating, deep and slow or deep and tight pulse
	Qi stagnation	Distended pain, paroxysmal, induced by emotional stress, a slight red tongue, and a wiry pulse
Heart vessels can be obstructed by one pathogen alone, such as blood stasis or phlegm, but also can be obstructed by multiple pathogenic factors, such as qi and blood stagnation, or qi stagnation with phlegm, or qi and blood stagnation with phlegm.		

Table 1.17 Clinical manifestation of Heart Vessels Obstruction

Key points: Palpitations, chest tightness and distress with pain.

Etiology and pathogenesis: External pathogenic attack, improper diet such as eating greasy cold foods, long-term emotional stress, or chronic illness, all can generate pathogenic cold, phlegm, blood stasis, or qi stagnation.

These pathogenic factors can obstruct vessels, preventing yang qi from performing its warming and promoting function, which leads to qi and blood circulation becoming blocked or unsmooth, causing palpitations, chest distress, and pain.

Depending on the etiological factor, pain can have different characteristics. If blood stasis obstructs the vessels there is a sharp and stabbing pain, which is worse in the evening and presents with a purple tongue and a choppy pulse. If phlegm obstructs the vessels there is a heavy and tight pain sensation in the chest and the patient usually presents with obesity, a thick greasy tongue coating, and a slippery pulse. When pathogenic cold obstructs the vessels it causes severe pain with sudden onset and pain relieved by warmth. And if qi stagnation obstructs the vessels it leads to distending pain and is usually induced or aggravated by emotional stress.

The Heart channel passes through the shoulder down to the arm, so when pathogenic factors obstruct the Heart vessels, pain may radiate to the shoulder and down to the arm.

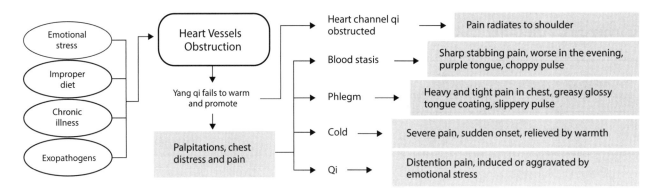

Chart 1.17 Etiology and pathogenesis of Heart Vessels Obstruction

Pathogenesis	Treatment Strategy	Herbal Formulas	Acupuncture	
Blood stasis	Promote blood circulation to remove blood stasis, remove obstruction in the channels to relieve pain	Xue Fu Zhu Yu Tang, Tong Qiao Huo Xue Tang	PC-6, BL-15, CV-17, HT-5, HT-7	BL-17, BL-18, SP-10
Phlegm	Activate yang and purge the turbid pathogens, eliminate phlegm and relieve stagnation	Gua Lou Xie Bai Ban Xia Tang		ST-40, CV-12
Cold	Warm and activate yang, expel cold, and relieve pain	Gua Lou Xie Bai Bai Jiu Tang		Moxa
Qi	Activate qi, relieve pain, calm *shén*	Mu Xiang Liu Qi Yin		LR-3, LI-4

Table 1.18 Diseases and treatments related to Heart Vessels Obstruction

Summary of Heart Disease Patterns

Key points: palpitations, sleep disorder, *shén* disorder, chest distress or pain, canker sores, pale or dark complexion, poor memory and concentration, tongue ulcers, irregular pulse				
	Patterns		**Clinical manifestations**	
			Common	**Different**
Deficiency	Heart Qi Deficiency		Palpitations, shortness of breath, chest distress or tightness, worse with exertion, somnolence, weak and/or irregular pulse	Fatigue, pale and sallow complexion, deficiency pulse
	Heart Yang Deficiency			Chest pain, cold limbs, intolerance to cold, dark lips, pale complexion, thin and faint pulse
	Heart Yang Collapse			Profuse cold oily sweat, severely cold limbs, severe palpitations, feeble breath, stupor or coma
	Heart Blood Deficiency		Palpitations, insomnia, dream-disturbed sleep	Pale, dizziness, blurry vision, poor memory and concentration, pale tongue, thin and weak pulse
	Heart Yin Deficiency			Low-grade fever in the afternoon and evening, five center heat, malar flush, night sweats, red tongue with scanty coating, thin rapid pulse
Excess	Heart Fire Blazing		Irritability, flushed face, restlessness, agitation, fidgeting, vexation, fever, insomnia, yellow urine, constipation, thirst, red tongue, rapid pulse	Canker sore or tongue ulcer, nosebleed, vomiting with blood
	Phlegm-Fire Harassing the Heart			Slurred speech, incoherent speech, uncontrolled laughing or crying, muttering, shouting, manic behavior, rattling sound in the throat, yellow sputum, thick, yellow, greasy tongue coating, slippery pulse
	Phlegm Misting the Heart	Yin mania (*diān*)	Abnormal behavior, cough with phlegm or breathing with phlegm sound, a thick greasy tongue coating, slippery pulse	Chronic depression, aversion to speaking, or mumbling to oneself, laughing or crying inappropriately
		Epilepsy (*xián*)		Sudden syncope with drooling saliva and spasms of the limbs. There is a short blackout or period of confused memory, odd changes in the way things look, sound, smell, or feel. After the symptoms pass, the patient manifests no abnormality.
		Phlegm collapse (*tán júe*)		Dim complexion, sense of fuzziness, ambiguous speech, breathing with phlegm sound, syncope, loss of consciousness
	Heart Vessels Obstruction	Blood Stasis	Continuous or fright palpitations, chest tightness and distress, chest pain, intermittent attack and pain that radiates to shoulder and arm	Sharp pain which is like a needle prick, purple tongue or purple spots on the tongue, a thin and choppy pulse
		Phlegm		Heavy and tight pain, obesity, heavy sensation of the body, tiredness, white greasy tongue coating, deep and slippery pulse
		Excess cold		Sudden onset, severe pain, relieved by warmth, cold limbs, pale tongue with white coating, deep and slow or deep and tight pulse
		Qi Stagnation		Distended pain, usually induced by emotional stress, a slight red tongue, and a wiry pulse

Table 1.19 Summary of Heart disease patterns

Chapter 2
Lung Disease Patterns

Physiological characteristics and functions of the Lung

Known as the 'florid canopy' (華蓋 *húa gài*), the Lung is located in the chest in the uppermost position of the *zàng fǔ* organs. It is also called a 'delicate organ' (嬌臟 *jīao zàng*) because it is a clear and empty organ and the pathological changes of other *zàng fǔ* organs frequently affect the Lung. Environmental changes easily affect the physiological function of the Lung because of its direct connection to the exterior through the Lung system (肺系 *fèi xì*), which includes the trachea, throat, and nose.

The Lung channel begins in the middle burner, goes through the Lung and emerges from the skin in the axilla, then runs down the arm to the end of the thumb, and is internally-externally connected with the Large Intestine. It controls and is associated with the body's surface (肌表 *jī biǎo*), which includes skin, sweat glands, body hair, and interstitial spaces (腠理 *còu lǐ*). It opens to the nose, manifests in the body hair, and its fluid is nasal mucus.

The Lung is a minister organ (相傅之官 *xiāng fù zhī guan*) in charge of cooperation and coordination, helping the Heart function normally. Its spirit is the corporeal soul (魄 *pò*) and its related emotions are sadness, worry, and grief. It belongs to the metal phase, governs qi, and is associated with the season of autumn and the climate of dryness.

Lung	Relationship
Spirit	Corporeal soul (魄 *pò*)
Internal-external connection	Large Intestine
Open orifice	Nose
Controls	Body's surface: skin, sweat glands, body hair, interstitial spaces
External manifestation	Body hair
Fluid	Nasal mucus
Fire	Minister
Emotion	Worry, grief, sadness
Season	Autumn
Five phase	Metal
Six climate factor	Dryness

Table 2.1 Lung and its related properties

1 | Governs and controls qi

(1) Governs the qi of respiration
- Responsible for respiratory movement (inhalation and exhalation)
- Air exchange site: inhales clear air and expels turbid air, normalizes the metabolic process

(2) Governs the qi of the whole body
- Governs and regulates *zàng fǔ* organs and vessels of the entire body.
- Generates and distributes gathering qi (宗氣 *zōng qì*)
- Inhalation and exhalation movement regulates the ascending and descending, exiting and entering movement of all qi in the body

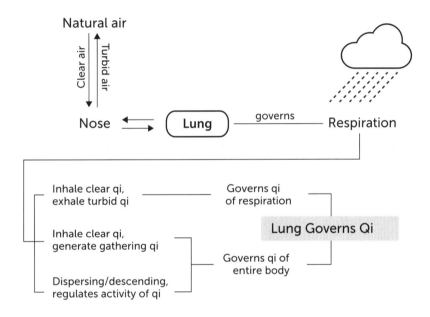

Chart 2.1 Physiology of Lung governing qi

2 | 'Lung governs the hundred vessels and is responsible for the coordinating function'

The 'Lung governs the hundred vessels and is responsible for the coordinating function' (肺朝百脈主治節 *fèi cháo bǎi mài zhǔ zhì jié*). The 'hundred vessels' refers to the blood vessels of the entire body all meeting in the Lung, carrying blood into the Lung, and conducting air exchange there. Normal blood circulation depends upon the distribution and regulation of Lung qi, thus the Lung plays an integral role as a coordinator of the *zàng fǔ* organs. *Simple Questions,* **Chapter 8** (素問, 靈蘭秘典論) states: "Lung is the premier who is responsible for the coordinating function" (肺主治節 *fèi zhǔ zhì jié*).

(1) Assists the Heart in promoting and regulating blood circulation
(2) The rhythmic inhaling and exhaling of the Lung regulates the ascending and descending movement of qi in the body
(3) Forms and distributes gathering qi and regulates the entire body's functional activities
(4) The distribution, circulation, and excretion of body fluids are regulated by the dispersing and descending function of the Lung

3 | Governs dispersing and descending function

(1) Dispersing (宣發 *xuān fā*) means diffusing and distributing, and is characterized by upward and outward movement.
- Dispersing and distributing protective qi (衛氣 *wèi qì*) to the body's surface, interstitial spaces (腠理 *còu lǐ*), and internal organs to warm, nourish and protect
- Disseminating qi, blood, and body fluids to the entire body; nourishing and moistening
- Expelling waste through air exchange and sweating

(2) Descending (肅降 *sù jiàng*) consists of two functions:
- *Sù* means to eliminate and refers to cleansing and purifying. *Sù* is a self-defense function of the human body, which includes clearing away toxins and foreign bodies.
- *Jiàng* means descending and downward. It mainly manifests in three functions:
  - Lung qi descending, which helps ensure deep, even, and smooth breathing
  - Promoting water metabolism and maintaining its balance
  - Distributing food and water essence to the entire body while sending waste down into the Urinary Bladder and Large Intestine to be excreted

4 | Regulates water metabolism: 'dredging and regulating'

(1) Through its dispersing function, the Lung regulates the excretion of sweat
(2) Through its descending function, the Lung ensures patency of the water passage, 'the Lung is the upper source of water'

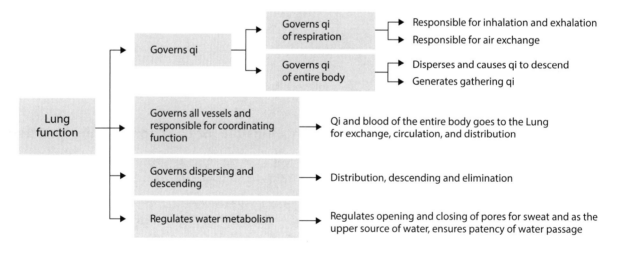

Chart 2.2 Lung function summary

Common etiological factors in Lung patterns

Exopathogenic factors are the major cause for Lung disease, but endopathogenic factors may also result in pathological changes to the Lung. The following are common etiological factors for Lung disease patterns:

(1) The six exopathogenic factors: wind, heat, cold, dryness, dampness, and summer-heat

(2) Improper diet: excessive consumption of raw, cold food, or sweet and greasy food, generating phlegm
(3) Long-term emotional stress: sadness, worry, and grief deplete Lung qi
(4) Smoking: consumes Lung yin and generates phlegm
(5) Chronic illness: damages Lung qi, impairs Lung yin

Pathological changes and major clinical manifestations of Lung disease

Pathological changes of the Lung are mostly due to disorders of its functions of governing qi and controlling respiration, as well as failure to disperse and descend. The major clinical manifestations of Lung function disorder include chills and fever, abnormal breathing, and coughing.

1 | Chills and fever

Definition: The condition in which the patient has a sensation of chills accompanied by an elevated body temperature, commonly referred to as 'simultaneous chills and fever.' It is seen in the initial stage of an exterior pattern caused by exogenous pathogens.

Etiology and pathomechanisms: Chills and fever reflect the struggle between protective qi and the pathogenic factor. When exogenous pathogens attack the body, protective qi will rise up against the pathogen. This process may weaken or impair the protective qi's warming function. Therefore, the patient feels an aversion to wind or cold. Meanwhile, the struggle between the protective qi and the exopathogen leads to the raising up of yang qi, which creates an elevated body temperature.

The Lung governs the body's surface, is responsible for the formation and distribution of protective qi, and regulates the entire body's functional activities. Therefore, chills and fever are the clinical manifestation of a pathological change in the Lung.

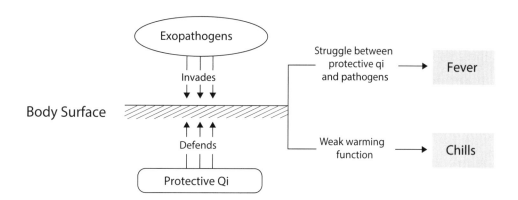

Chart 2.3 Etiology and pathomechanism of chills and fever

2 | Abnormal respiration

Definition: Abnormal respiration refers to changes in respiratory rate, rhythm, smoothness, strength, and sound quality (clear or turbid). Panting, wheezing, upper stifling breath, shortness of breath, and shortage of qi are the types of abnormal respiration commonly seen in the clinic. Abnormal respiration is the external manifestation of pathological changes in the Lung.

(1) Panting (喘 *chuǎn*): also called 'asthma,' is difficult, short, and rapid respiration. There is a sense of tightness, congestion, breathlessness or constriction in the chest, and difficulty inhaling. In severe cases, the patient gasps for breath with his mouth open, lifting his shoulders and flaring his nostrils to assist in respiration. During an attack, the patient is unable to lie flat.
(2) Wheezing (哮 *xiao*): respiration is rapid and makes a whistling sound. Recurrent attacks are likely. This condition is difficult to cure.
(3) Upper stifling breath (上氣 *shàng qì*): respiration is rapid with exhalation more evident than inhalation and may be accompanied by shortness of breath and edema of the face and eyes.
(4) Shortness of breath (短氣 *duǎn qì*): respiration is inconsistent, shallow, and rapid without sounds. It is like panting, but without lifting the shoulders to breathe.
(5) Shortage of qi (少氣 *shǎo qì*): respiration is feeble and short. It is difficult to produce the sound required for speech, but otherwise the breathing sounds normal.

Etiology and pathomechanisms: There are two major causes of abnormal respiration. The first is excess in nature and involves pathogens obstructing Lung qi. Pathogenic factors such as wind, heat, cold, dampness, or dryness may attack the Lung from the exterior. However, pathogenic factors such as phlegm, blood stasis, qi stagnation, or dampness can also be internally generated by dysfunction of the *zàng fǔ* organs. This dysfunction can be caused by an improper diet of over-consuming greasy, cold, sweet, or spicy foods; emotional stress; or smoking. When the Lung qi is obstructed, its descending function is impaired and the Lung qi rebels, which manifests as wheezing, panting, upper stifling breath, or shortness of breath.

The second cause of abnormal respiration is deficient in nature and involves the Lung and Kidney qi. Improper diet leading to malnutrition, smoking that damages Lung qi and yin, long-term emotional stress involving sadness or grief, or chronic illness can all lead to a deficiency in the Lung and Kidney. When the Lung qi is too weak to descend under its own power or when the Kidney qi is unable to aid the Lung in grasping qi, there may be accumulation or ascension of qi in the chest, leading to abnormal respiratory function.

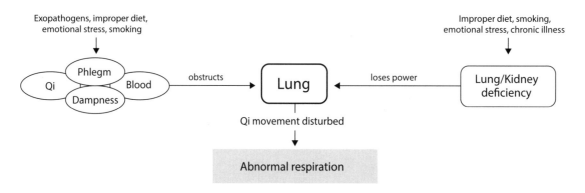

Chart 2.4 Etiology and pathomechanism of abnormal respiration

3 | Cough

Definition: Cough is a common symptom arising from pathological changes of the Lung. Expelling air from the Lung suddenly and noisily keeps the respiratory passages free of irritating material (phlegm or other). Therefore, coughing not only suggests pathological changes, but is also a response for self-protection.

Etiology and pathomechanism: The pathomechanism of coughing is rebellious Lung qi. The three major causes of cough are exopathogenic factors attacking the Lung, endopathogenic factors obstructing the Lung, and malnourishment of the Lung. Spasmodic contraction of the thoracic cavity causes the Lung qi to ascend, leading to a sudden closing of the glottis, which produces the sound of coughing.

When exopathogenic factors such as wind, heat, cold, dryness, or dampness attack the body, the Lung is often the first organ to be affected. Exopathogens disturb the movement of the Lung qi, causing rebellious qi, which leads to cough.

Endopathogenic factors such as phlegm, blood stasis, and qi stagnation arise from the dysfunction of internal *zàng fǔ* organs caused by improper diet such as overconsumption of cold, greasy, spicy, or raw foods; overconsumption of alcohol; emotional stress; or smoking. When pathogenic factors lodge in the Lung, qi circulation is disrupted, causing Lung qi counterflow and resulting in cough. In addition, cough is the body's natural attempt to expel the pathogens.

Improper diet leading to malnutrition, chronic illness, long-term emotional stress such as sadness and grief, and smoking can all cause qi and yin deficiency. If qi and yin are deficient there is an overall lack of nourishing and promoting in the body, which can lead to Lung qi failing to disperse and descend, resulting in cough.

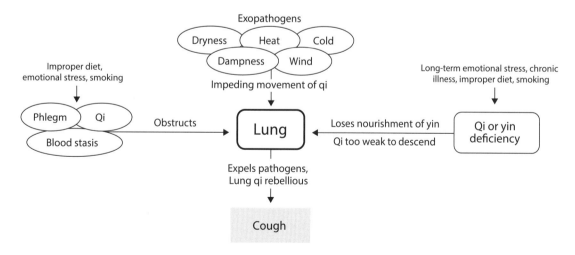

Chart 2.5 Etiology and pathomechanism of cough

4 | Other signs and symptoms related with the Lung

The following signs and symptoms can also appear in Lung patterns: nasal congestion, sneezing, edema, expectoration or hemoptysis, sore or itching throat, chest distress or pain, voice change, dry and withered body hair, abnormal sweating, and superficial pulse.

Physiological Function	Pathological Changes	Clinical Manifestation
Dominates qi, controls respiration	Reduced functional activity	Difficulty breathing, shortness of breath or shortage of qi, weak and low voice
Dispersing and descending	Failure to disperse and descend	Coughing, panting, wheezing, oppression or pain in the chest
Regulates water passage	Water metabolism disorder	Phlegm, edema
Correlation with the surface	Protective qi is impaired, fails to control interstitial spaces and skin pores	Spontaneous sweating, tendency to catch cold, aversion to wind
Correlation with the surface	Lack of nourishment and moisture of skin and hair	Dry and withered hair and skin
Opens into nose	Failure to disperse, leading to dysfunction of nose	Nasal congestion, runny nose, sneezing
Throat as a gateway of the Lung	Throat loses nourishment or is attacked by pathogens	Sore or itching throat, loss of voice, hoarseness

Table 2.2 Physiological functions, pathological changes, and clinical manifestations of the Lung

Common patterns in Lung disease

There are thirteen Lung patterns commonly seen in the clinic. These patterns can be divided into two categories according to their pathogenesis and clinical manifestation: excess patterns and deficiency patterns. Also, there are only two deficiency patterns: Lung qi deficiency and Lung yin deficiency.

Excess patterns can be subdivided into exterior excess patterns and interior excess patterns. Wind-cold invading the Lung, wind-heat invading the Lung, dryness invading the Lung, and wind-water invading the Lung are exterior excess patterns. Interior excess patterns include pathogenic heat congesting the Lung, pathogenic cold invading the Lung, cold-water shooting into the Lung, and phlegm obstructing the Lung. Phlegm obstructing the Lung can be divided into four sub-groups based on etiological factors and pathogenesis: heat-phlegm, cold-phlegm, phlegm-dampness, and phlegm-dryness.

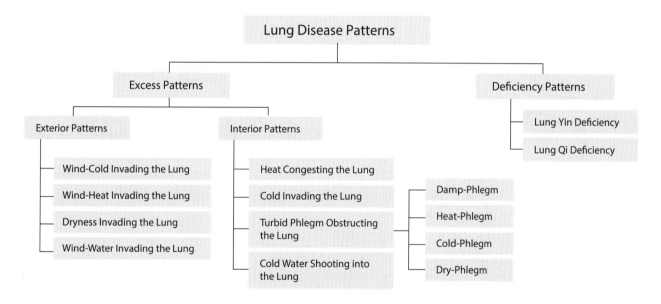

Chart 2.6   Common Lung disease patterns

	Etiology	Patterns
Deficiency	Congenital insufficiency, aging, chronic illness, improper diet, improper treatment, smoking, or long-term emotional stress	Lung Qi Deficiency, Lung Yin Deficiency
Excess	Exopathogens attacking, improper diet, improper treatment, smoking, or chronic illness	Wind-Cold Invading the Lung, Wind-Heat Invading the Lung, Dryness Invading the Lung, Wind-Water Invading the Lung, Cold Invading the Lung, Turbid Phlegm Obstructing the Lung, Heat Congesting the Lung, Cold-Water Shooting into the Lung

Table 2.3 Classification of common Lung patterns

1 Lung Qi Deficiency Pattern 肺氣虛証

Definition: A group of signs and symptoms that arises from hypofunction of the Lung.

Clinical manifestations: Feeble cough and panting that is worse with exertion, copious thin, clear sputum, shortage of qi, shortness of breath, aversion to speaking, weak voice, fatigue, low energy, spontaneous sweating, sensitivity to wind, easily catch cold, pale complexion, pale tongue with thin white coating, and a weak pulse.

Key points: Feeble cough and panting that is worse with exertion, plus qi deficiency signs and symptoms.

Etiology and pathogenesis: Insufficient production, excessive consumption, and aging are the three major causes of Lung qi deficiency.

Congenital insufficiency, chronic illness with Spleen and Stomach dysfunction, and improper diet all diminish generation and transformation, which results in lack of qi production. Disease, serious illness, injury to the vital qi, or long-term physical and mental overstrain excessively consume qi. Qi decline also follows the aging process.

The Lung governs qi, as well as dispersing and descending; therefore, if the Lung qi is deficient there is a low voice, feeble cough, or panting. When Lung qi is deficient, water metabolism is disrupted. Then pathological fluids accumulate inside, generating phlegm, which causes cough with thin white sputum. When qi is deficient, it may fail to protect the body's surface, causing susceptibility to catching colds.

Qi is the motive force of the body. When qi is insufficient, it fails to push and promote. Lack of qi manifests as shortness of breath, fatigue, aversion to speaking, and low voice, etc. When qi deficiency causes lack of blood generation, it may be reflected in a pale and tender tongue and a thin and deficient pulse. If qi is too deficient and unable to secure, the body surface will not be secured or contained, so there is spontaneous sweating. Activities consume qi; thus symptoms are worse after exertion.

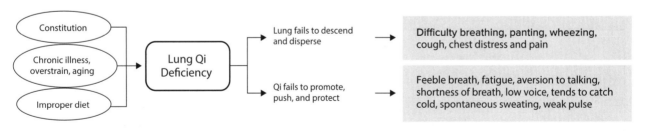

Chart 2.7 Etiology and pathogenesis of Lung Qi Deficiency

TCM Disease	Western Disease	Herbal Formulas		Acupuncture	
Cough (咳嗽)	Chronic bronchitis, emphysema, COPD, CHF, allergy asthma, lung TB, lung cancer	Bu Fei Tang	Wen Fei Tang	LU-7, LU-9, CV-6, CV-12, BL-13, GV-12, ST-36	CV-22, GV-14, ST-9, LU-1
Asthma and wheezing (哮喘)	Bronchial asthma, COPD, emphysema, pneumonia, CHF, silicosis, anxiety attack, lung TB		Sheng Mai San, Gui Zhi Jia Huang Qi Tang		Dingchuan, CV-17, CV-22, KI-1, GV-14, ST-9, LU-1
Spontaneous sweating (自汗)	Hyperthyroidism, vegetative nerve functional disturbance, HIV/AIDS, anxiety		Yu Ping Feng San		KI-7, LU-4, BL-13, BL-20, BL-43, CV-6, ST-6,
Fatigue (虛勞)	COPD, asthma, CHF, emphysema, Lyme disease, hypothyroidism		Si Jun Zi Tang		CV-4, GV-4, BL-20, BL-23

Table 2.4 Diseases and treatments related to Lung Qi Deficiency

2 Lung Yin Deficiency Pattern | 肺陰虛証 |

Definition: A group of signs and symptoms due to Lung yin deficiency, which leads to the Lung losing nourishment, generating deficiency heat, and failing to disperse and descend.

Clinical manifestations: Dry cough without sputum or with scanty sticky sputum or blood-stained sputum, difficult expectoration, dry mouth, emaciation, hoarse voice, low-grade fever in the afternoon and evening, malar flush, night sweats, five-center heat, a red tongue with scanty coating, and a thin rapid pulse.

Key points: Dry cough without sputum or with scanty sticky sputum, plus yin deficiency signs and symptoms.

Etiology and pathogenesis: Lung yin can be damaged by excess heat during the course of a febrile disease or by exopathogenic factors (especially heat, fire, and dryness). It can also be consumed by internal pathological conditions such as excessive emotional stimulation, sexual hyperactivity, aging, smoking, and over-consumption of spicy food or hot and acrid herbs. Sweating, vomiting, chronic illness and diarrhea can plunder yin fluids. Chronic illness with Kidney and Liver yin deficiency can also develop into Lung yin deficiency.

When yin fluids are damaged, yin and yang become imbalanced, with a relative excess of yang. This manifests as deficiency heat signs and symptoms: hot flashes, night sweats, five-center heat, malar flush; red tongue with scanty or no coating; thin and rapid pulse. The function of yin fluids is to nourish and moisten. Clinical manifestations of yin deficiency generally include dryness and malnutrition such as emaciation, dry mouth and throat, scanty and dark yellow urine, and constipation with dry stools.

Yin deficiency fails to nourish the Lung, causing rebellious Lung qi, which presents as coughing. The yin deficient heat condenses the phlegm and therefore the cough presents with dry sticky phlegm. If heat injures the blood vessels, the cough then presents with blood-stained sputum.

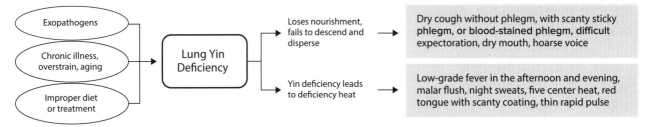

Chart 2.8 Etiology and pathogenesis of Lung Yin Deficiency

TCM Disease	Western Disease	Herbal Formulas		Acupuncture	
Cough (咳嗽)	Chronic bronchitis, emphysema, COPD, CHF, allergy asthma, lung TB, GERD, allergic rhinitis, lung cancer	Bai He Gu Jin Tang, Yang Yin Qing Fei Tang, Sheng Mai San	Sha Shen Mai Men Dong Tang, Mai Men Dong Tang	LU-9, LU-10, CV-4, CV-17, BL-13, BL-43, GV-12, KI-6, SP-6, LI-11	CV-22, BL-13, GV-14, ST-9, LU-1, LU-7
Consumptive disorder (肺痨)	Lung TB, lung cancer		Qing Hao Bie Jia San		LU-5
Hemoptysis (咳血)	Bronchitis, bronchiectasis, CHF, TB, lung cancer or lung tumors, pneumonia, pulmonary embolism		Bai He Gu Jin Tang		LU-6
Atrophic lung disease (肺痿)	Stiff lung disease, atrophic emphysema, atelectasis, pulmonary fibrosis		Qing Zao Jiu Fei Tang		BL-42

Table 2.5 Diseases and treatments related with Lung Yin Deficiency

3 Wind-Cold Invading the Lung Pattern | 風寒犯肺 |

Definition: A group of signs and symptoms caused by wind-cold disrupting the Lung's dispersing and descending functions. This pattern is also called wind-cold attacking, assailing, or insulting the Lung.

Clinical manifestations: Cough with thin clear sputum, aversion to cold, fever, headache, body ache, and nasal congestion and discharge with thin snivel, hoarseness or loss of voice, thin white tongue coating, and superficial and tight pulse.

Key points: Cough with thin clear sputum, plus exterior wind-cold signs and symptoms.

Etiology and pathogenesis: Exopathogenic wind-cold is the etiology of this pattern. The Lung is a 'delicate organ.' Located at the top of the body, it governs qi, controls the skin and hair, and opens to the nose. When exopathogens invade the body, the Lung is usually the first organ to be affected. Exopathogens compromise the Lung's dispersing and descending functions, causing cough, nasal congestion, and nasal discharge.

Exopathogenic wind-cold invasion disrupts the nutritive (營 *yíng*) and protective (衛 *wèi*) system, impairs protective qi, and leads to chills and fever. Exopathogens obstruct the channels and collaterals, qi and blood circulation is compromised, which leads to stagnation and results in headache, body aches, and a tight pulse. When the antipathogenic qi rises up against the exopathogens, it pushes the qi outward, causing a superficial pulse. Since the pathogens exist on the superficial level and have not entered the deep level of the *zàng fǔ* organs, the tongue's appearance will remain normal: a pink tongue body with a thin white coating.

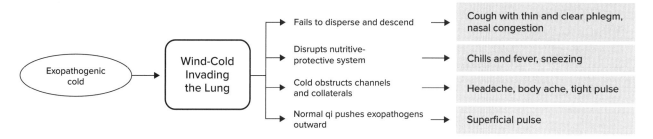

Chart 2.9 Etiology and pathogenesis of Wind-Cold Invading the Lung

TCM Disease	Western Disease	Herbal Formulas		Acupuncture	
Cough (咳嗽)	Acute bronchitis, pneumonia, URTI caused by common cold or flu	Ma Huang Tang, Xiao Qing Long Tang, Gui Zhi Tang	Xing Su San, Zhi Sou San	LU-7, LI 4, BL-12, BL-13, GB-20, GV-14, GV-16, TB-17	TB-5, ST-9, CV-22, LU-1, LU-5
Cold, flu (感冒)	Bronchitis, URTI caused by common cold or flu, such as sinusitis, rhinitis, pharyngitis, laryngitis		Ma Huang Tang		LI-20, SI-7
Asthma (喘証)	Bronchial asthma, URTI, LRTI such as bronchitis, pneumonia, lung abscess		San Ao Tang		LU-1, LU-3, LU-5, LU-9, BL-42, BL-44, CV-17, CV-22
Dysphonia (失音)	URTI caused by common cold or flu, such as pharyngitis, laryngitis		Xiang Yin Wan		LU-6, LU-10, LI-4, LI-10, ST-6, HT-6, HT-7

Table 2.6 Diseases and treatments related to Wind-Cold Invading the Lung

Comparison: Wind-Cold Invading the Lung vs. Exterior Wind-Cold

Wind-cold invading the Lung (風寒犯肺 *fēng hán fàn fèi*) and exterior wind-cold (風寒表証 *fēng hán biǎo zhèng*) share the same symptoms, etiology, and pathological location, but these two patterns are from different systems of pattern identification.

Wind-cold invading the Lung belongs to *zàng fǔ* pattern identification (臟腑辯證 *zàng fǔ biàn zhèng*), which emphasizes Lung function. The main symptoms involve disruption of the Lung's dispersing and descending function, resulting in coughing with thin clear sputum. Exterior wind-cold belongs to the eight principles pattern identification (八綱辯證 *bā gāng biàn zhèng*), which focuses on the pathological changes at the surface of the body, the protective qi, and the major symptom of chills and fever.

The key points to distinguish these two patterns are as follows:
1) Method of pattern identification: *zàng fǔ* vs. eight principles
2) Main symptoms: cough vs. chills and fever

38 Part 1: Zang Organs

Pattern	Wind-Cold Invading the Lung	Exterior Wind-Cold
Pathogenesis	Lung qi's dispersing and descending function is disrupted by wind-cold	Wind-cold attacks the body's surface, constricts protective qi
Diagnosis method	Zang Fu	Eight Principles
Location	Exterior and interior	Exterior
Symptoms — Common	Chills and fever, headache, body ache, cough with thin clear sputum, nasal congestion, thin clear discharge	
Symptoms — Main	Cough	Chills and fever
Symptoms — Other	Slight chills and fever, headache, mild exterior wind-cold signs and symptoms	With or without cough, very mild cough
Tongue & pulse	Normal tongue with thin white coating; superficial and tight pulse	
Treatment strategy	More focused on stopping cough	More focused on releasing the exterior
Herbal formulas	Xing Su San	Ma Huang Tang

Table 2.7 Comparison of Wind-Cold Invading the Lung and Exterior Wind-Cold

4 Wind-Heat Invading the Lung Pattern | 風熱犯肺 |

Definition: A group of signs and symptoms caused by wind-heat disrupting the Lung's dispersing and descending functions. This pattern is also called wind-heat attacking, assailing, or insulting the Lung.

Clinical manifestations: Cough with sticky yellow sputum, nasal congestion with thick yellow discharge, fever, slight aversion to wind or cold, slight thirst, and sore throat. Tongue has red tip with thin yellow coating. Pulse is superficial and rapid.

Key points: Cough with sticky yellow sputum, plus exterior wind-heat signs and symptoms.

Etiology and pathogenesis: Exterior wind-heat is the etiological factor for this pattern, although wind-cold can also be a factor if it transforms into heat. Wind-heat invading the Lung causes Lung qi to stagnate and rebel, resulting in nasal congestion and cough. Heat consumes fluids, causes thirst, and generates yellow sputum and discharge. Sore throat manifests when the throat lacks nourishment and is inflamed by heat toxins. Heat accelerates the blood circulation, resulting in a rapid pulse.

Wind-heat invasion causes imbalance between nutritive qi (營氣 *yíng qì*) and protective qi (衛氣 *wèi qì*). Protective qi is engaged in battle with the exopathogens and fails to warm the body's surface, which leads to chills and fever. Superficial pulse is the signature sign of exopathogen invasion.

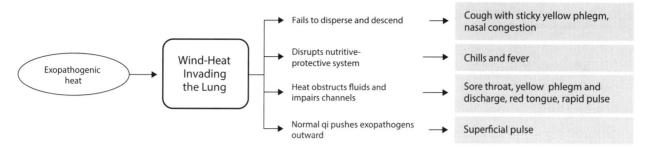

Chart 2.10 Etiology and pathogenesis of Wind-Heat Invading the Lung

TCM Disease	Western Disease	Herbal Formulas		Acupuncture	
Cough (咳嗽)	Acute bronchitis, pneumonia, URTI caused by common cold or flu	Sang Ju Yin, Yin Qiao San	Sang Ju Yin	LU-7, LI-4, LI-11, GV-14, GV-16, BL-12, GB-20, TB-5	LU-1, LU-5, L11, ST-9, CV-22, BL-13
Gan mao (感冒)	Bronchitis, URTI caused by flu or common cold, such as sinusitis, rhinitis, pharyngitis, laryngitis		Yin Qiao San		LI-20, SI-7
Asthma (喘証)	Bronchial asthma, LRTI such as lung abscess, pneumonia, bronchitis		Ma Xing Shi Gan Tang		LU-1, LU-3, LU-5, LU-9, BL-42, BL-44, CV-17, CV-22
Lung abscess (肺痈)	Suppurative pneumonia, lung abscess, bronchiectasis with infection		Wei Jing Tang		BL-13, CV-17, CV-22
Hemoptysis (咳血)	Acute bronchitis, pneumonia, bronchiectasis, URTI		Sang Xing Tang		LU-3, LU-5, LU-6, LU-9, ST-12, SI-2
Nosebleed (鼻衄)	Non-allergic rhinitis, sinusitis, common cold		Sang Ju Yin, Chai Ge Jie Ji Tang		LU-3, LU-5, L11, LI-2, LI-3, LI-5, LI-6, LI-20

Table 2.8 Diseases and treatments related to Wind-Heat Invading the Lung

Comparison: Wind-Cold Invading the Lung vs. Wind-Heat Invading the Lung

Wind-cold invading the Lung (風寒犯肺 *fēng hán fàn fèi*) and wind-heat invading the Lung (風熱犯肺 *fēng rè fàn fèi*) share the same location and pathogenesis, and therefore both exhibit cough along with mild exterior signs and symptoms. However, the clinical manifestations still differ because the two patterns have different etiologies, one being caused by wind-cold and the other by wind-heat.

Wind-cold disrupts the nutritive (*yíng*) and protective (*wèi*) system, cold impairs the protective qi and damages yang. Therefore, patients feel chills more than fever. Cold constricts and obstructs the channels and collaterals, compromising qi and blood circulation, which leads to stagnation and results in headache, body aches, low pitch, turbid and forceful cough, and tight pulse. Wind-heat invading the Lung causes Lung qi to stagnate. Thus patients feel more fever than chills. Heat consumes fluids, causes yellow sputum and discharge, thirst, hacking high-pitched cough, and a rapid pulse. Sore throat manifests when the throat lacks nourishment and is inflamed by heat toxicity.

The key points to distinguish these two patterns are as follows:
1) Cough sounds
2) Sputum quality and color
3) Presence of sore throat
4) Rapid vs. tight pulse

Pattern		Wind-Cold Invading the Lung	Wind-Heat Invading the Lung
Etiology	Common	Exopathogenic wind	
	Different	Cold	Heat
Pathogenesis	Common	Exopathogens' invasion disrupts Lung's descending and dispersing function	
	Different	Cold constricts and obstructs channels and collaterals	Heat impairs body fluids, heat toxin leads to inflammation of the throat
Symptoms	Common	Cough with mild exterior signs and symptoms	
	Cough	Harsh, coarse, low pitch, turbid, forceful	Hacking hoarseness, high-pitched
	Fever & Chills	Severe chills, mild fever	Severe fever, mild chills
	Sputum	Thin and clear	Sticky and yellow
	Other	Headache, body ache, itchy throat	Sore throat, thirst, slight sweating
Tongue & pulse		Normal tongue with thin white coating; superficial and tight pulse	Slight red tongue with thin yellow coating; superficial and rapid pulse
Treatment strategy		Warm and pungent herbs to promote sweating and release the exterior	Cool/cold and pungent herbs to promote sweating, clear heat, and relieve toxicity
Herbal formulas		Ma Huang Tang, Gui Zhi Tang, Xing Su San	Yin Qiao San, Sang Ju Yin

Table 2.9 Comparison of Wind-Cold Invading the Lung and Wind-Heat Invading the Lung

Comparison: Wind-Heat Invading the Lung vs. Exterior Wind-Heat

Wind-heat invading the Lung (風熱表証 *fēng rè fàn fèi*) and exterior wind-heat (燥邪犯肺 *fēng rè biǎo zhèng*) share the same symptoms, etiology, and pathological location, but these two patterns are from different systems of pattern identification.

Wind-heat invading the Lung belongs to *zàng fǔ* pattern identification, which emphasizes Lung function. The main symptoms are wind-heat disrupting the Lung's dispersing and descending function, leading to cough with a yellow sticky sputum. Exterior wind-heat belongs to eight principles pattern identification system, which focuses on the pathological changes at the surface of the body, the protective qi, and the major symptom of chills and fever.

The key points to distinguish these two patterns are as follows:
1) Method of pattern identification: *zàng fǔ* vs. eight principles
2) Main symptoms: cough vs. chills, fever, and sore throat

Pattern	Wind-Heat Invading the Lung	Exterior Wind-Heat
Pathogenesis	Wind-heat invades the Lung, disrupting its dispersing and descending function	Wind-heat invades the body's surface, disrupting the harmony of the nutritive and protective
Diagnosis Method	*Zàng Fǔ*	Eight Principles
Location	Exterior and interior co-exist	Exterior
Symptoms — Common	Cough with sticky yellow sputum, nasal congestion, thick yellow discharge, sore throat, thirst	
Symptoms — Main	Cough	Chills and fever
Symptoms — Other	Mild exterior wind-heat symptoms: slight chills and fever, sore throat	With or without cough; if there is cough, it is very mild
Tongue & pulse	Red tongue tip, thin yellow coating; superficial and rapid pulse	
Treatment strategy	Stop cough, clear heat	Release the exterior, clear heat
Herbal formulas	Sang Ju Yin	Yin Qiao San

Table 2.10 Comparison of Wind-Heat Invading the Lung and Exterior Wind-Heat

5 Dryness Invading the Lung Pattern | 燥邪犯肺 |

Definition: A group of signs and symptoms caused by exopathogenic dryness attacking the Lung and damaging Lung yin. This pattern is also called 'lung dryness' or 'exterior dryness.' Depending on the accompanying pathogens, it can manifest as warmth-dryness (溫燥 *wēn zào*) or coolness-dryness (涼燥 *liáng zào*).

Clinical manifestations: Dry cough, scanty sticky sputum or blood-stained sputum, difficult expectoration, dry mouth, throat and nose or nosebleeds, cough with blood, dry stool, scanty urine, thin and dry tongue coating. These symptoms are accompanied by fever, slight chills, and absent or slight sweating. Pulse is superficial and rapid or superficial and tight.

Key points: Dry cough with scanty sticky sputum, dry mouth, throat and nose, plus mild exterior signs and symptoms.

Etiology and pathogenesis: Exopathogenic dryness is the etiological factor for this pattern. The Lung is the organ that favors moisture and disfavors dryness. When dryness attacks the body, it first affects the Lung. When the Lung loses its moisture, it is unable to perform its dispersing and descending functions, resulting in Lung qi rebellion and stagnation, which gives rise to coughing.

Dryness impeding Lung function causes specific types of cough: cough without sputum, with scanty sticky sputum, or with blood-stained sputum. Sputum is difficult to expectorate and may arise with nasal congestion, or chest distress and pain. When dryness invades the superficial layer of the body, protective qi rises up to fight against the pathogen, resulting in fever, aversion to cold and a superficial pulse.

Dryness damages the body fluids. Signs and symptoms include dry mouth and lips, thirst with desire to drink, dry throat and nose, dry and chapped skin, dry hair, scanty urine, dry stools, and a dry tongue coating.

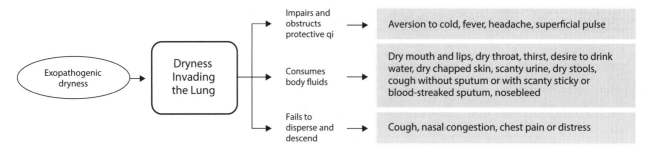

Chart 2.11 Etiology and pathogenesis of Dryness Invading the Lung

Pattern	Warmth-Dryness Invading Lung	Coolness-Dryness Invading Lung
Etiology	Dryness	
	Warmth	Coolness
Pathogenesis	Dryness leads to insufficient moistening and nourishing of the Lung, causing dysfunction of descending and dispersing	
	Warmth generates heat, damages more body fluid	Cold constricts and obstructs body's surface and channels
Season	Late summer and early autumn	Late autumn and early winter
Symptoms	Dry cough, possibly with scanty sputum, dry mouth, thirst, dry coating, superficial pulse	
	Yellow or blood-stained sputum, preference for cold drinks	Slight aversion to cold, no sweating, white sputum, headache
Tongue	Slightly red with thin, slightly yellow coating	Normal tongue with thin dry coating
Pulse	Rapid	Slightly tight
Treatment strategy	Clear and disperse warmth-dryness, moisten the Lung, stop cough	Gently disperse coolness-dryness, disseminate the Lung qi, transform phlegm
Herbal formulas	Sang Xing Tang, Qing Zao Jiu Fei Tang	Xing Su San

Table 2.11 Lung patterns caused by pathogenic dryness

TCM Disease	Western Disease	Herbal Formulas		Acupuncture	
Cough (咳嗽)	Chronic bronchitis, URTI, allergies, whooping cough, smoking, bronchospasm		Sang Xing Tang, Mai Men Dong Tang		LU-1, LU-5, LU-11, CV-22, BL-13, ST-9
Cold, flu (感冒)	Bronchitis, URTI caused by flu or common cold such as sinusitis, rhinitis, pharyngitis, laryngitis	Qing Zao Jiu Fei Tang, Bai He Gu Jin Tang, Sha Shen Mai Men Dong Tang	Jia Jian Wei Rui Tang	BL-13, BL-17, LU-1, LU-6, LU-7, KI-6	LI-20, SI-7
Asthma (喘证)	Bronchial asthma, URTI such as lung abscess, pneumonia, bronchitis		Bai He Gu Jin Tang		L1, L3, L5, L9, BL-42, BL-44, CV-17, CV-22
Hemoptysis (咳血)	Acute bronchitis, pneumonia, bronchiectasis, URTI		Xie Bai San		LU-3, LU-5, LU-6, LU-9, ST-12, SI-2
Nosebleed (鼻衄)	Non-allergic rhinitis, sinusitis, common cold		Sha Shen Mai Men Dong Tang		LU-3, LU-5, LU-11, LI-2, LI-3, LI-5, LI-6, LI-20

Table 2.12 Diseases and treatments related to Dryness Invading the Lung

Comparison: Dryness Invading the Lung vs. Exterior Dryness

Dryness invading the Lung (燥邪犯肺 *zào xié fàn fèi*) and exterior dryness (燥邪表証 *zào xié biǎo zhèng*) share the same symptoms, etiology, and pathological location, but these two patterns are from different systems of pattern identification.

Dryness invading the Lung belongs to *zàng fǔ* pattern identification, which emphasizes Lung function. Thus this pattern focuses on pathogenic dryness damaging Lung yin, disrupting the Lung's dispersing and descending function, and resulting in cough with white sticky sputum. Exterior dryness belongs to eight principles pattern identification, which focuses on pathological changes at the surface of the body, the protective qi, and the major symptom of chills and fever.

The key points to distinguish these two patterns are as follows:
1) Method of pattern identification: *zàng fǔ* vs. eight principles
2) Main symptoms: dry cough vs. chills and fever

Pattern		Dryness Invading the Lung	Exterior Dryness
Pathogenesis		Dryness impairs Lung yin and disrupts its dispersing and descending function	Dryness invades the body's surface, leading to ying and wei disharmony
Diagnosis Method		*Zàng Fǔ*	Eight Principles
Location		Exterior and interior co-exist	Exterior
Symptoms	Common	Cough without sputum or with scanty sputum, nasal congestion, dry mouth	
	Main	Dry cough	Chills and fever
	Other	Slight chills and fever, mild exterior signs and symptoms	With or without cough; if there is cough, it is very mild
Tongue & pulse		Normal or slightly red tongue with dry coating; superficial pulse	
Treatment strategy		Moisten the Lung to stop cough	Release the exterior, moisten
Herbal formulas		Xing Su San, Sang Xing Tang	

Table 2.13 Comparison of Dryness Invading the Lung and Exterior Dryness

Comparison: Dryness Invading the Lung vs. Lung Yin Deficiency

Dryness invading the Lung (燥邪犯肺 *zào xié fàn fèi*) and Lung yin deficiency (肺陰虛 *fèi yīn xū*) share many symptoms such as dry cough with little sputum, dry mouth and throat, and a dry tongue coating. However, there are differences in clinical presentation and treatment strategy because the etiology and pathogenesis of these two patterns are different.

Pathogenic dryness invading the Lung is an exterior excess condition caused by exopathogenic dryness, and is usually acute, mild, and short course. It usually occurs in autumn, with dry weather, or from overuse of dry room heaters. Dryness is the main symptom, but the patient may also experience mild chills and fever, cough, headache, and nasal congestion. Thus the treatment strategy is to moisten the Lung to relieve dryness and gently disperse to release the exterior.

Lung yin deficiency is an interior deficiency condition that is usually chronic and long course. It can develop during the course of a febrile disease or from dryness invading the Lung. It may also be caused by improper diet, improper treatment, excessive emotional stimulation, sexual hyperactivity, aging, or chronic illness. Besides dryness, patients also suffer from yin deficiency symptoms such as tidal fever, night sweats, and five-center heat. Thus the treatment strategy for Lung yin deficiency is to nourish Lung yin and clear deficiency heat.

The key points to distinguish these two patterns are as follows:
1) Course of illness: chronic and long vs. acute and short
2) Presence of exterior signs such as chills and fever
3) Presence of deficiency heat signs such as tidal fever, night sweats, and five-center heat
4) Tongue and pulse

Pattern		Dryness Invading the Lung	Lung Yin Deficiency
Etiology		Exopathogenic dryness or wind-heat attack	Dry heat impairs Lung, over-sweating, chronic illness, improper diet, improper treatment, long-term emotional stress, overstrain, and aging
Pathogenesis		Lung fluids impaired by exopathogenic dryness, leads to Lung dysfunction	Lung yin deficiency fails to nourish Lung, with yin deficiency heat
Characteristics		Acute onset, short course	Chronic onset, long course
Nature		Exterior, excess	Interior, deficiency
Symptoms	Common	Dry cough without sputum, with little sticky sputum, or with blood-streaked sputum, difficult to expectorate, dry mouth, throat, and nose, thirst, cough with blood, nosebleed, dry stools, scanty urine	
	Different	Exterior: fever, slight aversion to wind and cold, no sweating or little sweating	Deficiency heat: tidal fever, night sweats, feverish sensation in five centers, red cheeks
Tongue & pulse		Normal or slightly red tongue body with dry coating; superficial and rapid, or superficial and tight pulse	Red or red cracked tongue body with little coating; thin and rapid pulse
Treatment strategy		Moisten the Lung, release the exterior, stop cough	Nourish Lung yin, stop cough, clear deficiency heat
Herbal formulas		Xing Su San, Sang Xing Tang, Qing Zao Jiu Fei Tang	Bai He Gu Jin Tang, Bu Fei E Jiao Tang, Yang Yin Qing Fei Tang

Table 2.14 Comparison of Dryness Invading the Lung and Lung Yin Deficiency

Comparison: Exopathogenic Factors Invading the Lung

Wind-cold invading the Lung (風寒犯肺 *fēng hán fàn fèi*), wind-heat invading the Lung (風熱犯肺 *fēng rè fàn fèi*), and pathogenic dryness invading the Lung (燥邪犯肺 *zào xié fàn fèi*) are the most common Lung-related exopathogenic patterns. They have many similarities, including: (1) symptoms: cough, chills and fever, and superficial pulse; (2) pathological location: superficial level of the body and Lung; (3) etiological factors: external wind; and (4) pathogenesis: exopathogenic attack on the body's surface, protective qi failing to its job, pathogenic invasion leading to failure of the Lung's descending and dispersing function. However, there are also many differences, including the nature of the pathogens and characteristics of the pathological manifestations. Therefore, distinguishing one from the other is important.

Wind-cold disrupts the nutritive (*yíng*) and protective (*wèi*) system, cold impairs protective qi and damages yang. Patients therefore feel chills more than fever. Cold constricts and obstructs the channels and collaterals, qi and blood circulation is compromised, which leads to stagnation and results in headaches, body aches, low pitch, turbid, and forceful cough, and a tight pulse. Wind-heat invading the Lung causes Lung qi to stagnate. Thus the patient feels more fever than chills. Heat consumes fluids, causes yellow sputum and discharge, thirst, hacking cough, and rapid pulse. Sore throat manifests when the throat lacks nourishment and is inflamed by heat toxicity. When wind-dryness invades the Lung, dryness damages body fluids and disrupts Lung function. Therefore, in addition to exterior signs and symptoms, dryness is the major complaint.

The key points to distinguish these three patterns are as follows:
1) Nature of the illness
2) Sound of cough
3) Color and quality of sputum

Pattern		Wind-Cold Invading the Lung	Wind-Heat Invading the Lung	Dryness Invading the Lung
Etiology		Wind-cold	Wind-heat	Wind-dryness
Pathogenesis		Cold constricts Lung qi, obstructs channels and collaterals	Heat impairs Lung fluids, creates heat toxin, disrupts Lung function	Dryness impairs Lung fluids, disrupts Lung function
Symptoms	Common	Chills and fever, cough, nasal congestion, headache, superficial pulse		
	Cough	Harsh, coarse, forceful, low pitch, turbid	Hacking, hoarse	Dry hacking, high pitch, crisp
	Sputum	Thin, clear, easy to expectorate	Sticky, yellow, difficult to expectorate	Scanty, white, difficult to expectorate, may contain blood
	Chills & Fever	More chills than fever	More fever than chills	Possible fever more than chills
	Other	Headache, body aches	Sore throat, thirst	Dryness, thirst
Tongue & pulse		Thin white tongue coating; superficial and tight pulse	Red tongue tip, thin yellow coating; superficial and rapid pulse	Dry tongue coating, possibly yellow; superficial, possibly rapid pulse
Treatment strategy		Release the exterior, regulate Lung qi, stop cough	Release the exterior, clear heat, transform phlegm, stop cough	Release the exterior, moisten the Lung, stop cough
Herbal formulas		San Ao Tang, Zhi Sou San, Xing Su San	Sang Ju Yin	Qing Zao Jiu Fei Tang, Sha Shen Mai Men Dong Tang

Table 2.15 Comparison of exopathogenic factors invading the Lung

6 Wind-Water Invading the Lung Pattern │ 風水犯肺 │

Definition: A group of signs and symptoms caused by pathogenic wind attacking the Lung leading to dysfunction in the draining of water passages with water-dampness penetrating muscular interstices and the skin. It is called 'wind-water pattern' (風水証 *fēng shǔi zhèng*).

Clinical manifestations: Edema with acute onset and rapid development, starting from the eyelids and then spreading to the whole body with difficult urination; accompanied by fever, aversion to cold and no sweating. A white tongue coating with a superficial and tight pulse. There may also be a sore throat, red tongue and superficial and rapid pulse.

Key points: Acute onset, edema that starts from the eyelids, plus exterior wind-cold or wind-heat signs and symptoms.

Etiology and pathogenesis: This pattern is caused by exopathogenic factors such as wind-cold, wind-heat, or wind-dampness.

The Lung is in charge of dispersing and descending, and regulating the water passages to keep them free. The Lung distributes body fluids to the entire body. It is one of the most important organs and it cooperates and coordinates with the Spleen and Kidney for water metabolism.

When exopathogens attack the Lung it disables the Lung's function. Body fluids fail to be distributed, the water metabolism process is interrupted and the result is accumulation of water and dampness.

Wind is a yang type pathogen; it is light, its characteristics are upward and outward, and it changes quickly. If wind and water catch each other, the water will be brought upward, thus edema starts from the face. From there it spreads to the whole body. Overflowing of accumulated water to the muscles and skin develops into edema. Acute onset and rapid development are the characteristics of wind. Dysfunction of the Lung's ability to regulate the water passages and cause the fluids to descend to the Urinary Bladder disrupts qi transformation (氣化 *qì huà*) and results in scanty or difficult urination.

When exopathogens obstruct the channels and collaterals, qi and blood circulation is compromised, which leads to stagnation and results in headache and body aches. When the antipathogenic qi rises up against the exopathogens, it also pushes the qi outward, resulting in a superficial pulse.

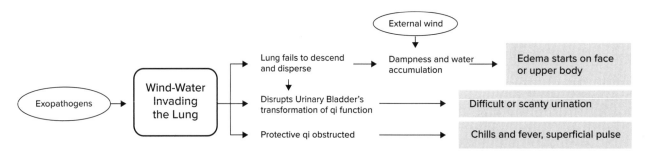

Chart 2.12 Etiology and pathogenesis of Wind-Water Invading the Lung

TCM Disease	Western Disease	Herbal Formulas		Acupuncture	
Wind-water (風水証)	Acute nephritis, acute attack of chronic nephritis, early stage pyelonephritis	Yue Bi Tang, Xiao Qing Long Tang	Yue Bi Jia Zhu Tang	LU-7, LI-4, LI-6, SP-9, BL-39	BL-13, BL-22, LU-5, TB-5, LI-4
Edema (水腫)	Allergic reactions, hypothyroidism		Wu Ling San, Wu Pi (San) Yin, Fang Ji Huang Qi Tang		
Wind-rash (風疹)	Atopic dermatitis, hives		Xiao Feng San		SP-10
Wind painful obstruction (風痹)	Rheumatoid arthritis		Huang Qi Gui Zhi Wu Wu Tang		BL-17, SP-10, GBL-20, GV-16

Table 2.16 Diseases and treatments related to Wind-Water Invading the Lung

7 Cold Invading the Lung Pattern |寒邪客肺|

Definition: A group of signs and symptoms caused by exopathogenic cold directly attacking the Lung, disrupting the Lung's dispersing and descending function.

Clinical manifestations: Coughing, panting, hoarseness or loss of voice, thin white or clear sputum, cold limbs and body, pale tongue with white coating, a deep and slow pulse.

Key points: Acute onset, coughing or panting, plus interior excess cold signs and symptoms.

Etiology and pathogenesis: This pattern is caused by exopathogenic cold directly attacking the Lung, which constricts the yang qi, leading Lung qi to rebel, resulting in coughing and panting. Cold is associated with yin; it coagulates and constricts, disrupts water metabolism, causes fluids to accumulate, and transforms accumulated fluids into phlegm, which is expectorated as sputum. Since yang qi is impaired by cold, it fails to warm, causing cold limbs. Cold slows down qi and blood circulation and makes the tongue pale and the pulse slow.

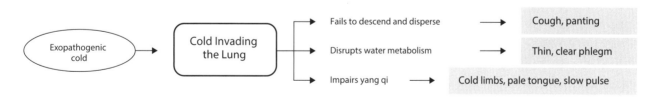

Chart 2.13   Etiology and pathogenesis of Cold Invading the Lung

48　Part 1: Zang Organs

TCM Disease	Western Disease	Herbal Formulas		Acupuncture
Cough (咳嗽)	Acute bronchitis, pneumonia, URTI caused by common cold or flu	Wen Fei Hua Yin Tang	Xiao Qing Long Tang	BL-13, TB-5, S9, CV-22, LU-1, LU-5
Cold, flu (感冒)	Bronchitis, URTI caused by common cold or flu such as sinusitis, rhinitis, pharyngitis, laryngitis			LI-20, SI-7, GB-20
Asthma (喘証)	Bronchial asthma, URTI, LRTI such as bronchitis, pneumonia, lung abscess		Xiao Qing Long Tang, Su Zi Jiang Qi Tang	LU-1, LU-3, LU-5, LU-9, BL-42, BL-44, CV-17, CV-22
Dysphonia (失音)	URTI caused by common cold or flu such as pharyngitis, laryngitis		Xiang Yin Wan	LU-6, LU-10, LI-4, LI-10, S6, HT-6, HT-7

Table 2.17 Diseases and treatments related to Cold Invading the Lung

8　Turbid Phlegm Obstructing the Lung Pattern　｜痰濁阻肺｜

Definition: A group of syndromes caused by phlegm accumulating inside the Lung, obstructing the Lung and disrupting its dispersing and descending function. According to the accompanying pathogens and pathogenesis, there are four major patterns:

(1) Phlegm-dampness Obstructing the Lung
(2) Heat-phlegm Obstructing the Lung
(3) Cold-phlegm Obstructing the Lung
(4) Phlegm-dryness Obstructing the Lung

Clinical manifestations: Productive cough, panting, wheezing, tightness and distress in the chest, phlegm in the throat, feeling of heaviness, thick tongue coating, and slippery pulse. Table 2.18 describes different types of phlegm patterns.

Key points: Productive cough, panting, wheezing, or phlegm sound in throat.

Etiology and pathogenesis: Phlegm is the pathological product of impaired water metabolism. It originates from conditions involving the accumulation of dampness. The main *zàng fǔ* organs involved in phlegm production include the Lung, Spleen, Kidney, and Triple Burner.

There are a variety of problems that can directly or indirectly affect the Lung, Spleen, and Kidney. Exo-pathogens, emotional stress, improper diet, and physical, sexual or mental overstrain can all cause pathological changes in the organs of water metabolism.

Known as the container of the phlegm, the Lung is the place where phlegm gathers after it has been generated. When phlegm enters the Lung, it obstructs and blocks the Lung qi, disrupting the Lung qi movement, leading to Lung's failure to disperse and descend, causing Lung qi counterflow, resulting in productive cough, panting or wheezing. The Lung qi's failure to disperse and descend causes the accumulation of phlegm to descend and causes tightness and distress in the chest. The nature of the phlegm is turbid and viscous, therefore the tongue coating is thick or greasy. Phlegm can also cause an increase in blood viscosity and a decrease in pulse wave flexibility, manifesting as a slippery pulse.

Patterns	Common Symptoms	Different Signs and Symptoms	
		Cough and Phlegm	Other
Dampness-Phlegm	Productive cough, wheezing, shortness of breath, distress and tightness in the chest, phlegm in the throat, feeling of heaviness, thick tongue coating, slippery pulse	Chronic paroxysmal cough with profuse white sticky sputum that is easy to expectorate, worse after eating	Obesity, aversion to lying down, nausea
Heat-Phlegm		Barking cough with profuse sticky yellow or green phlegm, difficult to expectorate	Thirst, agitation, insomnia, red tongue, rapid pulse
Cold-Phlegm		Cough with expectoration of thin white sputum, worse with exposure to cold or at night	Cold hands and feet, pale tongue, slow pulse
Dryness-Phlegm		Dry cough, occasionally difficult expectoration of scanty white or blood-streaked sputum	Dry throat and nose, dry coating

Table 2.18 Clinical manifestations of different types of phlegm

Phlegm Characteristics		Indications
Quantity	Scanty	Dryness, heat, yin deficiency
	Profuse	Dampness, deficiency, cold
Quality	White and clear	Cold
	White and thick, easy to expectorate	Dampness
	Yellow and thick	Heat
	White and thick, difficult to expectorate	Dryness, yin deficiency
	White, clear, and foaming	Deficiency, cold
	Blood	Excess heat in the Lung, or yin deficiency, or dryness
Smell & taste	Foul odor, fishing odor	Heat
	Sweet taste	Dampness
	Salty taste	Kidney deficiency

Table 2.19 Phlegm characteristics and indications

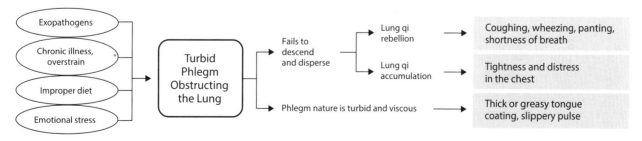

Chart 2.14 Etiology and pathogenesis of Turbid Phlegm Obstructing the Lung

Pattern	Treatment Strategy	Herbal Formulas	Acupuncture		
Dampness-Phlegm	Dry dampness, transform phlegm, regulate qi, harmonize the middle burner	Er Chen Tang, Dao Tan Tang	LU-5, LU-7, CV-12, CV-17, ST-40, BL-13	LU-1, PC-6, CV-9, CV-22, BL-20	SP-9
Cold-Phlegm	Expel cold, dissolve phlegm, warm yang, cause rebellious qi to descend	Ling Gui Zhu Gan Tang, She Gan Ma Huang Tang, San Zi Yang Qin Tang,			BL-23
Heat-Phlegm	Clear heat, dissolve phlegm, cause rebellious qi to descend	Ma Xing Shi Gan Tang, Qing Qi Hua Tan Tang		LU-1, LU-10, LI-11	
Dryness-Phlegm	Moisten the Lung, clear heat, regulate qi, transform phlegm	Bei Mu Gua Lou San		LU-9, KI-6, ST-36, SP-6,	
Phlegm and thin mucus	Warm the Lung, transform congested fluids	Ling Gan Wu Wei Jiang Xi Tang		LU-9, BL-20, BL-23, BL-43, ST-36, CV-9, SP-9	

Table 2.20 Diseases and treatments related to Turbid Phlegm Obstructing the Lung

Comparison: Wind-Cold Invading the Lung vs. Cold Invading the Lung vs. Cold-Phlegm Obstructing the Lung

Wind-cold invading the Lung (風寒犯肺 *fēng hán fàn fèi*), cold invading the Lung (寒邪客肺 *hán xié kè fèi*), and cold-phlegm obstructing the Lung (寒痰阻肺 *hán tán zǔ fèi*) all involve pathogenic cold impairing the Lung, which manifests with coughing, dyspnea, and expectoration of thin clear sputum. Although these three patterns share the same nature, they differ in depth and condition.

Wind-cold invading the Lung is an exterior excess condition that involves the presence of exopathogenic factors fighting with the protective qi (*wèi* qi) at the body's surface. Thus coughing with chills and fever and a superficial pulse are the major clinical symptoms. Cold invading the Lung is an interior excess condition caused by pathogenic cold directly invading the Lung and disrupting its function. Thus there are chills, but no fever. Cold phlegm obstructing the Lung is an interior deficiency condition and is caused by deficient yang failing to transform qi, which results in water metabolism dysfunction and phlegm accumulation in the Lung.

The key points to distinguish these three patterns are as follows:
1) Course of illness: chronic and long vs. acute and short
2) Presence of exterior signs and symptoms such as chills and fever
3) Presence of deficiency cold signs and symptoms such as intolerance of cold, loose stools, and clear copious urination
4) Tongue and pulse

Pattern	Wind-Cold Invading the Lung	Cold Invading the Lung	Cold-Phlegm Obstructing the Lung
Pathogenesis	Wind-cold attacks the body's surface, closes skin pores, Lung qi depressed, fails to disperse	Exopathogen directly attacks the Lung, constricts the yang qi, and causes Lung qi to rebel	Middle burner deficiency with cold creates phlegm, ascends and stores in the Lung, disrupts Lung's dispersing and descending function
Characteristics	Acute onset, short course, exterior, excess, cold	Sub-acute onset, longer course, interior, excess, cold	Chronic, long course, worse in the winter, common in the elderly, interior, deficiency and excess, cold
Symptoms — Common	Coughing, panting, thin and clear sputum		
Symptoms — Different	Chills and fever, nasal congestion, headache, body ache	Severe coughing, panting, cold limbs and body	Wheezing, asthma, dyspnea, chest oppression, condition induced or aggravated by exposure to cold
Phlegm source	Lung	Lung	Lung, Spleen or Kidney
Tongue & pulse	Thin white tongue coating; superficial tight pulse	Thin white tongue coating; deep, tight, and slow pulse	Pale and flabby tongue with greasy white coating; slippery or weak pulse
Treatment strategy	Regulate Lung qi, stop cough, release the exterior	Warm the Lung, stop cough	Warm the Lung, transform phlegm, stop cough
Herbal formulas	San Ao Tang, Zhi Su San	Xiao Qing Long Tang, Wen Fei Hua Tang Wan	San Zi Yang Qin Tang

Table 2.21 Comparison of Wind-Cold Invading the Lung, Cold Invading the Lung, and Cold-Phlegm Obstructing the Lung

9 Heat Congesting the Lung Pattern | 熱邪壅肺 |

Definition: A group of signs and symptoms brought about by excess heat congesting the Lung, disrupting the Lung's dispersing and descending function.

Clinical manifestations: Coughing, panting, high fever with flaring nostrils, sore throat, rapid breathing, thirst, pain in the chest, cough with foul pus and blood, dry stools, dark urine, a red tongue with yellow coating, and a rapid pulse.

Key points: Coughing, panting, plus interior excess heat signs and symptoms.

Etiology and pathogenesis: This pattern can be caused by exopathogenic heat attacking the Lung directly or by unresolved exopathogenic cold entering the interior and transforming into heat.

Excess heat congests in the Lung and disrupts its dispersing and descending function, leading to rebellious Lung qi, coughing, and panting. Heat-phlegm obstructing the airway gives rise to flaring nostrils. Heat scorches fluids, which condense into phlegm, so the sputum is yellow and sticky. If heat-phlegm accumulation rots flesh and injures blood vessels, there may be purulent and bloody sputum. When internal heat is excessive, it manifests as high fever. Heat consumes body fluids, causing thirst, dry throat, a dry tongue coating, yellow scanty urine, and constipation. Heat-phlegm obstructing the Lung causes chest pain and rapid breathing. Both the tongue and pulse will have signs of interior heat.

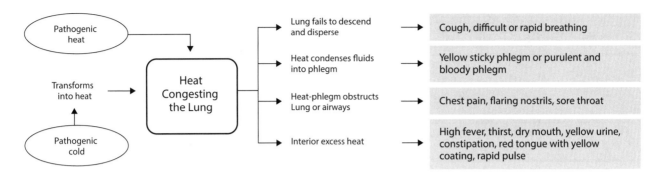

Chart 2.15 Etiology and pathogenesis of Heat Congesting the Lung

TCM Disease	Western Disease	Herbal Formulas		Acupuncture	
Cough (咳嗽)	Pneumonia, acute or chronic bronchitis, bronchiectasis	Qing Jin Hua Tan Tang	Bai Hu Tang, Xie Bai San	LU-1, LI-4, LU-7, LU-10, LU-11, BL-13	LU-1, LU-5, LU-11, CV-22, ST-9
Asthma (喘証)	Acute or chronic bronchitis, pneumonia, bronchi asthma	Ma Xing Shi Gan Tang			LU-3, LU-5, LU-9, BL-42, BL-44, CV-17, CV-22
Lung abscess (肺癰)	Suppurative pneumonia, lung abscess, bronchiectasis with infection	Qian Jin Wei Jing Tang			CV-17, CV-22

Table 2.22 Diseases and treatments related to Heat Congesting the Lung

Comparison: Wind-Heat Invading the Lung vs. Heat Congesting the Lung vs. Heat-Phlegm Obstructing the Lung

Wind-heat invading the Lung (風熱犯肺 *fēng rè fàn fèi*), heat congesting the Lung (熱邪壅肺 *rè xié yōng fèi*), and heat-phlegm obstructing the Lung (熱痰阻肺 *rè tán zǔ fèi*) all involve pathogenic heat impairing the Lung, which manifests with coughing, dyspnea, and expectoration of thick yellow sputum. Although these three patterns share the same nature, they differ in depth and condition.

Wind-heat invading the Lung is an exterior excess condition that involves the presence of exopathogenic factors fighting with the protective qi (*wèi* qi) at the body's surface. Thus coughing with chills and fever and a superficial pulse are the major clinical symptoms. Heat congesting the Lung is an interior excess condition caused by pathogenic heat directly invading the Lung, or by an unresolved exterior condition that transfers to the interior and disrupts Lung function; thus there is fever, but no chills. Heat-phlegm obstructing the Lung is also an interior excess condition, but it is combined with the presence of turbid phlegm. Water metabolism dysfunction, resulting from the Lung's failure to descend and disperse, along with the invasion of pathogenic heat condensing fluids can lead to the generation of phlegm. There may also be pre-existing phlegm that contributes to the development of this pattern.

The key points to distinguish these three patterns are as follows:
1) Course of illness: chronic and long vs. acute and short
2) Presence of exterior signs and symptoms, such as chills and fever
3) Tongue and pulse

Pattern		Wind-Heat Attacking the Lung	Heat Congesting the Lung	Heat-Phlegm Obstructing the Lung
Pathogenesis		Lung fails to descend and disperse		
		Wind-heat attacks the body's surface, nutritive and protective disharmony	Excess heat congests the Lung, damages body fluids	Heat-phlegm obstructs the Lung, causes Lung qi rebellion
Characteristics		Acute onset, short course, exterior, excess, heat	Sub-acute onset, longer course, interior, excess, heat	Sub-acute or chronic, long course, interior, excess, heat
Symptoms	Common	Coughing, panting, dyspnea, thick yellow sputum		
	Different	Chills and fever, headache, nasal congestion, sore throat	High fever with flaring nostrils, thirst, rapid breathing, pain in the chest	Productive cough, wheezing, difficult expectoration, distress in the chest
Tongue & pulse		Red tongue tip, thin yellow coating; superficial rapid pulse	Red tongue, yellow coating; forceful rapid pulse	Red tongue, thick, yellow, greasy coating; slippery rapid pulse
Treatment strategy		Release exterior wind-heat	Clear heat, generate body fluids	Clear heat, transform phlegm
Herbal formulas		Yin Qiao San	Bai Hu Tang	Qing Qi Hua Tang Wan

Table 2.23 Comparison of Wind-Heat Attacking the Lung, Heat Congesting the Lung, and Heat-Phlegm Obstructing the Lung

10 Cold-Water Shooting into the Lung Pattern | 寒水射肺 |

Definition: A group of signs and symptoms caused by pathogenic cold combining with water-thin mucus, invading the Lung, and causing Lung dysfunction.

Clinical manifestations: Cough with profuse white foamy sputum, panting or wheezing, chest pain with difficulty breathing, inability to lie down flat because of difficulty breathing, facial or body edema, scanty urine, intolerance of cold, cold limbs, stifling sensation in the chest, no thirst, a tongue coating that is white and greasy, and a pulse that is soft and slow, slippery, or wiry. This is a chronic condition and symptoms are often induced or aggravated by cold weather. If the pattern emerges with the appearance of exopathogenic cold, then it is accompanied by aversion to cold, fever, body aches, and a superficial pulse.

Key points: Cough with profuse white foamy sputum, panting or wheezing, and unable to lie down flat.

Etiology and pathogenesis: There are two main causes of this condition. The first is exopathogenic cold combined with water invading the Lung causing Lung dysfunction. The second is due to exopathogneic cold attacking while the patient already suffers from a chronic phlegm-thin mucus condition or edema. The pathogenic cold incites previously existing water-thin mucus, leading to cold-water shooting upward, which causes a failure in the Lung's descending function.

Cold-water shooting into the Lung pattern can be presented in different diseases. It is an acute critical condition and is commonly seen in the clinic. The root of this pattern is deficiency while symptoms are excess (本虛標實 běn xū biāo shí). Spleen and Kidney deficiency are the root (本虛 běn xū) while excess symptoms are water or thin mucus accumulating in the Lung and chest (標實 biāo shí).

When water or thin mucus obstructs and blocks the Lung qi, it disrupts its movement, leading to Lung's failure to disperse and descend, causing Lung qi counterflow, resulting in productive cough and panting or wheezing. Excessive phlegm-thin mucus or water accumulates in the Lung and chest, blocks qi, and causes pain, tightness, and distress in the chest. A supine position causes more severe accumulation, so the patient is unable to lie down.

When the Lung's distribution and dispersing function is disrupted, water metabolism is affected, causing water retention and edema. There is a cold sensation either because the invading exopathogenic cold damages yang qi or the Kidney and Spleen yang deficiency fails to warm the body. A white greasy tongue coating and a slippery pulse can also be expected with phlegm-thin mucus or water retention.

If the pattern emerges with the appearance of exopathogenic cold, it will be accompanied by aversion to cold, fever, body aches, and a superficial pulse.

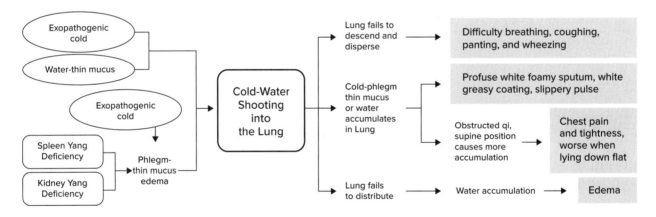

Chart 2.16 Etiology and pathogenesis of Cold-Water Shooting into the Lung

TCM Disease	Western Disease	Herbal Formulas		Acupuncture	
Asthma and wheezing (哮喘証)	Chronic asthmatic bronchitis, bronchial asthma, emphysema,	Xiao Qing Long Tang	Hei Xi Dan, Zhen Wu Tang	LU-5, LU-7, CV-17, ST-40, BL-13, SP-9	Ding Chuan, moxa BL-43
Propping thin mucus (支飲)	Congestive heart failure, pulmonary edema, cor pulmonale, emphysema		Ting Li Da Zao Xie Fei Tang		PC-6
Suspended thin mucus (懸飲)	Exudative pleurisy, tuberculosis pleurisy, pleural effusion		Shi Zao Tang		PC-4
Spillage thin mucus (溢飲)	Kidney failure, glomerulonephritis, uremia, nephrotic syndrome, congested heart failure		Ji Sheng Shen Qi Wan		BL-20, BL-23, ST-36

Table 2.24 Diseases and treatments related to Cold-Water Shooting into the Lung

Comparison: Cold-Phlegm Obstructing the Lung vs. Cold-Water Shooting into the Lung

Cold-phlegm obstructing the Lung (寒痰阻肺 *hán tán zǔ fèi*) and cold-water shooting into the Lung (寒水射肺 *hán shuǐ shè fèi*) are similar in etiology and pathogenesis, and may mutually influence. Both patterns exhibit coughing or panting, dyspnea, thin clear sputum, and chest oppression and both patterns are also induced or aggravated by exposure to cold.

Cold-water shooting into the Lung is either caused by exopathogneic cold combined with water-thin mucus invading the Lung, or by exopathogenic cold inciting internal pre-existing phlegm-thin mucus caused by Kidney and Spleen yang deficiency. On the other hand, cold-phlegm obstructing the Lung is usually caused by exopathogenic cold invading the Lung, generating cold-phlegm, or by Spleen yang deficiency failing to transform, leading to phlegm accumulation that moves upward and invades the Lung.

Cold-phlegm obstructing the Lung without proper treatment or care can develop into cold-water shooting into the Lung, therefore the latter pattern is considered more severe.

The key points to distinguish these two patterns are as follows:
1) Acute vs. chronic: cold-water shooting into the Lung is acute and severe, while cold-phlegm obstructing the Lung is sub-acute or chronic and relatively mild
2) Edema and an inability to lie down flat are the key symptoms for cold-water shooting into the Lung

Pattern		Cold-Water Shooting into the Lung	Cold-Phlegm Obstructing the Lung
Pathogenesis		Exopathogenic cold combined with water, or exopathogenic cold invasion inciting previously accumulated water-thin mucus	Exopathogenic cold invades the Lung, Spleen yang deficiency generates phlegm, which ascends and disrupts the Lung
Characteristics		Acute, severe clinical manifestation, pre-existing water-thin mucus condition	Chronic, long course, milder clinical manifestation
Symptoms	Common	Coughing, panting, thin and clear sputum, condition induced or aggravated by exposure to cold, white tongue coating, slippery pulse	
Symptoms	Different	Edema, severe dyspnea, inability to lie down flat, chest pain	Chest oppression, throat with phlegm sound
Phlegm source		Spleen and Kidney	Lung and Spleen
Tongue & pulse		White and slippery coating, wiry or superficial pulse	White greasy coating
Treatment strategy		Release the exterior, warm and transform phlegm, regulate rebellious Lung Qi	Warm Lung, transform phlegm, stop cough
Herbal formulas		Xiao Qing Long Tang, Hei Xi Dan	San Zi Yang Qin Tang

Table 2.25 Comparison of Cold-Water Shooting into the Lung and Cold-Phlegm Obstructing the Lung

Summary of Lung Disease Patterns

Key points: cough, abnormal breathing, panting, wheezing, shortness of breath, chills and fever, sneezing, nasal congestion, voice change, sore or itchy throat, superficial pulse

Patterns			Clinical manifestations	
			Common	Different
Deficiency	Lung Qi Deficiency			Feeble cough and panting that worsens with exertion, copious thin, clear phlegm, shortage of qi, shortness of breath, aversion to speaking, low voice, fatigue, low energy, spontaneous sweating, sensitivity to wind, easily catch cold, pale complexion, pale tongue with thin white coating, weak pulse
	Lung Yin Deficiency			Dry cough without sputum or with scanty sticky sputum or with blood-stained sputum, difficult expectoration, dry mouth, malar flush, hoarse voice, low-grade fever in the afternoon or evening, night sweats, five center heat, red tongue with scanty coating, thin rapid pulse
Excess	Exopathogens Invading the Lung	Wind-Cold	Mild chills and fever, superficial pulse	Harsh, coarse, forceful cough with thin clear sputum, easy to expectorate, headache, body aches, thin white tongue coating, tight pulse
		Wind-Heat		Hacking, hoarseness, cough, sticky yellow sputum, difficult expectoration, sore throat, slight thirst, red tongue tip, thin yellow tongue coating, rapid pulse
		Dryness		Dry hacking cough, scanty, white sputum, difficult to expectorate, or blood-stained, dry mouth, thirst, dry tongue coating, slight rapid pulse
		Wind-Water		Sudden swelling of eyes and face, gradually spreading to the whole body, bright shiny complexion, scanty and clear urine, cough, difficulty breathing
	Cold Invading the Lung		Cough, panting, thin white or clear phlegm, hoarseness or loss of voice, cold limbs and body, pale tongue with white coating, deep and slow pulse	
	Turbid Phlegm Obstructing the Lung	Dampness-Phlegm	Productive cough, wheezing, shortness of breath, distress and tightness in chest, phlegm in throat, a feeling of heaviness, thick or greasy tongue coating, and a slippery pulse	Chronic cough coming in bouts with profuse white sticky phlegm that is easy to expectorate, obesity, aversion to lying down, nausea
		Cold-Phlegm		Cough with expectoration of white water sputum, worse with exposure to cold or at night, cold hands and feet, pale tongue, slow pulse
		Heat-Phlegm		Barking cough with profuse sticky yellow or green sputum, difficult to expectorate, thirst, agitation, insomnia, red tongue, rapid pulse
		Dryness-Phlegm		Dry cough, but with occasional difficult expectoration of scanty white or blood-stained sputum, dry throat and nose, dry tongue coating
	Heat Congesting the Lung		Coughing, panting, high fever with flaring nostrils, rapid breathing, thirst, pain in the chest, cough with foul pus and blood, red tongue, surging rapid pulse	
	Cold-Water Shooting into the Lung		Cough with profuse white foamy sputum, panting or wheezing, chest pain with difficulty breathing, inability to lie down flat, edema, scanty urine, intolerance of cold, white greasy tongue coating, pulse is soft and slow, or slippery, or string-taut	

Table 2.26 Summary of Lung disease patterns

Chapter 3
Spleen Disease Patterns

Physiological characteristics and functions of the Spleen

The Spleen is a sickle-shaped organ located in the middle burner under the left side of the diaphragm. Its channel begins on the medial tip of the big toe, follows the inner aspect of the foot and leg and ascends the anterior thigh. From the groin, the Spleen channel enters the lower abdomen, penetrating the Spleen and Stomach, travels through the diaphragm, across the chest, up to the esophagus, and terminates under the tongue.

The Spleen and the Stomach are interior-exteriorly connected by a membrane in the abdomen. They are digestive organs that generate qi and blood to nourish the muscles. The Stomach receives food and decomposes it into chyme, sending it down to the intestines to be further separated, while the Spleen transforms it into food essence and transports it upward to the Lung to be distributed to the whole body. Thus, Spleen and Stomach form the pivot point of ascending and descending qi and are the root of post-natal qi.

The Spleen is a granary organ (食廩之官 shí lǐn zhī guān) in charge of food and nutrition supply. It controls the muscles and limbs, manifests on the lips, opens to the mouth, favors dryness, and disfavors dampness. Its fluid is saliva, its season corresponds to late summer, and its correlated emotions are worry and pensiveness.

Spleen	Relationship
Spirit	Intellect (意 yì)
Internal-external connection	Stomach
Orifice	Mouth
Controls	Muscles, limbs
External manifestation	Lips
Fluid	Saliva
Fire	Ministerial fire
Emotion	Thinking, worry
Season	Late summer
Five phase	Earth
Six climate factor	Dampness

Table 3.1 Spleen and its related properties

1 | Governs transformation and transportation

The Spleen transforms water and food into essences and transports them to the entire body, maintaining the body's normal physiological function.
   (1) Transportation means assimilation and distribution.
   (2) Transformation implies change, digestion, and absorption.

The Spleen's transforming and transporting function includes two aspects:
   (1) Transporting and transforming food and drink
   (2) Transporting and transforming water-dampness

2 | Controls blood

The Spleen controls and maintains blood circulation inside the blood vessels.

3 | In charge of 'sending up'
   (1) Sending the clear upward: ascending and distributing food and water essences to the Lung.
   (2) Stabilizing the internal organs in their proper positions.

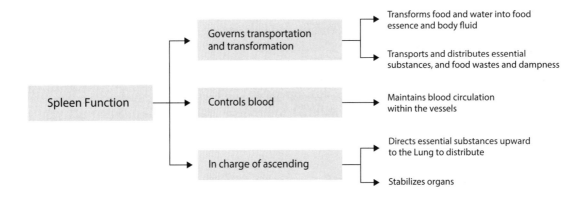

Chart 3.1   Spleen function summary

Common etiological factors in Spleen patterns

Spleen patterns are mainly caused by endopathogenic factors, but may also be caused by exopathogenic factors. The following are common etiological factors for Spleen disease patterns:
   (1) Exopathogenic cold or dampness invasion
   (2) Improper diet or malnutrition: overconsumption of raw, cold or greasy food or insufficient food intake
   (3) Improper treatment: overuse of cold, heavy or greasy herbs, or lack of proper treatment and care after severe illness
   (4) Emotional stress: excessive thinking and worry
   (5) Chronic illness impairs Spleen function
   (6) Constitution and aging

Pathological changes and major clinical manifestations of Spleen disease

Pathological changes of the Spleen are mostly caused by disorder of the Spleen's transformation and transportation function or an inability of the Spleen to control blood. There are four major clinical manifestations of Spleen function disorder: poor appetite, abdominal bloating and distention, loose stools, and bleeding.

1 | Poor appetite

Definition: The patient loses the desire to eat and might even develop an aversion to food.

Characteristics of poor appetite due to Spleen dysfunction: little sense of hunger or desire to eat, usually due to chronic illness, and may be accompanied by bloating and distention after meals.

Etiology and pathomechanisms: The underlying causes of poor appetite are slowed decomposition in the Stomach and disorder of the Spleen's ascending function. Improper diet or treatment, chronic illness, aging, and constitution can all impair Spleen function. When the Spleen is deficient or attacked by dampness, its ascending function will be compromised, which in turn will adversely affect the Stomach's descending function. A deficient Spleen and Stomach will fail to transport or transform, causing food to remain in the Stomach longer than usual, slowing the decomposition process.

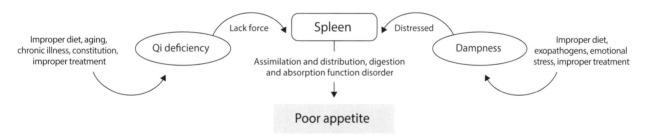

Chart 3.2   Etiology and pathomechanism of poor appetite

2 | Loose stools

Definition: An increased frequency of defecation with clear, dilute, or even watery stools.

Characteristics of loose stools due to Spleen dysfunction: soft stools or chronic loose stools that may contain undigested food. Stool is sometimes muddy or watery and rushes down. Severity of condition may fluctuate from mild to acute. When the patient overeats or consumes greasy food, bowel movement frequency will increase or the patient will experience abdominal bloating, distention, and borborygmus.

Etiology and pathomechanisms: Loose stools are usually due to too much fluid or dampness accumulating in the intestines with increased intestinal peristalsis. The Spleen is responsible for transforming and transporting water into essence and excreting water waste. If the Spleen's function of transformation and transportation fails, dampness will accumulate inside, and pour downward to the Large Intestine, which dilutes the stool, leading to loose stool.

There are two main causes for the failure of the Spleen's transformation and transportation function. The first is deficiency due to constitution; chronic illness; long-term emotional stress, such as overthinking or worrying; improper diet and lifestyle; improper treatment, such as overuse of cold, heavy herbs, or medication; or aging. When deficient, the Spleen lacks the power to perform its functions. The second is dampness besieging the Spleen, which usually results from improper diet, such as overconsumption of raw, cold, and greasy food; exopathogenic dampness invasion, such as living in a humid environment; or improper treatment, such as overuse of greasy herbs. The Spleen favors dryness and disfavors dampness. When dampness accumulates, the Spleen cannot perform its function.

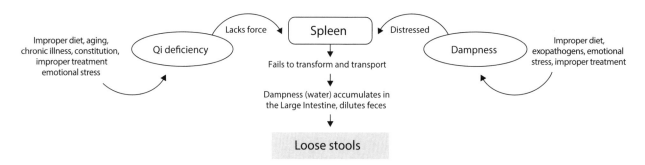

Chart 3.3 Etiology and pathomechanism of loose stools

3 | Bloating and distention

Definition: A sensation of bloating and distention in the abdomen. In severe cases there is enlargement of the abdomen. Bloating is a subjective sensation of fullness that is only felt by the patient. Distention is bloating that is both subjective and objective; it may be seen or felt by both the patient and the practitioner.

Characteristics of bloating and distention due to Spleen dysfunction: bloating and distention usually occurs after meals, and is worse with greasy, sweet, or cold food.

Etiology and pathomechanisms: Any disorder of qi circulation in the abdominal area can cause qi accumulation, resulting in bloating and distention. The Spleen and Stomach are located in the middle burner, serving as the pivot point of ascending and descending qi. When the Spleen qi fails to ascend, the Stomach qi is unable to descend, causing qi accumulation and leading to bloating and distention.

The Spleen may fail to ascend for two reasons. First, when Spleen qi is deficient, due to improper diet, improper treatment, chronic illness, aging, or constitution, the power to ascend is compromised, causing qi accumulation. Second, when dampness besieges the Spleen due to exopathogens, emotional stress, improper treatment, or improper diet, such as overeating greasy foods, the Spleen fails to transform and transport, leading to qi stagnation in the middle burner and more accumulation of dampness.

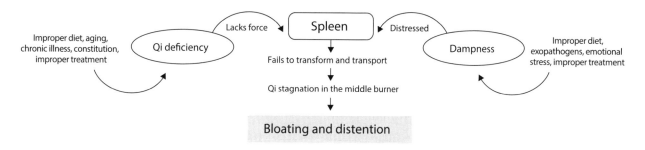

Chart 3.4 Etiology and pathomechanism of bloating and distention

4 | Bleeding

Definition: Process of losing blood from the body.

Characteristic of bleeding due to Spleen deficiency: chronic bleeding with mild, thin, light-colored blood, recurrent attacks, mostly subcutaneous bleeding, hematochezia, gum bleeding. For women, Spleen-related bleeding may involve preceded menstrual cycle, prolonged period, metrorrhagia, or metrostaxis.

Etiology and pathomechanisms: The Spleen has the function of controlling and maintaining blood inside blood vessels. Emotional stress, improper diet, aging, chronic illness, improper treatment, and constitution can all impair the Spleen. When Spleen qi is deficient, it fails to control blood and contain blood inside the vessels.

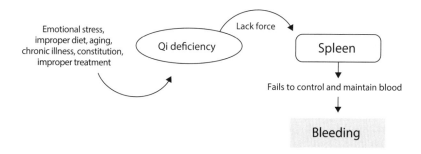

Chart 3.5 Etiology and pathomechanism of bleeding

5 | Other signs and symptoms related to the Spleen

Other signs and symptoms related to the Spleen patterns include abdominal pain, emaciation, edema, phlegm, prolapsed organs, hands and feet excessive sweating, flaccid muscles, poor muscle tone, weak and tired limbs, disabled wilted limbs, diminished sense of taste, and sweet and greasy taste in the mouth.

Physiological Function	Pathological Change	Clinical Manifestation
Governs transportation and transformation	Failure to transport and transform impairs digestion, absorption, and distribution	Abdominal bloating and distention, poor appetite, loose stools, emaciation
	Failure to transport and transform leads to water accumulation	Dampness, phlegm, edema
Ascends and lifts	Food essence unable to ascend to the Lung and Heart, which in turn fail to generate qi and blood	Fatigue, tiredness, dizziness, loose stools, shortness of breath, aversion to talking
	Failure to hold and support internal organs	Prolapse of internal organs such as the uterus or rectum
Controls blood	Failure to keep blood inside blood vessels	Bleeding, such as gum bleeding, subcutaneous bleeding, abnormal menstrual bleeding, hematochezia
Governs muscles and limbs	Failure to transport and transform reduces qi and blood production, leads to malnourished muscles and limbs	Emaciation, weak and tired limbs, muscle loss, or disabled atrophied limbs
Opens to the mouth	Failure to function	Tastelessness or sweet taste and greasy feeling inside mouth

Table 3.2 Physiological functions, pathological changes, and clinical manifestations of the Spleen

Common patterns in Spleen disease

There are seven Spleen patterns commonly seen in the clinic. According to their pathogenesis and clinical manifestation, these patterns can be divided into two groups: excess and deficiency. Deficiency patterns include Spleen qi deficiency, Spleen qi sinking, Spleen yang deficiency, and Spleen not controlling blood, all of which develop from Spleen qi deficiency.

Excess patterns are all caused by dampness besieging the Spleen. Based on the accompanying pathogens and clinical symptoms, excess patterns can be sub-classified into cold-dampness encumbering the Spleen, and damp-heat encumbering the Spleen.

	Etiology	Patterns
Deficiency	Congenital insufficiency, aging, chronic illness, improper diet, improper treatment, long-term emotional stress	Spleen Qi Deficiency, Spleen Qi Sinking, Spleen Yang Deficiency, Spleen Not Controlling Blood, Spleen Yin Deficiency (rare)
Excess	Exopathogenic dampness invasion, improper diet, improper treatment	Cold-Dampness Encumbering the Spleen, Damp-Heat Encumbering the Spleen

Table 3.3 Classification of common Spleen patterns

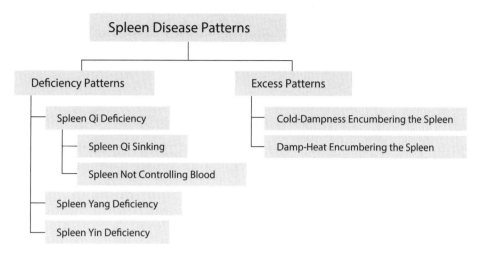

Chart 3.6 Common Spleen disease patterns

1 Spleen Qi Deficiency Pattern | 脾氣虛証 |

Definition: A group of signs and symptoms caused by the failure of the Spleen's transformation and transportation function.

Clinical manifestations: Sallow complexion, tiredness, lassitude, weak limbs, poor appetite, abdominal bloating and distention, loose stools, shortness of breath, aversion to speaking, low voice, a pale tongue with teeth marks and a thin white coating, and a weak or soft pulse. There may also be obesity and edema.

Key points: Poor appetite, abdominal bloating and distention, loose stools, plus qi deficiency signs and symptoms.

Etiology and pathogenesis: This pattern is mostly caused by constitutional deficiency, improper diet, physical overstrain, or excessive emotional stress, including long-term worry or overthinking. It may also be due to aging, severe illness, or improper care.

The Spleen is in charge of converting food and water into the essential substances used to generate qi and blood. It nourishes the muscles, governs the limbs, and maintains the body's physical and mental activities. When Spleen qi is deficient, it fails to transform and transport, so qi and blood production declines. Qi is the motive force of the human body; when qi is insufficient, it fails to push and promote. The lack of body energy manifests as shortness of breath, fatigue, aversion to speaking, weak limbs, low voice, sallow complexion, a pale tongue, and a weak pulse.

Impairment of the Spleen's transformation and transportation function disrupts the Stomach's reception and decomposition function, causing various digestive symptoms such as poor appetite, abdominal bloating and distention, and loose stool.

The Spleen is one of the most important organs responsible for water metabolism. Water or dampness pouring downward to the Large Intestine leads to loose stools or diarrhea. When the Spleen fails to transform and transport, water or dampness accumulates, which in turn stagnates in the tongue. This makes the tongue grow wider. When its edges press against the teeth, teeth marks develop.

64 Part 1: Zang Organs

TCM Disease	Western Disease	Herbal Formulas		Acupuncture
Diarrhea (泄瀉)	Chronic enteritis, Crohn's disease, chronic colitis, IBS, celiac disease, SIBO	Shen Ling Bai Zhu San	Si Jun Zi Tang	ST-21, SP-5, BL-32, ST-37, ST-49, ST-25
Epigastric pain (胃痛)	Peptic ulcer, chronic gastritis, IBS, pancreatitis, gastric neurosis, colitis	Huang Qi Jian Zhong Tang		CV-12, LR-13, PC-6, SP-4, ST-25
Abdominal pain (腹痛)	PID, diverticulitis, Crohn's disease, lead poisoning, celiac disease, IBS	Xiao Jian Zhong Tang		
Edema (水腫)	Hypothyroidism, kwashiorkor, chronic glomerulonephritis, myxedema, lymphedema	Shi Pi Yin, Fang Ji Huang Qi Tang, Wu Pi (San) Yin		SP-9, BL-22, BL-23, ST-28, CV-10, GV-23, LI-6
Phlegm and thin mucus (痰飲)	Meniere's disease, anorexia nervosa, dementia, depression, vertigo, motion sickness, numbness	Ling Gui Zhu Gan Tang, Ban Xia Bai Zhu Tian Ma Tang		ST-40, SP-9, TB-5
Atrophy disorder (痿証)	Sequelae of encephalitis or polio, MS, MG, tumors in the CNS, myelitis, progressive muscular dystrophy, progressive myodystrophy	Shen Ling Bai Zhu San, Bu Zhong Yi Qi Tang		Huatoujiaji, SP-9, ST-31, ST-32, ST-40, ST-41, GB-34, LI-2, LI-3, LI-4, LI-10, LI-11, LI-14, TB-5
Fatigue (虛勞)	Chronic hepatitis, anemia, lyme disease, mono, hypothyroidism, CFS, adrenal fatigue, fibromyalgia, malnutrition	Bu Zhong Yi Qi Tang		GV-4, BL-23, BL-24, BL-26
Childhood nutritional impairment (疳証)	Child malnutrition or vitamin deficiency, parasites, indigestion	Bu Dai Wan, Gan Ji San		CV-12, Sifeng, massage

(Acupuncture column also includes: ST-36, CV-4, CV-6, GV-24, SP-3, SP-6, BL-20, BL-21, BL-25)

Table 3.4 Diseases and treatments related to Spleen Qi Deficiency

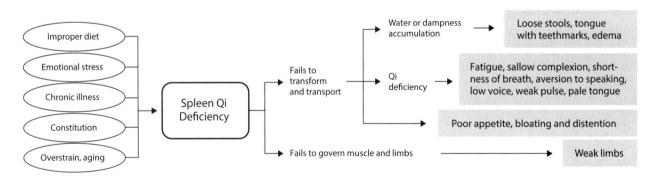

Chart 3.7 Etiology and pathogenesis of Spleen Qi Deficiency

2 Spleen Qi Sinking Pattern | 脾氣下陷 |

Definition: A group of signs and symptoms marked by prolapse of internal organs that is caused by severe Spleen qi deficiency, leading to failure of its supportive function. This pattern is also called 'middle qi sinking' (中氣下陷 *zhōng qì xià xiàn*).

Clinical manifestations: Poor appetite, abdominal bloating and distention with downbearing sensation, chronic loose stools, possibly with sagging sensation, listlessness, lassitude, low voice, emaciation, sallow complexion, pale tongue, weak pulse, prolapse of internal organs such as uterus, stomach, kidney, or rectum.

Key points: Prolapsed organs or chronic diarrhea and loose stools, plus qi deficiency signs and symptoms.

Etiology and pathogenesis: This pattern usually develops from Spleen qi deficiency. If treatment is delayed or improper, the qi deficiency worsens. Since Spleen has the function of lifting and supporting, deficient Spleen qi can prevent food and water essence from rising. This results in dizziness, chronic diarrhea or loose stools. If Spleen qi fails to support, the internal organs may prolapse, which may manifest as uterine prolapse, rectal prolapse, gastroptosis, renal ptosis, and hepatoptosis.

Fatigue, shortness of breath, low voice, spontaneous sweating, poor appetite, pale tongue, and deficient pulse are the general signs and symptoms of qi deficiency.

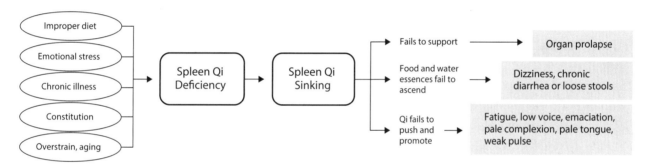

Chart 3.8 Etiology and pathogenesis of Spleen Qi Sinking

TCM Disease	Western Disease	Herbal Formulas		Acupuncture
Diarrhea (泄瀉)	Chronic enteritis, colitis, Crohn's disease, chronic colitis, IBS, celiac disease		Shen Ling Bai Zhu San	CV-3, CV-4, SP-3, ST-25, LR-13
Irregular uterine bleeding (崩漏)	Menorrhagia and metrostaxis cause hormonal imbalance, uterus fibroids, polyps, adenomyosis	Bu Zhong Yi Qi Tang	Gu Ben Zhi Beng Tang, Gui Pi Tang	SP-6, CV-4, SP-1
Rectum prolapse (直腸下垂)	Rectum prolapse		Bu Zhong Yi Qi Tang	ST-36, CV-6, CV-12, GV-20, BL-20, BL-25, Titou — GV-1, Erbai
Uterine prolapse (子宮下垂)	Uterine prolapse			GB-28, Zigongxue
Urinary incontinence (小便失禁)	Interstitial cystitis, BPH, overactive bladder		Suo Quan Wan	CV-2, CV-3, CV-4

Table 3.5 Diseases and treatments related to Spleen Qi Sinking

3 Spleen Not Controlling Blood Pattern | 脾不統血

Definition: A group of signs and symptoms due to Spleen qi failing to contain blood inside the vessels, resulting in various types of bleeding.

Clinical manifestations: All types of bleeding, including subcutaneous hemorrhage, gum bleeding, and hematochezia. In women: preceded menstrual cycle, prolonged period, menorrhagia, and metrostaxis. Sallow or pale complexion, poor appetite, abdominal bloating and distention, loose stools, a pale tongue, and a thin weak pulse.

Key points: Bleeding plus Spleen qi deficiency signs and symptoms.

Etiology and pathogenesis: This pattern also develops from Spleen qi deficiency, which may be caused by constitutional deficiency, improper diet, physical overstrain, or excessive emotional stress, including long-term worry or overthinking. It may also be due to aging, severe illness, or improper care.

The Spleen controls and maintains blood inside the vessels. When Spleen qi is deficient, this function is disrupted, and blood leaks out of the vessels and results in various types of bleeding such as menorrhagia and metrostaxis, hematochezia, easily bruised, etc.

The Spleen is in charge of converting food and water into the essential substances used to generate qi and blood. It nourishes the muscles, governs the limbs, and maintains the body's physical and mental activities. When the Spleen is deficient, it fails to transform and transport, so qi and blood production declines. Qi is the motive force of the human body; when qi is insufficient, it fails to push and promote. The lack of body energy manifests as shortness of breath, fatigue, aversion to speaking, weak limbs, low voice, pale complexion, pale tongue, weak pulse, etc.

Impairment of the Spleen's transformation and transportation function disrupts the Stomach's reception and decomposition function, causing various digestive symptoms such as poor appetite, abdominal bloating and distention, and loose stools.

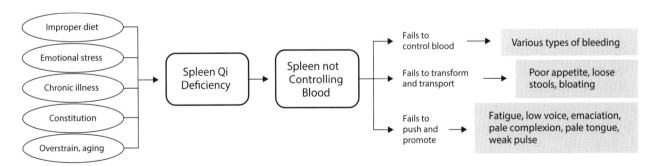

Chart 3.9 Etiology and pathogenesis of Spleen Not Controlling Blood

TCM Disease	Western Disease	Herbal Formulas		Acupuncture	
Hematochezia (便血)	IBD such as diverticulosis, Crohn's disease, Behcet's disease, colitis, hemorrhoid, rectum cancer	Huang Tu Tang	Gui Pi Tang	SP-1, SP-3, SP-4, SP-6, SP-10, ST-36, GV-20, BL-17, BL-20	BL-24, BL-36, BL-57, BL-58, KI-7
Bleeding (出血)	Thrombocytopenic purpura, chronic ITP, allergic purpura, aplastic anemia	Dang Gui Bu Xue Tang			BL-43, CV-6
Irregular uterine bleeding (崩漏)	Menorrhagia and metrostaxis caused by hormonal imbalance, uterine fibroids, polyps, adenomyosis	Gu Ben Zhi Beng Wan, Jiao Ai Tang, Ba Zhen Tang			CV-5, CV-6, CV-7, Zigongxue

Table 3.6 Diseases and treatments related to Spleen Not Controlling Blood

4 Spleen Yang Deficiency Pattern | 脾陽虛証 |

Definition: A group of signs and symptoms caused by deficiency of Spleen yang failing to warm the interior of the body.

Clinical manifestations: Poor appetite, abdominal bloating and distention, loose stools, dull and vague abdominal pain relieved by warmth and pressure, intolerance of cold, cold limbs, no desire to drink, edema, and scant urine. For women, copious clear vaginal discharge. Pale, flabby tongue with teeth marks. Tongue coating is white and greasy. Pulse is deep and slow.

Key points: Poor appetite, loose stools, plus yang deficiency signs and symptoms.

Etiology and pathogenesis: Spleen yang deficiency arises from chronic illness along with qi deficiency; the aging process in conjunction with Kidney deficiency; pathogenic cold attack, which damages yang; improper treatment; or overconsumption of cold, bitter food and herbs.

This pattern is substantially the same as Spleen qi deficiency with the addition of cold symptoms, which are caused by yang qi deficiency. Yang qi has the function of warming the body. When yang qi is insufficient, there is not enough power to warm the body. This gives rise to aversion to cold, cold limbs, preference for warm food and drink but no particular thirst, a pale tender tongue, and a slow pulse.

When Spleen yang is deficient, it lacks the power to perform its function of transforming and transporting fluids. As a result, fluids may accumulate inside, which causes edema or copious clear vaginal discharge in women and a greasy tongue coating.

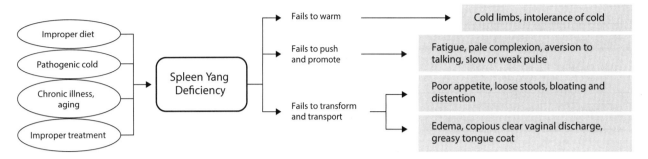

Chart 3.10 Etiology and pathogenesis of Spleen Yang Deficiency

TCM Disease	Western Disease	Herbal Formulas		Acupuncture	
Diarrhea (泄瀉)	Chronic enteritis, Crohn's disease, chronic colitis, IBS, celiac disease, SIBO		Zhen Ren Yang Zang Tang		CV-3, CV-4, ST-25, LR-13
Abdominal pain (腹痛)	PID, diverticulitis, Crohn's disease, lead poisoning, celiac disease, IBS, SIBO	Li Zhong Wan, Wu Zhu Yu Tang	Da Jian Zhong Tang	SP-3, SP-6, SP-9, CV-12, ST-28, ST-36, BL-20, BL-21, BL-22	LR-13, PC-6, SP-4, ST-25
Phlegm and thin mucus (痰飲)	Meniere's disease, anorexia nervosa, dementia, depression, vertigo, numbness		Ling Gui Zhu Gan Tang		ST-40, TB-5
Edema (水腫)	Nephrotic syndrome, CHF, Hypothyroidism, kwashiorkor, chronic glomerulonephritis, myxedema, lymphedema		Shi Pi Yin, Wu Ling San		BL-23, CV-10, GV-23, LI-6
Ascites (膨脹)	Cirrhosis, heart failure, constrictive pericarditis, nephrotic syndrome, kwashiorkor		Tiao Zhong Jian Pi Wan, Wu Ling San		LI-6, KI-7

Table 3.7 Diseases and treatments related to Spleen Yang Deficiency

Comparison: Spleen Qi Deficiency vs. Spleen Qi Sinking vs. Spleen Not Controlling Blood vs. Spleen Yang Deficiency

Spleen qi deficiency (脾氣虛 *pí qì xū*) is the most common pattern for Spleen dysfunction. Spleen qi sinking (脾氣下陷 *pí qì xià xiàn*) and Spleen not controlling blood (脾不統血 *pí bù tǒng xuè*) develop from Spleen qi deficiency, and therefore share many symptoms, including poor appetite, abdominal bloating and distention, loose stools, sallow complexion, weak limbs, a weak pulse, and a pale tongue.

Spleen qi sinking and Spleen not controlling blood manifest different aspects of Spleen qi deficiency. Spleen qi sinking focuses on a failure to support, causing organ prolapse; while Spleen not controlling blood focuses on a failure to keep blood inside the vessels, causing bleeding or easy bruising. Spleen yang deficiency (脾陽虛 *pí yáng xū*) also develops from Spleen qi deficiency and shares the same signs and symptoms, but manifests with cold, such as an intolerance of cold, cold limbs, and a slow pulse.

Chapter 3: Spleen Disease Patterns

The key points to distinguish these four patterns are as follows:
1) Chief complaints: fatigue vs. chronic loose stools vs. organ prolapse vs. bleeding vs. cold limbs

Pattern		Spleen Qi Deficiency	Spleen Qi Sinking	Spleen not Controlling Blood	Spleen Yang Deficiency
Pathogenesis		Spleen qi deficiency fails to transform and transport, reducing generation of qi and blood			
			Fails to support and lift	Fails to control blood	Fails to warm and promote
Symptoms	Common	Poor appetite, abdominal bloating and distention that is worse after eating, loose stools, sallow complexion, emaciation, weak limbs, aversion to speaking, edema, fatigue, pale tongue, and weak pulse			
	Different		Chronic loose stools or internal organ prolapse	Various types of bleeding	Cold extremities, edema, abdominal pain
Tongue & pulse				Thin pulse	Flabby tongue, greasy coating; slow pulse
Treatment strategy		Tonifies qi, strengthens the Spleen and Stomach			
			Raise sunken yang and counter prolapse	Nourish blood and nourish the Heart	Warm the middle burner
Herbal formulas		Si Jun Zi Tang	Bu Zhong Yi Qi Tang	Gui Pi Tang	Li Zhong Wan

Table 3.8 Comparison of Spleen Qi Deficiency, Spleen Qi Sinking, Spleen not Controlling Blood, and Spleen Yang Deficiency

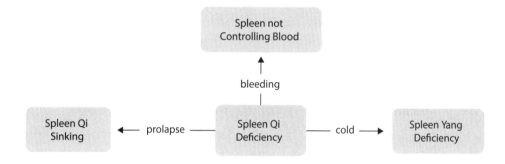

Chart 3.11 Spleen Qi Deficiency, Spleen Qi Sinking, Spleen Yang Deficiency, and Spleen Not Controlling Blood

5 Spleen Yin Deficiency Pattern | 脾陰虛証

Definition: A group of signs and symptoms caused by deficiency of Spleen yin fluids causing deficiency fire to flare up.

Clinical manifestations: Emaciation and lack of strength, hunger but no desire to eat, abdominal distention after eating, chapped lips and dry mouth, epigastric discomfort and pain, belching, reflux, five-center heat, yellow urine, dry stools, a red tongue with a thin yellow or scanty coating, and a thin rapid pulse. In some cases, there may also be abnormal bleeding such as hematochezia or hematemesis.

Key points: Poor appetite, abdominal bloating and distention after eating, chapped lips, plus yin deficiency signs and symptoms.

Etiology and pathogenesis: This pattern is usually caused by long-term mental and physical overstrain with internal organ deficiency. It may also be the result of malnutrition or febrile disease.

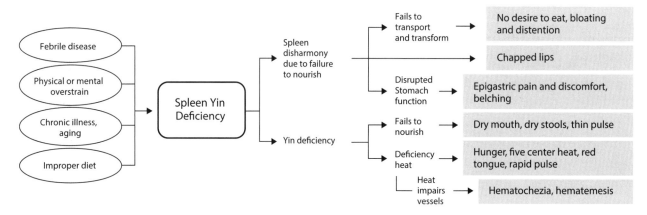

Chart 3.12   Etiology and pathogenesis of Spleen Yin Deficiency

Although the Spleen is the organ that favors dryness and disfavors dampness, in order to maintain normal function, the Spleen needs yin fluids to nourish and moisten. Spleen yin includes Spleen blood and body fluids. Long-term mental and physical overstrain or chronic illness consumes blood and body fluids, leading to insufficient nourishment of the Spleen. When in disharmony, the Spleen fails to transport and transform, which results in poor appetite, abdominal distention and bloating. The Spleen manifests in the luster of the lips, so when Spleen yin is deficient, the lips become dry and chapped. Failure of the Spleen's ascending function disrupts the Stomach's descending function, causing epigastric discomfort and pain, belching, and reflux.

Yin deficiency creates deficiency heat: five-center heat, dry mouth, dry stools, a red tongue with thin yellow or scanty coating, and a thin rapid pulse. If deficiency heat damages the blood vessels, there may be abnormal bleeding such as hematochezia or hematemesis.

TCM Disease	Western Disease	Herbal Formulas		Acupuncture	
Epigastrium pain (胃痛)	Atrophic gastritis, gastric neurosis, peptic ulcer, GERD, gastric carcinoma	Sha Shen Mai Men Dong Tang, Zhong He Li Yin Tang	Zhong He Li Yin Tang	CV-12, ST-36, SP-3, SP-6	CV-4, CV-6, PC-6, KI-3, ST-44
Constipation (便秘)	Diabetes mellitus, IBS, thyroid disease, dehydration		Ma Zi Ren Wan		ST-25, ST-44, BL-25, TB-6, KI-6, CV-6
Hematochezia (便血)	Hemorrhoids, colon cancer, IBD, diverticulosis, ulcerative colitis		Gui Pi Tang		BL-20, BL-24, BL-36, BL-57, BL-58, KI-7, SP-1, SP-3, SP-4, SP-6, SP-10
Hematemesis (吐血)	Peptic ulcer, gastritis, varices, esophagitis, hemorrhage		Mai Dong Yang Rong Tang		SP-1, SP-3, SP-4, SP-6, SP-10, BL-17, BL-20, CV-6

Table 3.9 Diseases and treatments related to Spleen Yin Deficiency

6 Cold-dampness Encumbering the Spleen Pattern | 寒濕睏脾 |

Definition: A group of signs and symptoms resulting from cold-dampness accumulating in the middle burner due to a dysfunction of the Spleen's transformation and transportation function. The character 睏 (*kùn*), translated here as 'encumbering,' can also mean to besiege, trap, or assail.

Clinical manifestations: Epigastric and abdominal bloating and distention, poor appetite, bland but slimy taste in the mouth, diarrhea or loose stools, nausea, vomiting, heaviness of the entire body and head, jaundice with smoky yellow skin, copious clear vaginal discharge, edema with scanty urine, pale flabby tongue with white greasy or white glossy coating, and a slow, moderate, or deep and thin pulse.

Key points: Epigastric and abdominal bloating and distention, poor appetite, diarrhea, loose stools, nausea, vomiting, plus interior cold-dampness signs and symptoms.

Etiology and pathogenesis: Exopathogenic cold-dampness invasion and improper diet are the two major etiologies for this pattern. Exopathogenic dampness invasion is usually related to the environment, including living or working in rainy or humid locations or near water, such as oceans, lakes, and rivers; wearing wet clothes; and overconsumption of energetically cold, raw, sweet, or greasy foods.

The Spleen is the organ that favors dryness and disfavors dampness. Cold-dampness invasion impairs the Spleen's transformation and transportation function, resulting in water metabolism disorder. This leads to more dampness accumulation that blocks qi circulation, causing bloating and distention or dull pain in the epigastrium and abdomen. Cold-dampness also affects the Spleen's ascending function. When the Spleen qi cannot ascend, the Stomach qi cannot descend, leading to poor appetite, nausea, vomiting, diarrhea, or loose stools. Furthermore, when dampness encumbers the Spleen, there can be a bland or slimy taste in the mouth because the Spleen opens into the mouth and is responsible for taste.

The nature of dampness is heavy and descending, thus it tends to cause pathological changes that feel heavy, including lassitude with sensations of heaviness and heavy limbs. Symptoms also tend to manifest in the lower part of the body, including diarrhea, loose stools, and abnormal vaginal discharge. Failure to transform and transport water and dampness impairs the qi transformation function, causing edema.

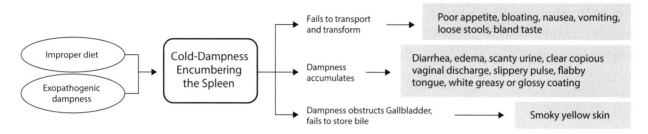

Chart 3.13 Etiology and pathogenesis of Cold-Dampness Encumbering the Spleen

TCM Disease	Western Disease	Herbal Formulas		Acupuncture	
Vomiting (嘔吐)	Food poisoning, stomach flu, gastro-enteritis, gastritis, motion sickness	Xiao Ban Xia with Ling Gui Zhu Gan Tang	Wei Ling San	PC-6	SP-3, SP-6, SP-9, CV-12, ST-8, ST-25, ST-36, BL-20
Diarrhea (泄瀉)	Bacterial, viral, or parasitic infection, acute gastroenteritis, ulcerative colitis, Crohn's disease	Huo Xiang Zheng Qi San, Bu Huan Jin Zheng Qi San		ST-25, ST-36, CV-6, BL-25	
Sudden turmoil disorder (霍亂)	Dysentery, cholera, typhoid, cryptosporidiosis, rotavirus, shigellosis			ST-25, ST-37, ST-44, CV-10, CV-12, LR-2, LR-3	
Epigastric pain (胃痛)	Peptic ulcer, GERD, pancreatitis, gastritis, gastric neurosis, gastric carcinoma	Ping Wei San		CV-13, ST-21, ST-34, ST-36, PC-6, SP-4,	
Jaundice (黃疸)	Chronic hepatitis, cirrhosis, Gilbert syndrome, baby jaundice, pancreas cancer, gallstone	Yin Chen Si Ni Tang		GV-6, GV-9, SI-4, BL-19, GBL-34, LR-3	
Edema (水腫)	Chronic nephritis, nephrotic syndrome, CHF, glomerulonephritis, myxedema, lymphedema	Shi Pi Yin		CV-9, CV-10, BL-23, GV-23, LI-6	
Phlegm and thin mucus (痰飲)	Cirrhosis, ascites, Meniere's disease, anorexia nervosa, SIBO, enteritis	Er Chen Tang, Ling Gan Wu Wei Jiang Xin Tang		ST-40, TB-5	

Table 3.10 Diseases and treatments related to Cold-Dampness Encumbering the Spleen

Comparison: Cold-Dampness Encumbering the Spleen vs. Spleen Yang Deficiency with Cold-Dampness

Cold-dampness encumbering the Spleen (寒濕困脾 *hán shī kùn pí*) and Spleen yang deficiency with cold-dampness (陽虛濕阻 *yáng xū shī zǔ*) share the same pathogens and pathological location, both exhibiting symptoms of Spleen dysfunction with aspects of cold and dampness. Thus they both manifest with abdominal cold pain, poor appetite, loose stools, clear copious vaginal discharge, a pale and flabby tongue, and a slow pulse. However, these two patterns require different treatment strategies because they are different in terms of excess and deficiency.

Cold-dampness encumbering the Spleen is usually caused by the invasion of exopathogenic cold-dampness or by the overconsumption of raw cold foods or unhygienic food and water, and thus it is acute, excessive, short course, and presents with severe diarrhea. Conversely, Spleen yang deficiency with cold-dampness develops from a weak constitution or chronic illness, and therefore is more chronic, long course, and presents with mild loose stools. Spleen yang deficiency fails to transform and transport, leading to dampness accumulation.

The key points to distinguish these two patterns are as follows:
1) Nature of onset and course of illness
2) Diarrhea vs. loose stools
3) Jaundice, edema, or scanty urine only appears in cold-dampness encumbering the Spleen pattern

Pattern		Cold-Dampness Encumbering the Spleen	Spleen Yang Deficiency with Cold-Dampness
Pathogenesis		Cold-dampness encumbers the Spleen, impairs Spleen and Stomach yang, disrupts ascending and descending function	Spleen yang deficiency, fails to warm and transform, generates dampness
Nature		External cold-dampness invades, excess, acute onset, short course, severe symptoms	Cold-dampess generated internally, deficiency, gradual onset, long course, mild symptoms
Symptoms	Common	Abdominal cold pain and preference for warmth, poor appetite, loose stools, clear copious vaginal discharge, pale tongue, slow pulse	
	Different	Severe abdominal pain averse to pressure, severe diarrhea, smoky yellow skin, edema, scanty urination	Dull chronic abdominal pain relieved by warmth and pressure, chronic loose stools, worse with exposure to cold or consumption of cold foods
Tongue & pulse		Pale flabby tongue with white greasy coating; deep, thin, slow pulse	Pale flabby tongue with teeth marks with white glossy coating; deep, slow, weak pulse
Treatment strategy		Dry dampness, strengthen the Spleen, regulate qi	Tonify Spleen, warm and tonify the middle burner
Herbal formulas		Huo Xiang Zheng Qi San, Ping Wei San	Shen Ling Bai Zhu San, Shi Pi Yin

Table 3.11 Comparison of Cold-Dampness Encumbering the Spleen and Spleen Yang Deficiency with Cold-Dampness

Comparison: Cold-Dampness Encumbering the Spleen vs. Water-Dampness Immersion

Pathologically, both cold-dampness encumbering the Spleen and water-dampness immersion have the same etiology and pathogenesis, which involves dampness invading the Spleen. Thus they share some signs and symptoms such as poor appetite, abdominal distention and bloating, nausea, clear copious vaginal discharge, edema, scanty urination, and a greasy tongue coating. However, the two patterns have different presentations.

Water-dampness immersion (水濕浸漬 *shuǐ shī jìn zì*), also called 'skin water pattern' (皮水証 *pí shuǐ zhèng*), which is from the qi, blood, and body fluids pattern identification system, is a type of yang edema, caused by water-dampness invasion. The Spleen has failed to transport and transform, leading to water and dampness infiltration and immersion to the skin and muscles. Entire body pitting edema is the major presentation, accompanied by other signs and symptoms related to dampness invasion of the Spleen such as abdominal distention, poor appetite, nausea or vomiting, and a greasy tongue.

Cold-dampness encumbering the Spleen (寒濕睏脾 *hán shī kùn fèi*) is a pattern caused by cold-dampness invasion that impairs yang qi and disrupts the Spleen's ascending and descending function, presenting mainly with gastrointestinal tract symptoms such as diarrhea or loose stools, abdominal pain, poor appetite, bloating, and distention.

The key points to distinguish these two patterns are as follows:
1) Nature of onset and course of illness: acute vs subacute; short course vs. long course
2) Chief complaints: gastrointestinal symptoms vs. pitting edema and scanty urine
3) Water-dampness immersion may present heat signs

Pattern	Cold-Dampness Encumbering the Spleen	Water-Dampness Immersion
Pathogenesis	Dampness invades the Spleen, which fails to transform and transport, disrupting the qi transformation of both the Triple Burner and Urinary Bladder	
	Impairs Spleen and Stomach yang, disrupts ascending and descending function	Leads to water and dampness infiltration and immersion to the skin and muscles, a type of yang edema
Characteristics	External cold-dampness invades, excess	
	Acute onset, short course	Acute or sub-acute onset, longer course
Symptoms — Common	Poor appetite, abdominal distention and bloating, nausea, clear copious vaginal discharge, edema, scanty urine, a greasy tongue coating	
Symptoms — Different	Severe abdominal cold pain, aversion to pressure, prefers warmth, severe diarrhea, smoky yellow skin	Entire body pitting edema, scanty urine
Tongue & pulse	Pale flabby tongue with white greasy coating; deep thin or slow pulse	Tongue may red with yellow coating; deep, maybe rapid, pulse
Treatment strategy	Dry dampness, strengthen the Spleen, regulate qi	Promote urination to reduce edema
Herbal formulas	Huo Xiang Zheng Qi San, Ping Wei San	Wu Pi Yin

Table 3.12 Comparison of Cold-Dampness Encumbering the Spleen and Water-Dampness Immersion

7 Damp-Heat Encumbering the Spleen Pattern | 濕熱睏脾

Definition: A group of signs and symptoms resulting from damp-heat accumulating in the middle burner due to a dysfunction of the Spleen's transformation and transportation function. The character 睏 (*kùn*), translated here as 'encumbering,' can also mean to besiege, trap, or assail.

Chapter 3 : Spleen Disease Patterns

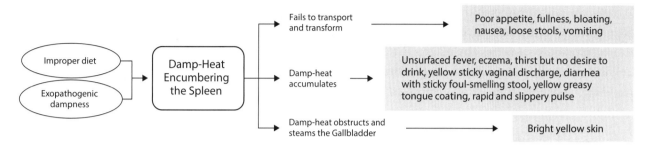

Chart 3.14 Etiology and pathogenesis of Damp-Heat Encumbering the Spleen

TCM Disease	Western Disease	Herbal Formulas		Acupuncture	
Diarrhea (泄瀉)	Bacterial, viral, or parasitic infection, acute gastroenteritis, ulcerative colitis, Crohn's disease		Lian Pu Yin, Xiang Lian Wan		ST-25, ST-37, ST-44, LI-4, BL-25, CV-12
Epigastric pain (胃痛)	Pancreatitis, peptic ulcer, IBS, GERD, gastritis, gallbladder infection	Yin Chen Wu Ling San	Zhong Man Fen Xiao Wan	SP-6, SP-9, GV-9, LI-11, BL-20, GB-34	CV-12, ST-21, ST-34, ST-36, PC-6, SP-4
Sudden turmoil disorder (霍亂)	Dysentery, cholera, typhoid, cryptosporidiosis, rotavirus, shigellosis		Lian Po Yin, Hong Xiang Zheng Qi San		ST-25, ST-37, ST-44, CV-10, CV-12, LR-2, LR-3
Jaundice (黃疸)	Acute cholecystitis, baby jaundice, Gilbert's syndrome, obstruction or inflammation of the bile duct		Yin Chen Hao Tang		GV-6, SI-4, BL-19, LR-3
Damp-warm (濕溫)	Typhoid, paratyphoid, Salmonella, stomach flu		Lian Pu Yin		CV-12, ST-21, ST-34, ST-36, PC-6, SP-4
Phlegm and thin mucus (痰飲)	Cirrhosis, ascites, Meniere's disease, anorexia nervosa, SIBO, enteritis		Er Chen Tang		ST-40, TB-5

Table 3.13 Diseases and treatment related to Damp-Heat Encumbering the Spleen

Clinical manifestations: Bloating and distention in the epigastrium and abdomen, poor appetite, diarrhea with sticky stinking stool, nausea and vomiting, heavy limbs, thirst but no desire to drink, unsurfaced fever that does not reduce after sweating, jaundice with bright yellow skin, eczema with skin itching, sticky yellow vaginal discharge, a red tongue with yellow greasy coating, and a slippery and rapid or soft pulse.

Key points: Fullness and distention, bloating, poor appetite, nausea and vomiting, plus internal damp-heat signs and symptoms.

Etiology and pathogenesis: Exogenous pathogenic damp-heat invades or damp-heat is interiorly generated by overconsumption of greasy, sweet or spicy foods, dairy, or alcohol.

When damp-heat stagnates in the middle burner, it disrupts Spleen and Stomach function. Damp-heat prevents the Spleen from transforming and transporting, causing Stomach qi to rebel. This causes fullness, distention, bloating, poor appetite, nausea and vomiting.

If damp-heat obstructs the Gallbladder, bile steams out, causing jaundice. Heat and dampness accumulate together, leading to unsurfaced fever that does not reduce after sweating. Although heat impairs the body fluids, which causes thirst, the accumulation of dampness inhibits desire to drink. If damp-heat obstructs in the skin, it can lead to eczema with skin itching. Sticky yellow vaginal discharge, yellow greasy coating, rapid and slippery pulse are all symptoms of damp-heat.

Comparison: Damp-heat Encumbering the Spleen vs. Cold-dampness Encumbering the Spleen

Damp-heat encumbering the Spleen (濕熱睏脾 shī rè kùn pí) and cold-dampness encumbering the Spleen (寒濕睏脾 hán shī kùn pí) share the same pathogen (dampness) and pathogenic location (Spleen), and therefore both exhibit fullness and distention, bloating, nausea and vomiting, diarrhea, a greasy tongue, and a slippery pulse. However, they have different clinical manifestations and treatment strategies because of the difference in the pathogenic nature of heat vs. cold.

Jaundice can appear in both patterns, but in damp-heat invading the Spleen it is yang jaundice, which presents with bright yellow skin and eyes, along with the presence of thirst. In damp-cold invading the Spleen it is yin jaundice, which presents with dim, smoky yellow skin and eyes, and no thirst. Additionally, in damp-heat invading the Spleen there is diarrhea with sticky and foul-smelling stools, while in cold-dampness invading the Spleen there is watery stools with abdominal pain that is relieved by warmth.

The key points to distinguish these two patterns are as follows:
1) Color of skin, urine, discharge, and tongue coating
2) Characteristics of phlegm, stools, and discharge
3) Tongue and pulse

Pattern		Damp-Heat Encumbering the Spleen	Cold-Dampness Encumbering the Spleen
Pathogenesis		Dampness besieges the Spleen, disrupting Spleen's transportation and transformation function	
		Dampness and heat accumulate, impairing body fluids	Dampness and cold accumulate, impairing Spleen and Stomach yang
Symptoms	Common	Abdominal distention and fullness, nausea, diarrhea, greasy coating, and slippery pulse	
	Different	Bright yellow jaundice, skin itching, diarrhea with sticky and foul-smelling stools, thirst but no desire to drink, unsurfaced fever that does not reduce after sweating	Smoky, dim yellow jaundice, abdominal pain, preference for warmth, copious and clear vaginal discharge
Tongue & pulse		Red tongue with yellow greasy coating; soft, slippery, rapid pulse	Pale flabby tongue with white greasy coating; soft, slippery, slow or moderate pulse
Treatment strategy		Clear heat, transform dampness, regulate qi, harmonize the middle burner	Dry dampness, strengthen the Spleen, regulate qi
Herbal formulas		Lian Po Yin, Zhong Man Fei Xiao Wan, Yin Chen Hao Tang	Ping Wei San, Huo Xiang Zheng Qi San

Table 3.14 Comparison of Damp-Heat Encumbering the Spleen and Cold-Dampness Encumbering the Spleen

Summary of Spleen Disease Patterns

Key points: poor appetite, abdominal distention and bloating, loose stools or diarrhea, bleeding, abdominal pain, emaciation, edema, phlegm, prolapse of organs, flaccid limbs, weak muscle tone, tastelessness or sweet and greasy taste in the mouth

	Patterns	Clinical manifestations	
		Common	Different
Deficiency	Spleen Qi Deficiency	Poor appetite, loose stools, abdominal bloating and distention that is worse after eating, emaciation, edema, sallow complexion, weak limbs, aversion to speaking, fatigue, pale tongue, and weak pulse	
Deficiency	Spleen Qi Sinking		Internal organ prolapse such as stomach, uterus, kidneys, or rectum, chronic loose stools
Deficiency	Spleen not Controlling Blood		Various kinds of bleeding
Deficiency	Spleen Yang Deficiency		Vague abdominal pain that is relieved by warmth and pressure, cold limbs, scanty urine, sensation of heaviness of limbs, edema, or copious vaginal discharge
Deficiency	Spleen Yin Deficiency	Emaciation and lack of strength, poor appetite, abdominal distention after eating, chapped lips, dry mouth, epigastric discomfort and pain, belching, reflux, five center heat, yellow urine, dry stools, red tongue with thin yellow or scanty coating, and thin rapid pulse	
Excess	Cold-Dampness Encumbering the Spleen	Abdominal distention and bloating, nausea, diarrhea, greasy coating, and slippery pulse	Smoky, dim yellow jaundice, edema with scanty urine, abdominal pain, preference for warmth, copious and clear vaginal discharge
Excess	Damp-Heat Encumbering the Spleen		Bright yellow jaundice or itchy skin, diarrhea with sticky and stinking stool, thirst but no desire to drink, un-surfaced fever that does not reduce after sweating

Table 3.15 Summary of Spleen disease patterns

Chapter 4
Liver Disease Patterns

Physiological characteristics and functions of the Liver

The Liver is located in the right hypochondriac region under the ribs. Its channel starts at the lateral aspect of the big toenail, courses up the inner leg, encircles the external genitals and bilateral lower abdomen, then distributes in the costal region and terminates at the top of the head. The Liver is internally-externally connected with the Gallbladder. It opens into the eyes and its related fluid are tears. It controls the tendons and sinews, and manifests on the nails. Its related emotion is anger. The ministerial fire (相火 xiàng huǒ) is associated with the Liver.

The Liver is called the commander organ (將軍之官 jiāng jūn zhī guan) and is in charge of strategy and planning. It is an unyielding organ (剛臟 gāng zàng), staunch and restless. "It takes blood as its body and qi as its function" (體陰用陽 tǐ yīn yòng yáng). Its nature is to grow and flourish. It favors soothing and dispersal and disfavors depression and constraint. It belongs to the wood phase, corresponding to growth-qi, and spring. The Liver governs strategic thinking. It is the origin (root) of tiredness (罷極之本 bà jí zhī běn): when the Liver undergoes pathological change, there is tiredness or easy fatigue.

Liver	Relationships
Spirit	Ethereal soul (魂 hún)
Internal-external connection	Gallbladder
Orifice	Eyes
Controls	Tendons, sinews
External manifestation	Nails
Fluid	Tears
Fire	Ministerial fire
Emotion	Anger
Season	Spring
Five phase	Wood
Six climate factor	Wind

Table 4.1 Liver and its related properties

1 | Governs coursing and discharging

The Liver governs coursing and discharging or conducting and dispersing (疏泄 *shū xiè*). *Shū* means to dredge while *xiè* means to discharge or release. Under this function, the Liver:

(1) Regulates emotional activities: when qi circulation is smooth, people feel calm, happy and at ease.
(2) Assists digestion and absorption: by ensuring the smooth flow of qi, the Liver promotes harmony between the ascending function of the Spleen and the descending function of the Stomach, and stimulates the Gallbladder to secrete bile.
(3) Promotes smooth flow of qi, blood, and water: when qi moves smoothly, then blood moves without stagnating.
(4) Assists in water metabolism: qi movement maintains normal water metabolism process (distribution and excretion).
(5) Regulates reproductive function: normal menstruation cycle for women and seminal ejaculation for men depends on the Liver's coursing and discharging function.

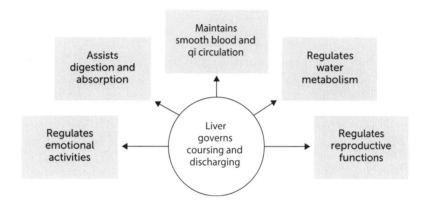

Chart 4.1   Liver governs coursing and discharging

2 | Stores blood, retains blood, and regulates its volume in circulation

(1) Stores blood, nourishes Liver, controls Liver yang, and prevents bleeding
(2) Regulates blood volume: according to the body's activities, the Liver increases or decreases blood volume inside the body to nourish organs and tissues as needed.

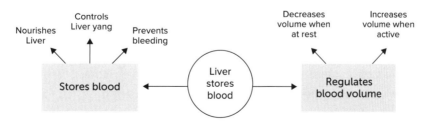

Chart 4.2   Liver stores blood

The Liver's blood storage function and its coursing and discharging function are mutually restraining and complementary. The Liver is called the 'sea of blood' and 'takes blood as its body and qi as its function.' The extra blood stored inside the Liver nourishes and supplies the Liver, ensuring that Liver yang is controlled, and yin and yang are balanced. When the Liver is nourished, it performs its coursing and discharging function, allowing qi and blood to circulate smoothly.

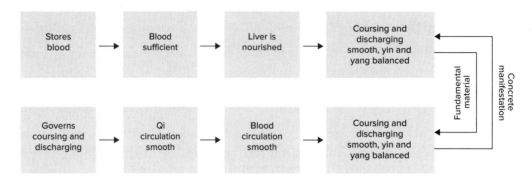

Chart 4.3   Relationship between Liver functions

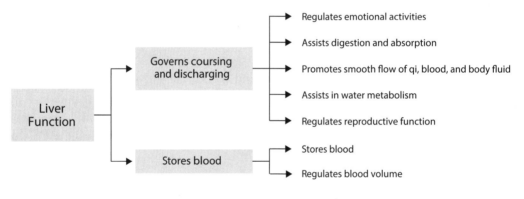

Chart 4.4   Liver function summary

Common etiological factors in Liver patterns

Emotional stress is one of the major causative factors for Liver disease, but other factors also result in Liver pathological changes such as invasion by exopathogenic factors, diet, or lifestyle. The following are common etiological factors for Liver disease patterns:
   (1) Exopathogenic factors: wind, cold, heat, dryness, dampness, summer-heat, or pestilence (癘氣 lì qì)
   (2) Emotional stress: anger, depression, anxiety, worry, fear, sadness, fright
   (3) Improper diet: overconsumption of hot spicy or pungent foods and alcohol
   (4) Improper treatment or medications
   (5) Congenital defect
   (6) Chronic illness

Pathological changes and major clinical manifestations of the Liver

Failure to course and discharge and failure to store blood are the main causes of pathological changes in the Liver. There are four major clinical manifestations of Liver function disorder: emotional stress (anger, depression), hypochondriac pain or distention, internal wind, and menstrual disorders.

1 | Emotional disorder

Definition: A group of disorders characterized by prolonged, pervasive disturbance of mood coupled with a full or partial manic or depressive response that is not caused by a separate physical or mental disorder.

Characteristics of emotional disorder due to Liver dysfunction include depression, mood swings, worry, unhappiness, irritability, quick temper, and anxiety. The symptoms are usually induced or aggravated by emotional stress.

Etiology and pathomechanisms: The Liver's coursing and discharging function balances emotions. Emotions develop from the *shén*, which needs to be nourished by qi and blood. Thus normal emotional health depends on the harmony of qi and blood. When the Liver keeps qi flowing smoothly, a relaxed internal emotional environment is created.

Emotional imbalance leads to disturbances of the qi and blood, yin and yang imbalance, compromised *zàng fǔ* organ function, and other pathological changes. Emotional imbalance can be caused by sudden, severe, or exceptionally long-term and repeated emotional stimulation. Alternatively, emotionally hypersensitive people with low endurance and low adaptability may be unable to adjust to changing circumstances and may become imbalanced.

Sudden or long-term emotional stress such as anger or frustration; improper diet such as overconsumption of alcohol or greasy foods; invasion of exopathogenic factors; and chronic illness can all disrupt the Liver's coursing and discharging function. When the Liver lacks coursing, it can lead to qi stagnation, resulting in depression, worry, melancholy, paranoia, and frequent sighing. When the Liver over discharges, it can lead to qi counterflow, resulting in irritability, short temper, and anxiety.

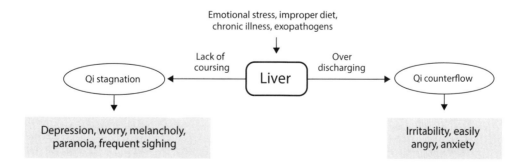

Chart 4.5 Etiology and pathomechanism of Liver-related emotional disorders

2 | Hypochondriac distention, pain, or masses

Definition: Distention, pain, or mass(es) under the ribcage margin on one or both sides, or beneath the ribs in the back.

Etiology and pathomechanisms: The hypochondrium is the house of the Liver and Gallbladder, whose channels traverse the hypochondriac region. Exopathogenic factors, emotional stress, improper diet, or chronic illness with internal *zàng fǔ* organ dysfunction all can result in qi and blood deficiency, phlegm, and/or blood stagnation. When the Liver and Gallbladder channels are obstructed by stasis, the organs may become undernourished or produce distention, pain, or masses.

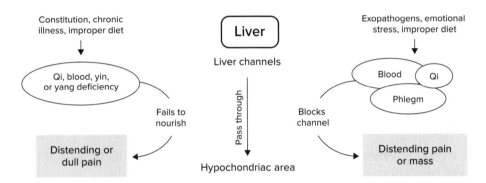

Chart 4.6 Etiology and pathomechanism of hypochondriac distending pain and/or masses

3 | Wind syndrome

Definition: Liver wind, also called Liver wind stirring internally, is a group of signs and symptoms caused by Liver dysfunction manifesting with either involuntary movement or stiffness such as spasms, tremors, tics, convulsion, muscle twitching, numbness, tingling, or hemiplegia.

Characteristics of wind syndrome due to Liver dysfunction include sudden or chronic onset, induced or aggravated by emotional stress.

The main signs and symptoms of Liver wind include all uncontrolled or involuntary movements such as spasms, tremors, tics, convulsions, paralysis, tingling or numbness in the limbs, muscle twitching, seizures, and hemiplegia. It also involves dizziness and vertigo, headache with a pulling sensation, tension and stiffness in the neck, or sudden loss of consciousness.

Etiology and pathomechanisms: This condition may be caused by emotional stress, exopathogenic attack, chronic illness, or improper diet such as a lack of nourishment or overconsumption of alcohol and greasy foods.

There are two groups of wind symptoms. The first group—dizziness, vertigo, headache with a pulling sensation, and/or loss of consciousness —is due to disturbance of sensory orifices of the head and brain, referred to as the 'clear orifices' (清竅 *qīng qiào*), by pathogenic factors or a lack of nourishment. The second group—tense and stiff neck, tremors, tics, convulsions, paralysis, tingling or numbness in the limbs, seizures, hemiplegia, deviated or stiff tongue, and wiry pulse—is caused by spasms of the tendons, sinews, and muscles.

Dizziness can result from the stirring up of pathogenic heat that disturbs the clear orifices or from a lack of nourishment to the brain. According to *The Divine Pivot*, Chapter 33, "all wind, shaking, and dizziness pertain to the Liver" (靈樞海論) and "deficiency of the brain leads to dizziness." Deficiency of the brain can be caused by a lack of nourishment due to qi, blood, or essence deficiency; or it may be due to pathogenic factors such as blood stasis or phlegm obstructing the channels and collaterals. In either case, qi and blood cannot adequately circulate, leading to a lack of nourishment in the head.

Spasms of the tendons, sinews, and muscles are usually caused by a lack of nourishment. Therefore, any cause of blood or yin deficiency may also generate Liver wind.

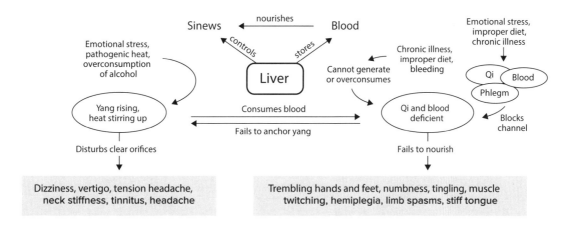

Chart 4.7 Etiology and pathomechanism of Liver wind

4 | Menstrual disorder

Definition: Any form of abnormal menstruation, including abnormal menstrual cycle, abnormal menstrual bleeding flow, and abnormal accompanying symptoms during, pre- or post-menstruation. Conditions include irregular menstrual cycle, menorrhagia, dysmenorrhea, and amenorrhea.

Characteristics of menstrual disorder due to Liver dysfunction: irregular menstrual cycle, abnormal menstrual bleeding flow, dysmenorrhea or amenorrhea accompanied by emotional distress, mood swings, irritability, breast distention and wiry pulse, the symptoms related to Liver qi stagnation.

Etiology and pathomechanisms: The Liver regulates the Penetrating vessel (冲 *chōng*) and the Conception vessel (任 *rèn*). The Liver's free coursing allows blood to fill and refill these vessels. When the Liver is over-coursing, menstruation comes early; when Liver coursing is insufficient, menstruation is delayed. The Kidney and Liver have a common source. The Liver stores blood and the Kidney stores essence. Essence and blood mutually replenish each other and transform into each other. The Liver is the root of the Penetrating vessel and the Kidney is the root of the Conception vessel. When there is Liver and Kidney dysfunction, the filling and refilling of these vessels is compromised, which causes irregular menses.

Smooth qi and blood circulation is a prerequisite for normal menstruation. Dysfunction of the Liver's coursing and discharging function causes qi and blood stagnation, which may result in dysmenorrhea, scanty bleeding, delayed menstrual cycle, or even amenorrhea. If qi and blood stagnation generate heat, the heat will accelerate blood circulation and impair the vessels, which causes preceded menstrual cycle and profuse bleeding.

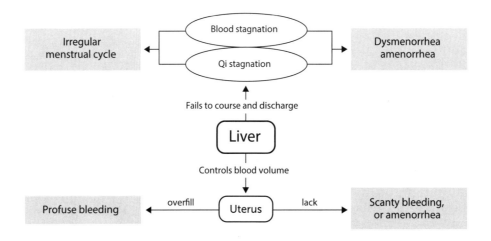

Chart 4.8   Etiology and pathomechanism of Liver-related menstrual disorder

5 | Other signs and symptoms related to the Liver

The following signs and symptoms are all closely related to Liver pathology: inguinal hernia, scrotum or testicular pain, abnormal ejaculation, erectile dysfunction, frequent sighing, eye or vision disorders, and wiry pulse.

Physiological Function		Pathological Change	Clinical Manifestation
Govern coursing and discharging	Regulate emotional activities	Lack of discharging leads to Liver qi stagnation	Depression, suspicion, anxiety, frequent sighing
		Over coursing causes hyperactivity of Liver qi	Irritability, anger, quick temper, headache, insomnia
	Assist digestion	Liver qi counterflow attacks the Stomach	Epigastric pain, vomiting, poor appetite, belching, hiccups, acid regurgitation
		Liver and Spleen disharmony	Distending abdominal pain, loose stool, poor appetite
		Liver and Gallbladder disharmony	Pain in hypochondrium, bitter taste in the mouth, aversion to food, jaundice
	Maintain smooth blood circulation	Qi stagnation leading to blood stagnation	Pain or masses in the hypochondrium, dysmenorrhea
		Rebellious qi damages blood vessels	Bleeding, vomiting with blood, cough with blood, profuse menstrual bleeding, metrorrhagia and metrostaxis
	Regulate water metabolism	Qi fails to distribute and excrete water	Phlegm, edema
	Regulate reproductive function	Coursing and discharging disorder	Women: irregular menstruation, dysmenorrhea, amenorrhea, pms, infertility Men: difficult ejaculation or abnormal frequency of ejaculation
Store blood	Store blood	Failure to store blood	Bleeding, vomiting with blood, epistaxis, cough with blood, profuse menstrual bleeding or metrorrhagia and metrostaxis
	Regulate blood volume	Blood insufficiency fails to nourish organs and tissues	Dizziness, blurry vision, trembling hands and feet, numbness of limbs, scanty menstruation or amenorrhea

Table 4.2 Physiological functions, pathological changes, and clinical manifestations of the Liver

Common patterns in Liver disease

There are eleven Liver patterns commonly seen in the clinic. According to pathogenesis and clinical manifestation, these patterns are divided into three groups: excess, deficiency, and combination of excess and deficiency.

Liver blood deficiency and Liver yin deficiency are the most common deficiency patterns; Liver qi deficiency and Liver yang deficiency are rare. Liver qi deficiency is usually congenital or due to chronic illness. Liver yang deficiency develops from Liver qi deficiency.

Excess patterns include Liver qi stagnation, Liver fire blazing, Liver blood stagnation, cold stagnating in the Liver channel, and Liver wind agitating within. Based on etiology and pathogenesis, Liver wind is subdivided into four patterns: extreme heat generating wind, Liver yang transforming into wind, blood deficiency generating wind, and yin deficiency generating wind. Liver yang rising is a pattern which belongs to excess above and deficiency below.

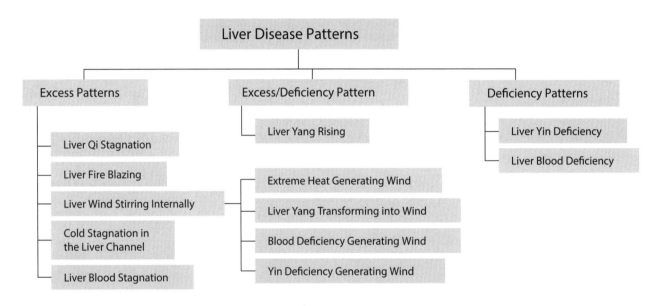

Chart 4.9 Common Liver disease patterns

	Etiology	Patterns
Deficiency	Congenital insufficiency, aging, chronic illness, improper diet and treatment or medication, long-term emotional stress	Liver Blood Deficiency, Liver Yin Deficiency, Liver Qi Deficiency (rare), Liver Yang Deficiency (rare)
Excess	Exopathogenic factors invasion, emotional stress, improper diet (overconsumption of hot spicy foods or alcohol), improper treatment or medications	Liver Qi Stagnation, Liver Fire Blazing, Liver Wind Stirring Internally, Liver Yang Transforming into Wind, Extreme Heat Generating Wind, Blood Deficiency Generating Wind, Yin Deficiency Generating Wind, Cold Stagnated in the Liver Channel, Liver Blood Stagnation
Excess with Deficiency	Emotional stress, improper diet, sexual overstrain, aging	Liver Yang Rising

Table 4.3 Classification of common Liver patterns

1 Liver Blood Deficiency Pattern | 肝血虛証 |

Definition: A group of signs and symptoms caused by the Liver and other organs lacking nourishment due to insufficient blood.

Clinical manifestations: Dizziness, tinnitus, blurry vision, dry eyes, night blindness, floaters, pale brittle or withered nails, numbness of limbs, muscle twitching, joint stiffness, and trembling of hands and feet. In women: scanty menses with light-colored bleeding, dysmenorrhea or amenorrhea, pale lips and tongue, and a thin wiry pulse.

Key points: Signs and symptoms due to malnourishment of tendons, eyes, and nails, plus blood deficiency signs and symptoms.

Etiology and pathogenesis: Since the Liver is the organ that stores blood, blood deficiency affects the Liver first. The causes of blood deficiency include: profuse bleeding; improper diet; parasites; compromised Spleen and Stomach unable to generate sufficient blood; mental overstrain, which consumes blood; blood stagnation causing lack of space to generate new blood; or chronic or severe illness damaging blood.

Blood nourishes and moistens. When deficient, it fails to nourish the muscle, tendons, and sinews. This causes numbness and twitching of hands and feet with pale, brittle, and fragile nails, since nails are the surplus of tendons and sinews. Failure to nourish tendons causes tremors and stiffness of the limbs. Failure to nourish the head and face results in dizziness, blurred vision, and pale complexion, tongue, and lips.

Blood also fills the vessels and channels. Failure to fill the Penetrating and Conception vessels may cause delayed menstruation, scanty/light periods, or amenorrhea. Failure to fill the vessels results in dysmenorrhea and a thin and weak pulse.

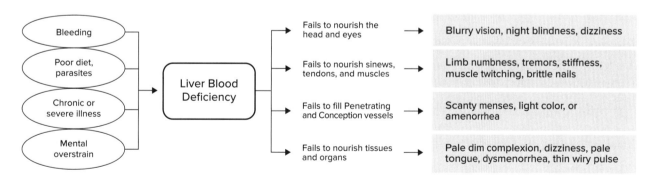

Chart 4.10 Etiology and pathogenesis of Liver Blood Deficiency

TCM Disease	Western Disease	Herbal Formulas		Acupuncture	
Fatigue (虛勞)	Adrenal fatigue, CFS, Lyme disease, EBV hypothyroidism, chronic hepatitis, anemia		Ba Zhen Tang		CV-4, CV-6
Insomnia (不寐)	Neurosis, menopause syndrome, depression, anxiety		Suan Zao Ren Tang		HT-5, HT-6, HT-7, Anmian, BL-15
Numbness (麻木)	Peripheral neuropathy, diabetes, MS, Lyme disease, amyloidosis, Sjoren's syndrome, stroke	Si Wu Tang, Bu Gan Tang	Bu Gan Tang	LR-3, LR-8, SP-6, KI-3, BL-17, BL-18, BL-20, BL-23, ST-36	GB-34, GV-9, GV-14, LI-11, BL-14, BL-16, BL-60
Blurry vision (視物不清)	Night blindness, presbyopia, diabetes, glaucoma, cataracts		Si Wu Tang		BL-1, BL-2, SP-10, ST-1
Irregular menses (月經不調)	Perimenopause, PCOS, anorexia, malnutrition, or caused by stress, D&C., miscarriage		Dang Gui Si Wu Tang		CV-4, CV-6, SP-10
Amenorrhea (閉經)	Anorexia, malnutrition, PCOS, hypothyroidism, bulimia		Sheng Yu Tang		
Dysmenorrhea (痛經)	Endometriosis, fibroids, PID, STI, adenomyosis, or use IUD		Tao Hong Si Wu Tang		SP-4, SP-8, CV-4, LI-4

Table 4.4 Diseases and treatments related to Liver Blood Deficiency

2 Liver Yin Deficiency Pattern | 肝陰虛証 |

Definition: A group of signs and symptoms due to insufficient yin fluid in the Liver.

Clinical manifestations: Dizziness, tinnitus, dry eyes, blurry vision, hypochondria pain with burning sensation, hot flashes, low-grade fever in the afternoon or evening, five-center heat, night sweats, trembling hands and feet, a red tongue with dry coating, and a thin, wiry, and rapid pulse.

Key points: Malnourishment of eyes, sinews, and nails, plus yin deficiency signs and symptoms.

Etiology and pathogenesis: Long-term and excessive emotional stress causes qi stagnation that generates heat, which in turn impairs yin. In the later stages of febrile disease, yin can also become damaged. Additionally, yin deficiency can result from chronic illness, especially in elderly patients with Kidney yin deficiency or 'water failing to nourish wood.'

When Liver yin is deficient, it cannot nourish the clear orifices such as the brain, eyes, and ears, resulting in dizziness, dry eyes with blurry vision, poor vision, tinnitus, dry mouth, and thirst. It also cannot nourish the sinews, tendons, and muscles, causing tremors of the hands and feet. A deficiency of yin means a relative excess of yang, which manifests with deficiency heat such as night sweats, hot flashes, five-center heat, a red tongue with scanty coating, and a rapid pulse. This deficiency heat along with a failure to nourish the Liver channel results in burning pain in the hypochondria and a wiry pulse.

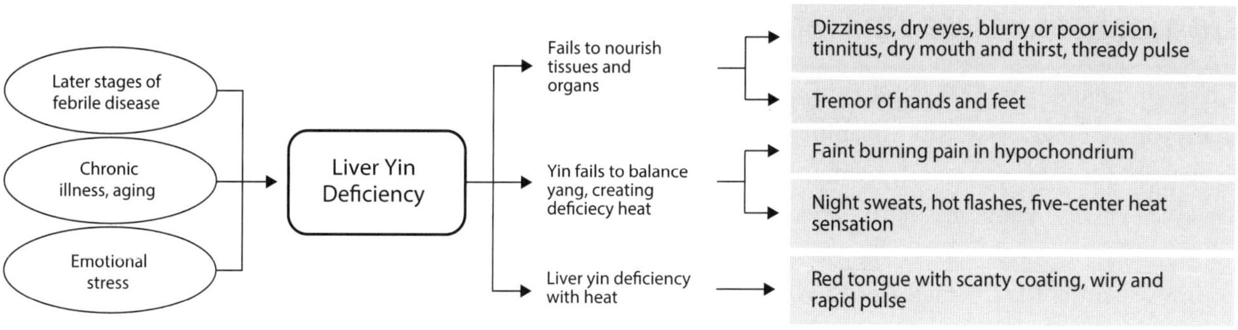

Chart 4.11 Etiology and pathogenesis of Liver Yin Deficiency

<table>
<tr><th>TCM Disease</th><th>Western Disease</th><th colspan="2">Herbal Formulas</th><th colspan="2">Acupuncture</th></tr>
<tr><td>Dizziness and vertigo (眩暈)</td><td>Hypertension, hypotension, BPPV, vestibular migraine, anemia, anxiety, hypoglycemia</td><td rowspan="10">Yi Guan Jian</td><td>Yi Guan Jian with Tian Ma Gou Teng Yin</td><td rowspan="10">LR-2, LR-8, SP-6, ST-36, CV-6, KI-3, KI-6</td><td>GV-20, GB-20, GB-34</td></tr>
<tr><td>Hypochodriac pain (脇痛)</td><td>Hypochondriasis, costochondritis, pleurisy, arthritis, osteoporosis, Intercostal neuralgia</td><td>Yi Guan Jian</td><td>TB-5, GB-34, GB-40, LR-3, BL-19</td></tr>
<tr><td>Headache (頭痛)</td><td>Hypertension, migraine or cluster headache, glaucoma, sinusitis, tension headache</td><td>Ren Shen Yang Yong Tang</td><td>GB-20, GV-20, LI-4</td></tr>
<tr><td>Fatigue (虛勞)</td><td>Chronic hepatitis, Addison's disease, hypothyroidism, Lyme disease, cancer</td><td>Bu Gan Tang</td><td>CV-4, GV-14</td></tr>
<tr><td>Endogenous fever (内傷發熱)</td><td>Chronic virus or bacterial infections, malignant tumor, rheumatoid arthritis, AIDS</td><td>Qing Gu San, Zhi Bai Di Huang Wan</td><td>LI-11, GV-13</td></tr>
<tr><td>Sweating (汗証)</td><td>Menopause syndrome, autonomic neuropathy, HIV/AIDS, carcinoid syndrome</td><td>Dang Gui Liu Huang Tang</td><td>LR-4, KI-7, SI-3</td></tr>
<tr><td>Insomnia (不寐)</td><td>Neurosis, menopause syndrome, depression, anxiety</td><td>Suan Zao Ren Tang</td><td>HT-5, HT-7, PC-6 Anmian</td></tr>
<tr><td>Dysmenorrhea (痛經)</td><td>Endometriosis, fibroids, PID, STI, adenomyosis, IUD use</td><td>Tiao Gan Tang</td><td>SP-4, SP-8, CV-4, LI-4</td></tr>
<tr><td>Amenorrhea (閉經)</td><td>PCOS, menopause, excessive exercise, anorexia or bulimia, stress, thyroid malfunction</td><td>Xiao Yao San with Si Wu Tang</td><td>SP-6, CV-3, CV-4, SP-10, LR-3, BL-23</td></tr>
<tr><td>Night blindness (雀盲)</td><td>Eye disease, Vitamin A insufficient</td><td>Qi Ju Di Huang Wan</td><td>BL-1, BL-2, ST-1</td></tr>
</table>

Table 4.5 Diseases and treatments related to Liver Yin Deficiency

Comparison: Liver Yin Deficiency vs. Liver Blood Deficiency

Liver yin deficiency (肝陰虛 gān yīn xū) and Liver blood deficiency (肝血虛 gān xǔe xū) both have symptoms of dizziness, tinnitus, blurry vision, dry eyes, trembling hands and feet, and a wiry thin pulse. However, Liver blood deficiency manifests as malnourishment of the Liver, while Liver yin deficiency involves yin and yang imbalance, and yin deficiency heat.

Malnourishment is the major presentation in Liver blood deficiency, exhibiting pale facial complexion, pale tongue and nails, withered and dry hair and nails, and fatigue. Liver yin deficiency is caused by yin and yang imbalance, yin deficiency leading to a relative yang excess, and therefore heat signs appear such as tidal fever, low-grade fever, five-center heat, night sweats, and a rapid pulse.

The key points to distinguish these two patterns are as follows:
1) Facial and tongue color: red vs. pale
2) Heat signs: Liver yin deficiency includes yin deficiency heat

Pattern		Liver Yin Deficiency	Liver Blood Deficiency
Pathogenesis		Liver yin deficiency fails to control yang, leading to deficiency heat	Blood deficiency fails to nourish the Liver
Symptoms	Common	Dizziness, tinnitus, blurry vision, dry eyes, trembling hands and feet, wiry and thready pulse	
Symptoms	Different	Deficiency heat: tidal fever, hot flashes, low-grade fever in the afternoon or evening, five-center heat, night sweats, bitter taste in the mouth	Blood fails to nourish: pale face, nails, and tongue, night blindness; in women: scanty or light-colored menses, delayed cycle, or amenorrhea
Tongue & pulse		Red or red cracked tongue with little or no coating; wiry, thin, rapid pulse	Pale tongue with dry coating; wiry, thin, or weak pulse
Treatment strategy		Nourish Liver yin	Tonify Liver blood
Herbal formulas		Yi Guan Jian	Si Wu Tang, Bu Gan Tang

Table 4.6 Comparison of Liver Yin Deficiency and Liver Blood Deficiency

3 Liver Qi Stagnation Pattern | 肝鬱氣滯証 |

Definition: A group of signs and symptoms caused by the Liver's failure to course and discharge, which inhibits the smooth flow of qi.

Clinical manifestations: Distending pain in the hypochondria or lateral abdomen (少腹 shào fù), sensation of chest oppression, frequent sighing, depression, short temper, irregular menstrual cycle, premenstrual syndrome, distending breast pain, dysmenorrhea, and a wiry pulse. There may possibly be plum-pit syndrome (globus hystericus) or goiter.

Key points: Depression, distending pain in the hypochondria or lateral abdomen, irregular menstrual cycle, wiry pulse, plus qi stagnation signs and symptoms.

Etiology and pathogenesis: The Liver is an unyielding organ that favors smooth, easy movement and disfavors constraint and depression. "It takes blood as its body and qi as its function." Emotions develop from the *shén*, which needs to be nourished by qi and blood. Therefore, normal emotional health depends on the Liver's coursing and discharging to keep qi flowing smoothly, and to ensure sufficient blood will store and nourish the Liver.

The Liver's function of maintaining the free flow of qi can be disrupted by emotional stress, such as sudden, severe, or exceptionally long-term emotional stimulation; improper diet, such as overconsumption of alcohol or greasy food; or exopathogens, such as wind-cold and wind-dampness, which can cause phlegm, dampness, or blood stasis that obstructs the Liver channel, leading to qi stagnation. Chronic illness can also lead to qi and blood deficiency, which deprives the Liver of nourishment and impairs its coursing and discharging function.

When the Liver lacks coursing, it can lead to qi stagnation, resulting in depression, worry, melancholy, paranoia, and frequent sighing. When the Liver overly discharges, it can lead to qi counterflow, resulting in irritability, short temper, and anxiety. When qi stagnation affects the qi circulation in the Liver channel, it causes distention and pain in the hypochondria or lateral abdomen, breast distention, and dysmenorrhea or amenorrhea.

The filling and refilling of the Pentrating and Conception vessels requires qi regulation. When the Liver fails to course and discharge, these two vessels are not filled and refilled regularly, resulting in an irregular menstrual cycle and dysmenorrhea. Thus the Liver is fundamental in women.

Additionally, when Liver dysfunction leads to qi and phlegm accumulation in the throat area, it can result in plum-pit syndrome (globus hystericus) or goiter. When qi stagnation lodges in the abdomen, it can cause an abdominal mass. Qi stagnation strongly pushes the blood, which increases vasotonia and gives rise to a wiry pulse.

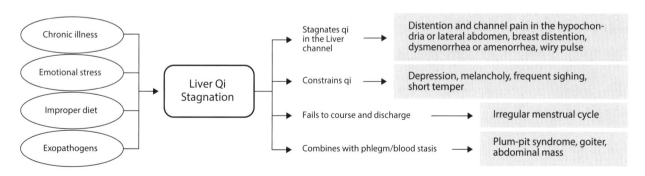

Chart 4.12 Etiology and pathogenesis of Liver Qi Stagnation

TCM Disease	Western Disease	Herbal Formulas		Acupuncture
Hypochondriac pain (脇痛)	Chronic hepatitis, costochondritis, chronic cholecystitis, intercostal neuralgia, hypochondriasis	Xiao Yao San, Chai Hu Shu Gan Wan	Chai Hu Shu Gan Wan	GB-40, ST-36, BL-19
Epigastric pain (胃痛)	Chronic gastritis, gastric ulcer, duodenal ulcer, GERD, gallstone, pancreatitis			CV-12, ST-21, ST-34, ST-36, PC-6, SP-4
Plum-pit syndrome (梅核氣)	Hyperthyroidism, throat-esophagus neurosis, globus hystericus, post nasal drip		Ban Xia Hou Po Tang	LR-2, LR-5, CV-17, CV-22, CV-23, ST-40, SP-9
Constraint presentations (鬱証)	Depression, anxiety, menopause syndrome, neurosis, hysteria, PMS		Chai Hu Jia Long Gu Mu Li Tang	GV-20, Yintang, PC-6
Dysmenorrhea (痛經)	Endometriosis, fibroids, PID, STI, adenomyosis, IUD use		Ge Xia Zhu Yu Tang	LR-2, CV-3, CV-6, GB-34, SP-6, SP-8
Irregular menses (月經不調)	Perimenopause, PCOS, eating disorder, malnutrition, or caused by stress, D&C, miscarriage		Xiao Yao San	LR-14, ST-25, SP-8, KI-14

Acupuncture column common points: LR-3, LR-13, LR-14, LI-4, GB-34, TB-6, PC-6

Table 4.7 Diseases and treatments related to Liver Qi Stagnation

4 Liver Fire Blazing Pattern | 肝火上炎証 |

Definition: A group of signs and symptoms caused by the flaring up of qi and fire in the Liver channel.

Clinical manifestations: Dizziness, vertigo, distending headache, flushed face, conjunctival congestion, bitter taste and dryness in the mouth, irritability, burning pain in the chest and hypochondrium, insomnia, dream-disturbed sleep, sudden tinnitus and deafness, dry stool and yellow urine, nosebleed or hematemesis. Red tongue with yellow coating. Wiry and rapid pulse.

Key points: Dizziness, vertigo, distending headache, tinnitus or deafness, plus interior excess heat signs and symptoms.

Etiology and pathogenesis: This is the condition of 'excessive qi accumulation transferring to fire' (氣有餘便是火 *qì yǒu yú biàn shì huǒ*). Extra qi can be caused by long-term emotional stress, exopathogenic heat invasion, and excessive consumption of spicy and aromatic food or alcohol.

There are two main components of this pattern: excessive heat and the flaring up of that fire, especially when it occurs suddenly. When Liver fire flares up following the Liver channel, it passes the hypochondria and reaches the head, eyes, and ears, causing burning pain in the hypochondria, a red face, and red eyes. When the fire disrupts the clear orifices, it leads to tinnitus, deafness, dizziness, and distending pain of the head. When it affects the Gallbladder, bile overflows and causes a bitter taste in the mouth. And, when heat disrupts *shén*, there are symptoms of irritability, short temper, and dream-disturbed sleep.

Excess heat can impair the blood vessels and accelerate the blood, causing bleeding. This heat can also impair the body fluids, causing thirst and a desire to drink fluids, constipation, and scanty yellow urine. A red tongue with yellow coating and a rapid pulse can be expected as signs of this internal heat.

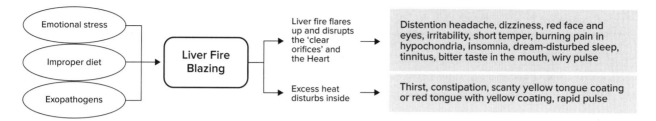

Chart 4.13 Etiology and pathogenesis of Liver Fire Blazing

TCM Disease	Western Disease	Herbal Formulas		Acupuncture
Xiao Pi (消痞)	Hyperthyroidism	Dang Gui Long Hui Wan with Xia Ku Cao	Jia Wei Xiao Yao San, Long Dan Xie Gan Tang	TB-13, ST-9, ST-40, PC-6, LI-4, SP-6, HT-7, GB-40
Hu Hou Bing (狐惑病)	Behcet's syndrome	Long Dan Xie Gan Tang		KI-3, LI-4, BL-18, BL-23
Insomnia (不寐)	Menopause syndrome, anxiety, neurosis, ADD/ADHD	Xie Qing Wan		HT-5, HT-6, HT-7, Anmian
Headache (頭痛)	Cerebral arteriosclerosis, migraines, hypertension	Long Dan Xie Gan Tang		GV-20, LI-4, Taiyang
Manic behavior (狂躁)	Schizophrenia, manic depression, bipolar disorder, hypomania, psychosis	Dang Gui Long Hui Wan with Meng Shi Gun Tan Wan		BL-15, BL-18, BL-20, ST-40, HT-7, PC-6, PC-7, SP-6, LI-1, Yintang, GV-16, GV-26
Acid reflux (吞酸)	GRED, hiatal hernia	Zuo Jin Wan	LR-2, LR-3, GB-13, GB-20, GB-34, LI-11	CV-12, ST-36, SP-6, PC-6
Ear bleeding (耳衄)	Ear infection, ruptured eardrum, otitis externa, folliculitis	Long Dan Xie Gan Tang with Si Shen Wan		GB-2, GB-8, GB-43, TB-3, LI-4, SI-19, LI-4
Red eye (赤帶抱紅)	Conjunctivitis, acute optic neuritis, fascicular keratitis, glaucoma, acute congestive, acute iridocyclitis	Long Dan Xie Gan Tang		LI-4, BL-2, Taiyang, GB-43
Tinnitus (耳鳴)	Hypertension, Meniere's disease, TMJ disorder, atherosclerosis			GB-2, GB-8, GB-43, TB-3, LI-4, SI-19
Face wind (面風)	Trigeminal neuralgia, TMJ, migraine	San Cha Tang		TB-5, TB-17, TB-21, GB-2, SI-18, ST-2, ST-3, ST-7, ST-36, ST-44, ST-45, GV-26, LI-20

Table 4.8 Diseases and treatments related to Liver Fire Blazing

Comparison: Liver Fire Blazing vs. Heart Fire Blazing

Both Liver fire blazing (肝火上炎 gān huǒ shàng yán) and Heart fire blazing (心火上炎 xīn huǒ shàng yán) are caused by excess fire flaring up. Thus they share many signs and symptoms such as insomnia, irritability, dream-disturbed sleep, bitter taste in the mouth, red face, thirst with a preference for cold water, yellow urine, dry stools, red tongue with a yellow coating, rapid pulse, nosebleed, and hematemesis. However, the location of the pathology is different, and therefore there are differences in clinical manifestation, treatment strategy, and herbal formula selection.

Liver fire blazing shows excess heat in the Liver or its channel, manifesting in red eyes, tinnitus or deafness, and a burning sensation in the hypochondrium. There may also be 'wind' symptoms such as dizziness and tension headache. Conversely, Heart fire blazing indicates an excess in the Heart or its channel, and therefore its main presentation is *shén* disturbance such as manic behavior, irritability, agitation, vexation, delirium, and even coma. There may also be tongue ulcers, canker sores, and burning or painful urination.

The key points to distinguish these two patterns are as follows:
1) Location: eyes and ears vs. chest, mouth, and tongue
2) Wind symptoms vs. *shén* disturbance symptoms

Pattern		Liver Fire Blazing	Heart Fire Blazing
Pathogenesis		Qi stagnation transforms into fire and flares up following Liver channel	Internal excess heat disrupts Heart
Symptoms	Common	Insomnia, irritability, dream-disturbed sleep, bitter taste in the mouth, red face, thirst and preference for cold water, yellow urine, dry stool, red tongue with yellow coating, rapid pulse, or nosebleed, hematemesis	
	Different	Dizziness, distending headache, conjunctival congestion, burning pain in hypochondrium, sudden tinnitus and deafness	Vexation, hot sensation in the chest, palpitations, tongue ulcers, rapid and forceful pulse, manic behavior, delirium, burning painful urination
Tongue & pulse		Red tongue with yellow coating, rapid pulse	
Treatment strategy		Clear Liver fire	Clear Heart fire
Herbal formulas		Jia Wei Xiao Yao San, Chai Hu Qing Gan Wan	Xie Xin Tang, Dao Chi San

Table 4.9 Comparison of Liver Fire Blazing and Heart Fire Blazing

5 Liver Yang Rising Pattern | 肝陽上亢証 |

Definition: A group of signs and symptoms caused by hyperactivity of Liver yang with Liver and Kidney yin deficiency.

Clinical manifestations: Dizziness, vertigo, tinnitus, distending pain in the head and eyes, flushed face, congested eyes, vexation, lassitude in the loins and legs, feeling heavy in the head 'top-heavy,' tendency to fall, insomnia and dream-disturbed sleep, poor memory, red tongue, wiry and rapid pulse.

Key points: Distending pain in the head and eyes, dizziness, and vertigo, 'top-heavy' feeling, lumbar and knee soreness and weakness.

Etiology and pathogenesis: This pattern can be caused by emotional stress, especially anger, which stagnates qi that can then transform into fire and flare up to disrupt the clear sensory orifices. In addition, chronic illness, aging, or sexual overstrain causes yin deficiency, which cannot anchor yang, leading to yang rising.

Liver yang rising disrupts the clear orifices of the head, causing tinnitus, dizziness, and vertigo. Yang is heat; heat disturbs *shén*, causing dream-disturbed sleep, insomnia, irritability, and anger. Deficient Liver and Kidney yin fails to nourish the bones, leading to soreness and weakness in the lower back and knees. Yin deficiency generates deficiency heat, which gives rise to a red tongue with scanty coating, and a thin rapid pulse. Yang rising upward with Liver and Kidney deficiency below causes a top-heavy sensation and a tendency to fall.

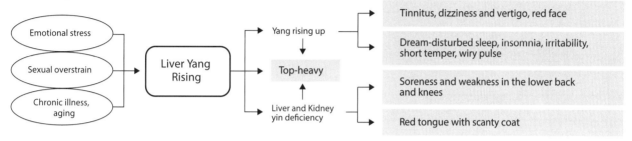

Chart 4.14 Etiology and pathogenesis of Liver Yang Rising

TCM Disease	Western Disease	Herbal Formulas		Acupuncture	
Headache (頭痛)	Cerebral arteriosclerosis, hypertension, migraine or tension headache	Tian Ma Gou Teng Yin	Ling Jiao Gou Teng Tang	LR-3, LR-8, LI-4, TB-5, BL-18, SP-6, KI-3, KI-6, GV-16, BL-20, BL-34, BL-38	GB-20, GB-34, GV-20, Taiyang
Dizziness (眩暈)	Parkinson's disease, SCA, hypertension, Meniere's syndrome, anxiety		Tian Ma Gou Teng Yin		LR-2, GB-20, GV-20
Tinnitus (耳鳴)	Meniere's syndrome, manic depression, hypertension		Long Dan Xie Gan Tang		LR-2, GB-8, GB-20, GB-43, TB-3
Wind-stroke (中風)	CVA		An Gong Niu Huang Wan		GV-26, PC-6, ST-36, LI-11

Table 4.10 Diseases and treatments related to Liver Yang Rising

Comparison: Liver Fire Blazing vs. Liver Yang Rising

Liver fire blazing (肝火上炎 *gān huǒ shàng yán*) and Liver yang rising (肝陽上亢 *gān yáng shàng kàng*) both manifest with symptoms of heat and excess above: dizziness, tinnitus, distending pain in the head and eyes, red face and eyes, irritability, and a quick temper. However, the etiology and pathogenesis, as well as the clinical manifestations and treatment strategies, are different.

Liver fire blazing is due to emotional stress and qi stagnation transforming into fire. It is usually acute onset and short course. Clinical manifestation involves interior excess heat, such as a red face and eyes, thirst with desire to drink cold water, and a bitter taste in the mouth. Liver yang rising can be caused by emotional stress, improper diet, sexual overstrain, and aging. It has a gradual onset with a longer course and is usually due to Liver and Kidney yin deficiency failing to control yang. This leads to yang excess above and deficiency below or 'root deficiency, branch excess,' which manifests with distention headache, dizziness, top-heavy feeling, tendency to fall, and soreness and weakness in the lower back and knees.

The key points to distinguish these two patterns are:
1) Nature of onset and course of illness: acute and short course vs. gradual onset and longer course
2) Key symptoms:
    - Liver fire blazing: excess heat, red face and eyes, thirst with desire to drink cold water, a bitter taste in the mouth
    - Liver yang rising: distending headache, dizziness, top-heavy feeling, tendency to fall, and soreness and weakness in the lower back and knees

Pattern		Liver Fire Blazing	Liver Yang Rising
Pathogenesis		Qi stagnation transforms into fire and flares up following Liver channel	Liver and Kidney yin deficiency fails to control yang, yang rising disrupts "clear orificies"
Characteristics		Acute onset, short course, excess, heat	Gradual onset, long course, heat, excess above, deficiency below, branch excess, root deficiency
Symptoms	Common	Fire and yang all tends to move upward, so symptoms are mostly related with the head and face, such as dizziness, tinnitus, distending pain in the head and eyes, red face and eyes, irritability and quick temper	
	Different	Red eyes, painful burning sensation in the hypochondrium, bitter taste in the mouth, constipation, yellow urine	Top-heavy feeling, tendency to fall, soreness and weakness in the lower back and knees
Tongue & pulse		Red tongue with yellow coating; wiry, rapid, forceful pulse	Red tongue with thin yellow or dry coating; wiry, thready pulse
Treatment strategy		Clear Liver fire	Calm the Liver, subdue the Yang
Herbal formulas		Zuo Jin Wan, Chai Hu Qing Gan Tang, Jia Wei Xiao Yao San	Tian Ma Gou Teng Yin

Table 4.11 Comparison of Liver Fire Blazing and Liver Yang Rising

Comparison: Liver Yin Deficiency vs. Liver Yang Rising

Liver yin deficiency (肝陰虛 gān yīn xū) is part of Liver yang rising (肝陽上亢 gān yáng shàng kàng), and therefore both patterns present with dizziness, tinnitus, distending pain in the hypochondrium, a red tongue, and a wiry thin rapid pulse.

However, Liver yin deficiency is purely a deficiency pattern, involving yin deficiency leading to relative yang excess that causes deficiency heat, five-center heat, hot flashes, night sweats, hectic fever, dry mouth, thirst, dry eyes, and trembling hands and feet. Conversely, Liver yang rising is a pattern of excess above and deficiency below, because it involves the deficiency of Liver and Kidney yin, which fails to control excess Liver yang, leading to distending headaches, a top-heavy sensation, red face and eyes, irritability, quick temper, and soreness and weakness of the lower back and knees. Thus the root for both patterns is yin deficiency, but Liver yin deficiency presents with mainly yin deficiency signs and symptoms, whereas Liver yang rising presents mainly with yang rising.

The key points to distinguish these two patterns are:

- Liver yin deficiency: deficiency heat, five-center heat, hot flashes, night sweats, hectic fever, dry mouth, thirst, dry eyes, and trembling hands and feet
- Liver yang rising: distending headache, irritability, quick temper, red face and eyes, and Kidney deficiency signs and symptoms

Pattern		Liver Yin Deficiency	Liver Yang Rising
Pathogenesis		Yin deficiency cannot nourish yang	
		Deficiency heat	Heat above
Characteristics		Deficiency	Root deficiency, branch excess; excess above, deficiency below
Symptoms	Common	Dizziness, tinnitus, distending pain in hypochondria, red tongue, wiry, thready and rapid pulse	
	Different	Five center heat, hot flashes, night sweats, hectic fever, dry mouth, thirst, dry eyes, trembling hands and feet	Distending headache, red face and eyes, irritability, quick temper, low back and knee weakness, top-heavy feeling
Tongue & pulse		Dry, scanty, or peeling coating	May be slight yellow coating; forceful pulse
Treatment strategy		Nourish Liver yin, soothe Liver qi	Calm the Liver, subdue yang
Herbal formulas		Yi Guan Jian	Tian Ma Gou Teng Yin

Table 4.12 Comparison of Liver Yin Deficiency and Liver Yang Rising

6 Liver Wind Stirring Internally Pattern | 肝風內動 |

Liver wind agitating within generalizes pathogenesis and clinical manifestations of internal wind. It is a series of patterns that are characterized by swinging symptoms like vertigo, poor balance, tendency to fall, tremors, and contractions. 'Internal wind' is generated by internal organ(s), especially Liver dysfunction, and yin/yang imbalance. According to etiology and pathogenesis, it can be classified into four sub-patterns:

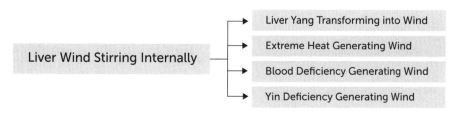

Chart 4.15 Liver Wind Stirring Internally subpatterns

6.1 Liver Yang Transforming into Wind Pattern | 肝陽化風 |

Definition: A group of signs and symptoms related to uncontrollable and involuntary movement or spasm caused by hyperactive Liver yang.

Clinical manifestations: Dizziness and vertigo, tendency to fall, shaking head, headache, neck stiffness, slurred speech, numbness of limbs, trembling hands and feet, staggering, or sudden loss of consciousness, deviated mouth and eyes, hemiplegia, and difficult speech. There may be a red tongue with yellow or greasy coating and a wiry, thin, and forceful pulse; or a red tongue and a wiry pulse; or a red tongue with peeled coating and a wiry, rapid, thin pulse.

Key points: A history of dizziness and headaches with Liver yang rising signs and symptoms, sudden onset of wind signs and symptoms, or sudden collapse combined with hemiplegia.

Etiology and pathogenesis: This pattern is a combination of deficiency and excess, usually caused by emotional stress, especially a continuous state of anger, resentment or frustration which stagnates qi, transforms into fire, and consumes yin. Chronic illness, aging, and sexual overstrain can also consume yin. When deficient Liver and Kidney yin are unable to constrain Liver yang, hyperactive Liver yang can cause wind. Therefore, this pattern is marked by 'root deficiency, apparent excess' as well as deficiency below and excess above.

Liver and Kidney yin deficiency fails to nourish, leading to tendon, sinew and muscle spasm, headache, shaking head, neck stiffness, tingling or numbness in the limbs, trembling hands and feet, staggering, abnormal gait, or hemiplegia, deviated or stiff tongue with slurred speech, and a wiry pulse. Yin deficiency fails to constrain yang, which rises and disturbs the clear orifices, leading to dizziness, distending headache, red face and eyes. Liver yang rising leads to qi and blood inverse and chaos, and can lead to sudden collapse or loss of consciousness.

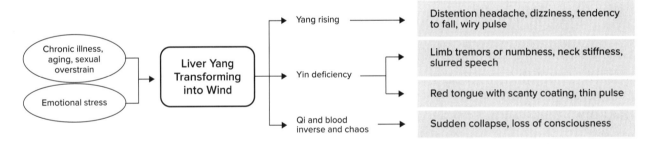

Chart 4.16 Etiology and pathogenesis of Liver Yang Transforming into Wind

TCM Disease	Western Disease	Herbal Formulas	Acupuncture
Headache (頭痛)	Cerebral arteriosclerosis, hypertension, migraine or tension headache, CVA	Zhen Gan Xi Feng Tang, Tian Ma Gou Teng Yin	GB-20, GB-34, GV-20, Taiyang
Dizziness (眩暈)	Parkinson's disease, hypertension, Meniere's syndrome, anxiety, CVA		LR-2, GB-20, GV-20
Faint (昏撲)	Epilepsy, hypertension, CVA, vasovagal syncope, arrhythmia		GV-20, GV-26
Wind-stroke (中風)	CVA		GV-26, PC-6, ST-36, LI-11, KI-3
Warm disease (溫病)	Encephalitis B, cerebrospinal, scarlet fever, meningitis, epidemic hemorrhagic fever, puerperal infection		GV-8, GV-14, GV-20, LI-11

(Acupuncture common points: LR-3, BL-20, LI-4, TB-5, GV-19, SP-6)

Table 4.13 Diseases and treatments related to Liver Yang Transforming into Wind

6.2 Extreme Heat Generating Wind Pattern | 熱極生風

Definition: A group of signs and symptoms caused by extreme heat consuming body fluids, causing sinews to spasm due to malnourishment; or due to extreme heat invading the pericardium during the course of exogenous febrile disease.

Clinical manifestations: High fever, irritability, fidgeting, coma, spasms and convulsions, stiff neck, opisthotonus, lockjaw, upward or straight staring eyes, deep red crimson tongue with dry yellow coating, wiry and rapid pulse.

Key points: High fever plus signs and symptoms of wind.

Etiology and pathogenesis: This is an excess pattern related to acute febrile diseases in which exopathogens attack and transform into heat that penetrates deeply into the Pericardium. The Liver is the organ related to wind; it governs the sinews and stores blood. When pathogenic heat penetrates inside, it scorches the Liver channel, causes the sinews and vessels to lose nourishment, and stirs wind.

Pathogenic heat is internally exuberant, resulting in high fever with thirst, red face, and red eyes. Extreme fever engenders wind, which rises and harasses the clear orifices and the brain, disturbs the *shén*, and results in dizziness and distending pain in the head. Rigid limbs, lockjaw, upward gazing eyes, and opisthotonus are also manifestations of stirred wind. When pathogenic heat penetrates the Pericardium and disturbs the *shén*, it causes irritability and mania. Red tongue with yellow coating and rapid pulse are signs of heat. This pattern is more common in children.

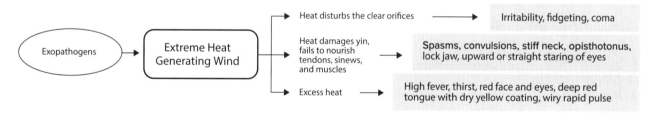

Chart 4.17 Etiology and pathogenesis of Extreme Heat Generating Wind

TCM Disease	Western Disease	Herbal Formulas	Acupuncture
Convulsions in children (小兒驚風)	Epidemic encephalitis B, epidemic cerebrospinal meningitis, brain abscess, tuberculosis encephalitis, epidemic hemorrhagic fever, scarlet fever, puerperal infection	Ling Jiao Gou Teng Tang	LR-3, Shixuan, GV-8, GV-14, GV-20, LI-4, LI-11
Warm febrile disease (溫熱病)			

Table 4.14 Diseases and treatment related to Extreme Heat Generating Wind

6.3 Blood Deficiency Generating Wind Pattern | 血虛生風 |

Definition: A group of signs and symptoms caused by the malnutrition of sinews, tendons, muscles, and channels due to blood deficiency and resulting in twitching, spasms, and numbness.

Clinical manifestations: Numbness of the limbs, stiff joints, muscle spasms or twitching, tremors of hands and feet, itching, dizziness accompanied with symptoms of Liver blood deficiency.

Key points: Tremors in extremities, muscle twitching, numbness, or itching, plus blood deficiency signs and symptoms.

Etiology and pathogenesis: There are three commonly observed causes of Liver blood deficiency. First is the damage to yin and blood during the course of an enduring illness, which deprives the Liver of blood for storage and adequate nourishment. Second is blood loss due to acute or chronic hemorrhage or other types of bleeding. And third is an improper diet or overstrain that causes a lack of nutritive qi to generate blood. Deficiency of Liver blood deprives the sinews of nourishment and gives rise to spasms, numbness, twitching, or itching.

Besides the main signs of Liver wind, this pattern presents with general blood deficiency signs with symptoms that get worse as the day goes on: functional weakness, dryness, and difficulty sleeping. Since blood is deficient it cannot ascend to nourish the head and face, manifesting in dizziness, tinnitus, lusterless complexion, unclear vision, dry eyes, night blindness, scanty menstrual flow or amenorrhea, pale tongue, and thin weak pulse.

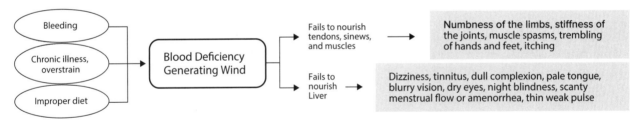

Chart 4.18 Etiology and pathogenesis of Blood Deficiency Generating Wind

TCM Disease	Western Disease	Herbal Formulas		Acupuncture
Dizziness (眩暈)	Anemia, hypotension, BPPV, Meniere's disease, vestibular migraine	E Jiao Ji Zi Huang Tang	Gui Pi Tang	LR-3, 8, GB-20, LI-4, TB-5, GV-19, SP-6, KI-3, BL-17, CV-4	SIS8, BL-2, BL-6, BL-62, TB-5, TB-16, GB-19, GV-17, CV-4
Numbness (麻木)	Raynaud's syndrome, VB-12 deficiency, Lyme disease, peripheral neuropathy, etc.		Shao Yao Gan Cao Tang		ST-38 TB-14, GB-32, GB-34
Itching (搔癢)	Eczema (dermatitis), psoriasis, celiac disease, iron deficiency anemia, thyroid problems		Dang Gui Yin Zi		ST-15, BL-16, BL-28, BL-34, SP-10
Wind-stroke (中風)	CVA		Da Qin Jiao Tang		GV-26, PC-6, ST-36, LI-11, KI-3

Table 4.15 Diseases and treatments related to Blood Deficiency Generating Wind

6.4 Yin Deficiency Generating Wind Pattern | 陰虛生風 |

Definition: A group of signs and symptoms caused by deficient Liver and Kidney yin fails to nourish sinews, tendons, muscles, and channels.

Clinical manifestations: Trembling or flaccid hands and feet, dizziness, tinnitus, low-grade fever in the afternoon or evening, five-center heat, steaming bone disorder, malar flush, hot flashes, emaciation, dry mouth and throat, a small red tongue or cracked tongue with scanty or peeled coating, and a thin rapid pulse.

Key points: Hands and feet tremor, flaccidity, dizziness, plus yin deficiency signs and symptoms.

Etiology and pathogenesis: This pattern is usually caused by consumption of yin fluid at the later stage of exogenous febrile disease. It is also seen when *zàng fǔ* impairment, chronic illness, overstrain, or improper treatment consumes yin fluids, causing malnutrition of tendons, channels, and muscles, resulting in internal wind. Oversweating, vomiting, or diarrhea also consumes yin fluids, as does improper diet, which fails to generate blood and body fluids.

Deficient Liver and Kidney yin is unable to nourish the sinews, tendons, muscles, and channels causing spasms due to malnutrition, tremors, or flaccidity of hands and feet. Kidney and Liver yin deficiency also fails to nourish and replenish the organs and their respective orifices, leading to dizziness, tinnitus, dry eyes, dry mouth and throat, and cracked tongue. Yin deficiency generates deficiency heat: low-grade fever in the afternoon or evening, malar flush, hot flashes, five-center heat, steaming bone disorder, red tongue, and thin rapid pulse.

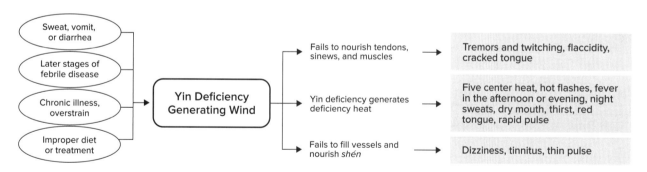

Chart 4.19 Etiology and pathogenesis of Yin Deficiency Generating Wind

TCM Disease	Western Disease	Herbal Formulas		Acupuncture
Wind-warmth (風溫)	Later stage of some infectious diseases such as epidemic encephalitis B, epidemic cerebrospinal meningitis and scarlet fever as well as at the later stage of some chronic and consumptive diseases such as hematopathy and malignant tumor	Di Huang Yin Zi, Yi Guan Jian	San Jia Fu Mai Tang, Da Ding Feng Zhu	LR-3, 8, GB-20, LI-4, TB-5, GV-19, SP-6, KI-3, BL-17, CV-4
Spring warmth (春溫)				
Summerheat-warmth (暑溫)				
Wind-stroke (中風)	Parkinson's disease, stroke, essential tremor, MS, anxiety, dehydration, B12 deficiency		Shao Yao Gan Cao Tang, Zuo Gui Wan, Da Bu Yuan Jian, Zhen Gan Xi Feng Tang	
Atrophy disorder (痿証)	Myelitis, polyradiculitis, progressive myotropy, MS, ALS, myasthenia gravis		Hu Qian Wan	

Table 4.16 Diseases and treatments related to Yin Deficiency Generating Wind

Pattern	Extreme Heat	Liver Yang	Blood Deficiency	Yin Deficiency
Pathogenesis	Heat consumes yin, tendons spasm due to insufficient nourishment	Kidney and Liver yin deficiency, rising yang stirs wind	Blood and yin deficiency deprive tendons of nourishment and cause spasm	
Nature of disease	Excess, heat	Heat, excess above with deficiency below	Deficiency, heat/cold	Deficiency, heat
Main symptoms	Convulsions, stiff neck, opisthotonus, lockjaw, eyes staring upward or straight	Severe vertigo, distending headache, tremors, slurred speech, top-heavy sensation, sudden coma, hemiplegia	Numbness, tremor, twitching, itching, stiff joints	Twitching, tremors
Other symptoms	High fever, fidgeting, coma	Headache, stiff tongue, staggering	Pale face and lips, dizziness, fatigue	Tidal fever, night sweats
Tongue	Red or deep red, yellow coating	Red, yellow coating	Pale and tender, thin white coating	Red, cracked, little coating
Pulse	Forceful, rapid	Wiry, maybe thin	Thin, weak	Thin, rapid

Table 4.17 Summary of Liver Wind Stirring Internally patterns

Comparison: Liver Yang Rising vs. Liver Yang Transforming into Wind

Liver yang rising (肝陽上亢 *gān yáng shàng kàng*) and Liver yang transforming into wind (肝陽化風 *gān yáng huà fēng*) are both caused by deficient Liver and Kidney yin failing to constrain Liver yang, which rises upward. They are both patterns of excess combined with deficiency or excess above with deficiency below, and thus both exhibit dizziness, tinnitus, distention pain in the head and eyes, red face and eyes, and a wiry pulse.

The etiology and pathogenesis of these two patterns are the same. Liver yang transforming into wind develops from Liver yang rising. Thus they differ mainly in severity and clinical manifestation. In Liver yang transforming into wind, the major presentation involves wind symptoms such as vertigo, severe neck stiffness, headache worsens with movement, trembling of the hands and feet, numbness of the limbs, slurring speech, or sudden coma.

The key point to distinguish these two patterns is the presence of wind symptoms.

Pattern		Liver Yang Rising	Liver Yang Transforming into Wind
Pathogenesis	Common	Kidney and Liver yin deficiency leads to Liver yang failing to be constrained, yang rises upward, excess combined with deficiency (excess above, deficiency below)	
	Different		Hyperactive Liver yang stirs up wind
Symptoms	Common	Dizziness, tinnitus, distention pain in the head and eyes, red face and eyes, top-heavy sensation, tendency to fall	
	Different		Vertigo, severe neck stiffness, headache worse with movement, trembling hands and feet, numbness of limbs, slurred speech, sudden coma
Tongue & pulse		Red tongue; rapid pulse or wiry, thready, rapid pulse	
Treatment strategy		Calm Liver, subdue yang	Calm Liver, subdue yang, extinguish wind
Herbal formulas		Tian Ma Gou Teng Yin	Zhen Gan Xi Feng Tang

Table 4.18 Comparison of Liver Yang Rising and Liver Yang Transforming into Wind

Comparison: Liver Yang Transforming into Wind vs. Wind-Phlegm Disturbing Upward

Wind-phlegm disturbing upward (風痰上擾 *fēng tán shàng rǎo*) develops from Liver yang transforming into wind (肝陽化風 *gān yáng huà fēng*). Thus both patterns present with wind sympoms such as dizziness and vertigo, staggering or a tendency to fall, head shaking, headache, neck stiffness, slurred speech, numbness of the limbs, and trembling hands and feet.

Wind-phlegm disturbing upward involves internal wind combining with turbid phlegm that upwardly disrupts the "clear orifice" (清竅 *qīng qiào*) or obstructs the channels. Thus, besides wind symptoms, there are phlegm symptoms such as sudden loss of consciousness, deviated mouth and eyes, hemiplegia, difficult speech, rattling sounds in the throat, a thick greasy tongue coating, and a slippery pulse.

The key point to distinguish these two patterns is the presence of phlegm symptoms.

104 Part 1: Zang Organs

Pattern	Liver Yang Transforming into Wind	Wind-Phlegm Disturbing Upward
Pathogenesis	Develops from Liver yang rising that stirs up wind	Develops from Liver yang rising transforming into wind, Liver wind combines with phlegm, upward disrupts the "clean orifice," obstructs channels
Symptoms – Common	Vertigo, severe neck stiffness, headache worse with movement, trembling of the hands and feet, numbness of the limbs, slurred speech, or sudden coma, wiry pulse	
Symptoms – Different		Deviated mouth and eyes, hemiplegia, difficult speech, rattling sound in the throat, thick greasy tongue coating and slippery pulse
Tongue & pulse	Red tongue or red tongue with thin or peeled coating; wiry rapid or thin pulse	
Treatment strategy	Calm the Liver, subdue yang, extinguish internal wind	Calm the Liver, subdue yang, extinguish internal wind, transform phlegm
Herbal formulas	Zhen Gan Xi Feng Tang	Ban Xia Bai Zhu Tian Ma Tang

Table 4.19 Comparison of Liver Yang Transforming into Wind and Wind-Phlegm Disturbing Upward

7 Cold Stagnation in Liver Channel Pattern | 寒滞肝脉

Definition: A group of signs and symptoms due to pathogenic cold attacking the Liver channel, which manifests as pain and spasms.

Clinical manifestations: Cold pain in bilateral lower abdomen or genitals, or contracture of scrotum, pain aggravated by cold and relieved by warmth, cold limbs, vomiting of clear mucus, moist white tongue coating, deep, slow, or tight and wiry pulse.

Key points: Cold pain in the lower abdomen, pudendum, vertex headache, plus internal excess cold signs and symptoms.

Etiology and pathogenesis: This pattern is usually caused by pathogenic cold invasion, stagnation of qi and blood in the Liver channel, inhibited circulation of qi and blood as well as spasms of channels and collaterals.

The Liver channel circuits the external genital area, passing the lateral abdomen and hypochondria, and ends at the top of the head. Pathogenic cold causes contraction and constriction, and impairs yang. Thus, when it invades the Liver channel, there is lower abdominal cold pain, sagging distention and pain of the pudendum, cold pain in the vertex, or contraction and pain of the scrotum. Cold pain is aggravated by cold and alleviated by warmth. Cold limbs, pale tongue, and a deep, slow, and tight pulse are additional signs of this internal cold.

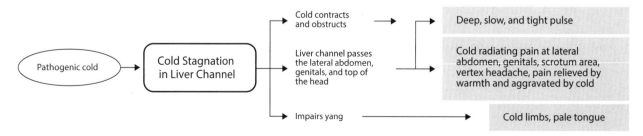

Chart 4.20 Etiology and pathogenesis of Cold Stagnation in Liver Channel

TCM Disease	Western Disease	Herbal Formulas		Acupuncture	
Hernia (疝氣)	Inguinal hernia, umbilical hernia	Tian Tai Wu Yao San	Tian Tai Wu Yao San	LR-1, LR-4, CV-3	CV-6, SP-6
Abdominal pain (腹痛)	Orchitis, varicocele, intestinal adhesion, PID, diverticulitis, lead poisoning, celiac disease, IBS		Wu Zhu Yu Tang, Nuan Gan Jian		CV-12, LR-13, PC-6, SP-4, ST-25
Headache (頭痛)	Tension headache, migraine headache, brain freeze, hypertension		Wu Zhu Yu Tang		GV-20, GB-20
Dysmenorrhea (痛經)	Endometriosis, fibroids, PID, STI, adenomyosis, or use IUD		Wen Jing Tang		CV-6, ST-29, SP-6, SP-10

Table 4.20 Diseases and treatments related to Cold Stagnation in Liver Channel

8 Liver Blood Stagnation Pattern | 肝血瘀滯 |

Definition: A group of signs and symptoms involving pain or masses caused by blood stagnation in the Liver or blood stasis obstructing the Liver channel.

Clinical manifestations: Sharp pain or masses in hypochondrium or lateral abdomen, vomiting blood, epistaxis, dysmenorrhea with dark blood and clots, irregular cycle, infertility, purple nails and lips, purple or dark complexion, dry skin (in severe cases), purple petechiae, purple tongue, especially or only on the sides, in severe cases, purple spots on the sides, wiry, choppy, and/or irregular pulse.

Key points: Sharp pain or masses along Liver channel, plus blood stagnation signs and symptoms.

Etiology and pathogenesis: This pattern usually develops from Liver qi stagnation, since qi is the motive force for blood circulation. Emotional stress, excessive consumption of cold and greasy food or alcohol, overstrain, and chronic illness all may result in blood stagnation.

When blood stasis obstructs the Liver and its channels, qi movement is impeded, and blood and qi fail to nourish the tissues resulting in stabbing, sharp pain in a fixed location that resists pressure. Since blood stagnation accumulates more at night, pain is worse at that time. Accumulation of stagnated blood can cause formation of lumps, masses, or inflammation. When blood stasis takes up space inside there is less room for generation of new blood. This causes the skin color to turn green, blue or purple and the lips and nails to turn dark purple. If blood stasis obstructs the vessels it will appear as distended veins. Eruption of distended veins causes vomiting of blood. The choppy and irregular pulse arises from impeded blood circulation.

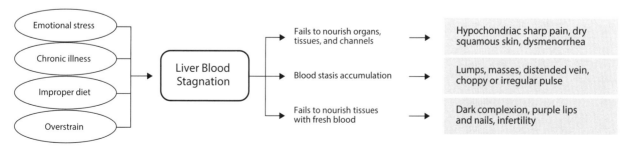

Chart 4.21 Etiology and pathogenesis of Liver Blood Stagnation

TCM Disease	Western Disease	Herbal Formulas		Acupuncture	
Hypochondriac pain (脇痛)	Cholelithiasis, acute cholehepatic carcinoma	Ge Xia Zhu Yu Tang, Shao Fu Zhu Yu Tang, Shi Xiao San	Ge Xia Zhu Yu Tang	LR-3, GB-34, BL-17, 18, SP-10	GB-40, ST-36, BL-19, LR-14
Jaundice (黃疸)	Chronic cholecystitis, chronic hepatitis, cirrhosis, pancreatic cancer, gallstone		Xiao Shi Fan Shi San		GV-6, GV-9, SI-4, SP-9
Masses (積聚)	Cirrhosis, ovarian tumor, pancreatic cancer, splenomegaly, aortic aneurysm, cholecystitis		Jin Ling Zi San, Shi Xiao San		ST-36, PC-6, SP-6
Ascites (膨脹)	Cirrhosis, heart failure, constrictive pericarditis, nephrotic syndrome, kwashiorkor		Gui Zhi qu Shao Yao Jia Ma Xin Fu Zi Tang		LI-6, LR-14, CV-12, ST-36, GB-34
Dysmenorrhea (痛經)	Endometriosis, fibroids, PID, STI, adenomyosis, IUD		Tao Hong Si Wu Tang, Ge Xia Zhu Yu Tang		CV-6, ST-29, SP-6, SP-10
Amenorrhea (閉經)	PCOS, menopause, excessive exercise, anorexia or bulimia, stress, thyroid malfunction				CV-3, ST-29, SP-6, SP-10, LI-4

Table 4.21 Diseases and treatments related to Liver Blood Stagnation

Liver disease patterns relationship and development

Usually caused by emotional stress, Liver qi stagnation is the most common of the Liver disease patterns. It can develop into Liver fire blazing pattern if qi stagnation transforms into fire. When Liver fire consumes yin, then Liver yin deficiency pattern develops. Liver yin deficiency failing to constrain yang leads to Liver yang rising pattern. Liver yin deficiency can also stem from Liver blood deficiency when long-term blood deficiency fails to replenish yin. Liver blood deficiency, Liver yin deficiency, and Liver yang rising all can generate Liver wind.

In addition to Liver qi stagnation developing to Liver fire blazing pattern, Liver qi stagnation also can develop into Liver blood stagnation pattern if qi fails to promote blood circulation.

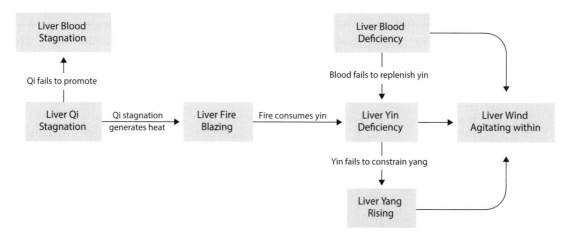

Chart 4.22 Liver disease pattern relationships and development

Summary of Liver Disease Patterns

Key points: emotional disorder, hypochondriac pain, distention, or masses, menstruation disorder, wind syndrome, wiry pulse			
	Patterns	Clinical manifestations	
		Common	Different
Deficiency	Liver Blood Deficiency	Dizziness, tinnitus, blurry vision, dry eyes, trembling hands and feet, wiry and thin pulse	Pale face, nails and tongue, night blindness. In women, scanty or light menses, amenorrhea. Pale tongue, dry coating, weak pulse
Deficiency	Liver Yin Deficiency	Dizziness, tinnitus, blurry vision, dry eyes, trembling hands and feet, wiry and thin pulse	Tidal fever or low fever, heat sensation in five centers area, night sweats, bitter taste in mouth, red or cracked tongue with little or no coating, rapid pulse
D/E	Liver Yang Rising	Dizziness, tinnitus, distending pain in the head and eye, red face and eyes, irritability, short temper	Excess above with deficiency below; knee and back weakness, with 'top-heavy' feeling
Excess	Liver Fire Blazing	Dizziness, tinnitus, distending pain in the head and eye, red face and eyes, irritability, short temper	Excess heat: Headache, burning pain sensation in hypochondrium, bitter taste, constipation, yellow urine
Excess	Liver Qi Stagnation	Depression, distending pain in the hypochondrium or lateral abdomen, irregular menstrual cycle, wiry pulse	
Excess	Liver Wind Stirring Internally — Yang Rising	Dizziness, trembling, twitching, wiry pulse	Severe vertigo, tremor, headache, difficult speech, sudden coma, hemiplegia, wiry pulse
Excess	Liver Wind Stirring Internally — Extreme Heat	Dizziness, trembling, twitching, wiry pulse	Convulsions, stiff neck, opisthotonus, lockjaw, upward or straight staring eyes, high fever, rapid pulse
Excess	Liver Wind Stirring Internally — Yin Deficiency	Dizziness, trembling, twitching, wiry pulse	Twitching or flaccid hands and feet, night sweats, tidal fever, red and cracked tongue, thin and rapid pulse
Excess	Liver Wind Stirring Internally — Blood Deficiency	Dizziness, trembling, twitching, wiry pulse	Numbness, trembling, twitching, stiff joints, pale face, dizziness, pale tongue, thin weak pulse
Excess	Liver Blood Stagnation	Sharp pain or masses in the hypochondrium or lateral abdomen, dysmenorrhea with dark blood and clots, infertility, purple or dark complexion, purplish tongue, wiry and firm pulse	
Excess	Cold Stagnation in Liver Channel	Cold pain in lateral abdomen, external genitalia, or top of the head, wiry and tight pulse	

Table 4.22 Summary of Liver disease patterns

Chapter 5
Kidney Disease Patterns

Physiological characteristics and functions of the Kidney

Located on either side of the lower back, the Kidney comes as a pair and occupies the lowermost position of the five *zàng* organs. The lower back is known as the 'residence of the Kidney.' The Kidney organs are bean-shaped, hence kidney beans. The main pathway of the Kidney channel starts at the inferior aspect of the small toe, courses along the medioposterior aspect of the lower extremities, spinal column, abdomen, chest, throat, and tongue, and ends at the chest.

The distinguishing physiological function of the Kidney is 'sealing and hibernating' (主蟄守位 *zhǔ zhé shoù wèi*). Also translated as 'dormancy,' this function involves preserving, storing, and housing. The Kidney stores *jīng*, or essence, ensuring that essence is full and retained. The Kidney also governs *mìng mén* fire (命門之火 *mìng mén zhī huǒ*); while *mìng mén* fire lies dormant within Kidney water, it is unable to be dispersed. Kidney function provides the foundation for essence qi (精氣 *jīng qì*) to play its physiological role in the body.

The Kidney is a power organ (作強之官 *zuò qiáng zhī guān*) in charge of the body's strength and intelligence. It is internally-externally connected with the Urinary Bladder. It corresponds to winter and water, and is the yin within yin organ. Hair is the manifestation of the Kidney, and spittle is the Kidney-related fluid. The Kidney opens to the ears and controls the opening and closing of the two lower yin orifices (urethra and anus). It governs bones and teeth, correlates with the emotions of fear and fright, belongs to the water phase, and is related to the winter season and cold climate.

Kidney	Relationship
Spirit	Wisdom (智 *zhì*)
Internal-external connection	Urinary Bladder
Orifice	Ears, genitalia, anus
Dominates	Bones, teeth
External manifestation	Hair
Fluid	Spittle
Fire	*Mìng mén* fire
Emotion	Fear, fright
Season	Winter
Five phase	Water
Six climate factor	Cold

Table 5.1 Kidney and its related aspects

1 | Stores essence

The Kidney preserves and stores essence (精 *jīng*), which includes congenital essence and acquired essence. Congenital essence, also known as pre-heaven or prenatal essence, comes from the parents and is the basic material constituting the human body. Acquired essence, also known as post-heaven or postnatal essence, is derived from food essence and is generated by the Spleen and Stomach.

Congenital essence and acquired essence are inseparable. To generate acquired essence, the Spleen and Stomach draw upon the vitality of congenital essence. Acquired essence nourishes and reinforces congenital essence. Since the Kidney stores essence, it performs the following physiological functions:

(1) Governs reproduction: reproductive functions include sexual activity and procreation. Kidney stores essence, which provides the material basis for the origin of life. The 'heavenly dew' or *tiān kúi* (天癸 *tiān kúi*) is an aspect of congenital essence and is responsible for menarche and menopause. It comes from the parents, relies on acquired essence for nourishment and reinforcement, and increases and decreases following Kidney qi. *Tiān kúi* stimulates development of secondary sexual characteristics and maturation of sexual instinct during puberty, and maintains exuberant sexual ability.

(2) Governs growth and development: growth and development of the human body depends on the Kidney essence. Female, from birth to age 7: essence qi of the Kidney develops gradually, allowing the body to grow and develop rapidly with exuberant vitality. Age 7 to 14: baby teeth are replaced and hair grows fast. Age 14 to 21: onset of puberty and secondary sexual characteristics develop; females begin menstruating and are able to conceive; sperm is formed in males. Age 21 to 35: prime of life, *tiān kúi* reaches a threshold, Kidney qi flourishes, the body is healthy and strong. Age 35 to 42: Kidney qi declines, sexual and reproductive ability decreases. Age 42 to 49: premenopause or menopause, loss of reproductive ability. Age 49 and above: body degenerates, hair grays, teeth loosen, humpback develops, hearing impairs, and walking becomes difficult. The growth and development cycle of males starts at 8 years old and each stage is an 8-year interval.

(3) Generates marrow, fills the brain, and engenders blood: marrow includes bone marrow, spinal marrow, and brain marrow. The brain is called the 'sea of marrow.' The Kidney stores essence, which manufactures marrow. Marrow has three main functions: nourish the brain, supplement the bones, and engender blood.

(4) Transforms essence to Kidney yin and Kidney yang, governs and regulates yin and yang of the entire body. Kidney essence and Kidney qi are the same substance in different forms. Kidney essence is the substance in a liquid state and Kidney qi is the substance in a gaseous state. Under certain circumstances, they transform into one another and supplement each other. Together they are called essence qi (精氣 *jīng qì*). Essence qi provides the motive force for the body's metabolic and physiological functions.

Kidney essence qi transforms into Kidney qi, which can be divided into Kidney yin and Kidney yang. The Kidney is called the 'root of yin and yang' (陰陽之根 *yīn yáng zhī gēn*) and the 'house of water and fire' (水火之宅 *shuǐ huǒ zhī zhái*) because Kidney yin and Kidney yang are the root of the five *zàng*'s yin and yang.

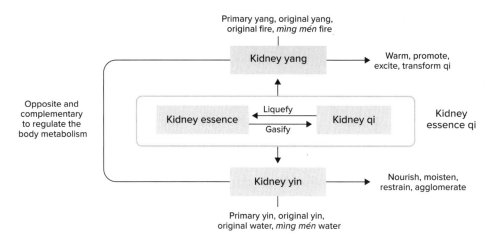

Chart 5.1 Kidney is the root of yin and yang

Kidney yang is also called original yang (元陽 *yuán yáng*), true yang (真陽 *zhēn yáng*), or true fire (真火 *zhēn huǒ*), and *mìng mén* fire (命門之火 *mìng mén zhī huǒ*). It has the functions of warming, promoting, exciting, and transforming qi. Kidney yin is also called original yin (元陰 *yuán yīn*), true yin (真陰 *zhēn yīn*), true water (真水 *zhēn shuǐ*), and *mìng mén* water (命門之水 *mìng mén zhī shuǐ*). It has the functions of nourishing, moistening, restraining, and agglomerating. Kidney yin and Kidney yang are mutually dependent, promoting and restraining each other, leading to the internal harmony of yin and yang and the healthy functioning of the body's organs. The dynamic interaction between the two maintains normal life activities.

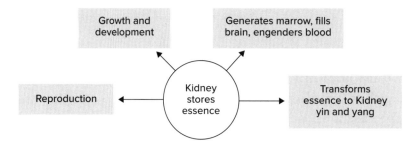

Chart 5.2 Kidney stores essence

2 | Governs water metabolism

Since the Kidney is the major organ involved in water metabolism, it is also known as the 'water organ.' Qi transformation (氣化 *qì huà*) refers to the evaporation and distillation functions of Kidney yang. Kidney yang evaporates body fluids, transforming and gasifying them into qi. In turn, Kidney yang accumulates, condenses and liquifies qi into body fluids. This process ensures ascending, descending, exiting and entering, as well as distribution and excretion of water in the body. The Kidney's governance of water metabolism manifests in the following three aspects:

(1) Ascending the clear and descending the turbid: 'Clear' refers to fluids that are nutritive, such as water essence and body fluids; 'turbid' implies fluids containing metabolic waste.
(2) Controls the opening and closing of the Urinary Bladder: the Urinary Bladder stores and discharges urine, which is closely related to the qi transformation function of the Kidney.
(3) Promotes the functional activities of *zàng fǔ* organs involved in water metabolism: Kidney is the root of yang, which provides the motive force for the Lung, Spleen, Liver, Small Intestine, Large Intestine, and Triple Burner in water metabolism.

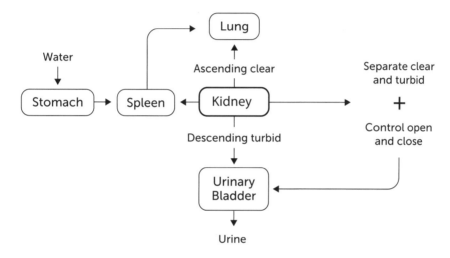

Chart 5.3   Kidney and water metabolism process

3 | Controls the reception of qi

The Kidney regulates respiration in order to prevent shallow breathing and to maintain normal gas exchange. The Kidney's 'sealing, storing, and preserving' function helps Lung qi to descend, because the Kidney receives clear qi inhaled by the Lung. The Kidney's reception of qi during respiration is a manifestation of its 'dormant' nature.

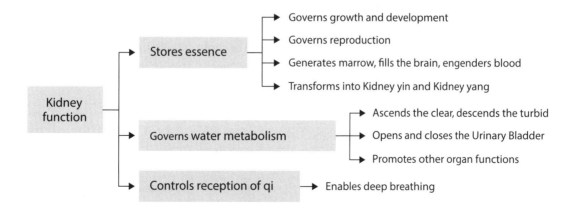

Chart 5.4   Kidney function summary

112 Part 1: Zang Organs

Common etiological factors in Kidney disease

Kidney patterns are mostly caused by endopathogenic factors such as congenital insufficiency, chronic illness, malnutrition, or sexual and physical overstrain. Aging is another major factor leading to Kidney deficiency. However, exopathogenic factors also may result in pathological changes of the Kidney. The following are common etiological factors for Kidney disease patterns:

(1) Weak constitution: prenatal deficiency, which includes premature and congenital disorders; and postnatal deficiency, which includes malnutrition and chronic illness
(2) Improper diet, malnutrition
(3) Sexual and physical overstrain
(4) Aging

Pathological changes and major clinical manifestations of the Kidney

Pathological manifestations of Kidney disease are usually due to Kidney essence deficiency, Kidney failing to receive qi, or Kidney failing at qi transformation to promote water metabolism. Symptoms manifest in the following groups:

(1) Soreness and weakness of the lower back and knees
(2) Growth, development, and reproductive ability disorder
(3) Water metabolism disorder: edema, difficult urination or frequent urination
(4) Respiratory disorder: panting or asthma
(5) Symptoms related with brain, marrow, bone, hair, ear or bowl movement and urination

1 | Soreness and weakness in the lower back and knees

Definition: Chronic achy pain or dull pain in the lower back and knees, which may be relieved by warmth and pressure.

Etiology and pathomechanisms: "The lower back is the residence of the Kidney." The Kidney transforms blood, governs the bones, and stores essence, which generates marrow. Chronic illness, overstrain, especially sexual overstrain, long-term panic and fear, improper diet, improper treatment, and aging are the main factors that contribute to a decline in the Kidney. When the Kidney is deficient, it may fail to store essence, which leads to a deficiency of marrow. In turn, bones will lack nourishment, leading to soreness and weakness, especially of the lower back. The knee joint carries the majority of body weight and requires strong support from the bones, muscles, and ligaments. Thus essence insufficiency failing to nourish results in knee pain or weakness.

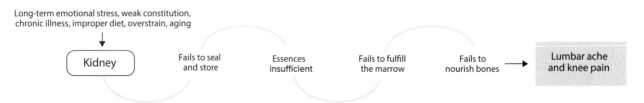

Chart 5.5 Etiology and pathomechanism of soreness and weakness in the lumbar and knees

2 | Abnormal growth and development

Definition: Growth and developmental delays such that children do not reach milestones by the expected age, including 'five types of developmental delay' (五遲 *wǔ chí*) (delayed hair growth, teeth eruption, and ability to stand, walk, and speak) and 'five types of flaccidity' (五軟 *wǔ ruǎn*) (weakness and softness of the head, neck, extremities, muscles and mastication). In adults, this pathology manifests as premature aging.

Etiology and pathomechanisms: Kidney stores essence, the essential material and substance that constitutes the human body, forms the *zàng fǔ* organs, tissues, skin, hair, tendons and muscles, and provides the material basis for growth, development and physiological activities. Embryonic formation and fetal growth and development both require Kidney essence. Essence fills marrow, manufactures blood to nourish and moisten *shén*, tissues, and organs, and transforms into qi to provide original life-force energy. If Kidney essence is insufficient, there will be insufficient nutritive foundation for physical growth and brain development. When tissues, organs, and muscles fail to be nourished, abnormal growth and development occurs in children and premature aging occurs in adults.

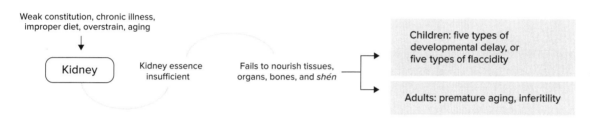

Chart 5.6 Etiology and pathomechanism of abnormal growth and development

3 | Reproductive and sexual function disorder

Definition: Any disorder that impairs the ability to reproduce or engage in sexual activities including impotence, low libido, premature ejaculation, spermatorrhea, and infertility.

Etiology and pathomechanisms: *Tiān kúi*, or reproductive essence, which is stored in the Kidney, is the aspect of congenital essence that deals with growth and reproduction. It is responsible for puberty, development of secondary sexual characteristics, menarche, sperm production, maturation of sexual instinct, and maintaining exuberant sexual ability. Congenital weakness, chronic illness, improper diet, overstrain, aging, and long-term emotional stress can all impair the Kidney. When Kidney deficiency fails to secure and store, essence becomes deficient and is unable to perform its reproductive function.

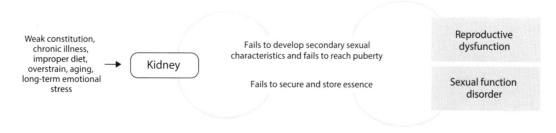

Chart 5.7 Etiology and pathomechanism of reproductive and sexual function disorder

4 | Water metabolism disorder

Definition: Disorder of the process by which water passes in and out of the body that includes water intake, generating and distributing body fluids, and expelling and excreting water waste.

Etiology and pathomechanisms: The Kidney is the root of yang, the motive power of the *zàng fǔ* organs involved in water metabolism. If the Kidney does not function properly, the Lung may fail to distribute and descend, the Spleen may fail to transport and transform, the Triple Burner may fail to transport and transmit, and the Small Intestine and Large Intestine may fail to transport and reabsorb. In turn, water may not be transformed into body fluids, distributed, or excreted.

The Kidney is in charge of qi transformation (氣化 *qì huà*), which ensures the ascent of the clear and the descent of the turbid. It also controls the opening and closing of the Urinary Bladder. A weak constitution, chronic illness, improper diet, overstrain, and aging can all impair the Kidney. Dysfunction of the Kidney prevents the transformation of water into body fluids.

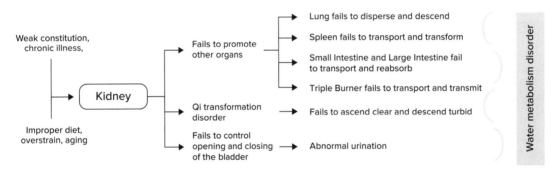

Chart 5.8 Etiology and pathomechanism of water metabolism disorder

5 | Other symptoms and signs related to Kidney

The following signs and symptoms are also closely related to Kidney dysfunction: dizziness, poor memory, dull thinking, tinnitus, hearing loss, premature gray hair or thin hair, loose teeth, and loss of teeth.

Physiological Function		Pathological Change	Clinical Manifestation
Stores essence	Governs growth and development	Essence deficiency	Infant: delayed development of physique and intelligence, five types of developmental delay, and five types of flaccidity. Adult: senility, premature graying of hair
	Governs reproduction	Diminished reproductive function	Male: sterility, impotence Female: infertility, amenorrhea, scanty menses
	Generates marrow, fills brain, manufactures blood	Deficient brain marrow	Dizziness, poor memory, dull thinking, disorientation
		Bone loses nourishment	Soreness and weakness of legs and feet, loose teeth
	Transforms into Kidney yin and Kidney yang	Kidney yang deficiency	Aching and cold sensation in the lumbar and knees, intolerance of cold, impotence, cold uterus
		Kidney yin deficiency	Night sweats, five center heat, hot flashes, tidal fever, spermatorrhea, irregular menstruation
Governs water metabolism		Failure in qi transformation	Edema, dampness, phlegm, abnormal urination
Receives qi		Unable to grasp qi	Panting, exhaling more than inhaling
Opens into ear		Kidney essence and qi fail to ascend and nourish	Tinnitus and deafness
Controls anterior and posterior yin orifices		Failure to control the closing and opening of the yin orifices	Frequent nighttime urination, enuresis, oliguria, anuria, seminal emission, impotence, premature ejaculation and infertility. Diarrhea, constipation, or even rectal prolapse
Manifests in the hair		Insufficient nourishment	Premature gray hair, withering hair, or hair loss

Table 5.2 Physiological functions, pathological changes, and clinical manifestations of the Kidney

Common patterns in Kidney disease

Clinically, the most common Kidney patterns are Kidney qi deficiency, Kidney failing to secure, Kidney failing to grasp, Kidney yang deficiency, Kidney deficiency with water effusion, Kidney yin deficiency, and Kidney essence deficiency. Since the Kidney stores essence, which can never be over-produced, the Kidneys generally do not have excess patterns, only deficient ones. There is, however, a rare exception to this rule: acute damp-heat can occasionally affect the Urinary Bladder and Kidneys, leading to damp-heat accumulating in the Kidney pattern.

Depending on the pathological changes and clinical manifestation, Kidney qi deficiency can be subcategorized as Kidney qi failing to secure, and Kidney failing to grasp qi.

116 Part 1: Zang Organs

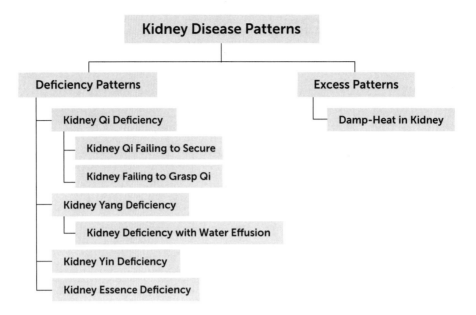

Chart 5.9 Common Kidney disease patterns

	Etiology	Patterns
Deficiency	Congenital insufficiency, aging, chronic illness, improper diet and treatment, physical or sexual overstrain	Kidney Qi Deficiency, Kidney Qi Failing to Consolidate, Kidney Failing to Grasp Qi, Kidney Yang Deficiency, Kidney Yang Deficiency with Water Effusion, Kidney Yin Deficiency, Kidney Essence Deficiency
Excess	Improper diet, exopathogenic factor invasion	Damp-Heat in Kidney (rare)

Table 5.3 Classification of common Kidney patterns

1 Kidney Qi Deficiency Pattern | 腎氣虛証 |

Definition: A group of signs and symptoms caused by the hypofunction of the Kidney.

Clinical manifestations: Soreness and weakness of the lower back and knees, dizziness, fatigue, hearing loss, tinnitus, frequent or difficult urination, loose stools, panting, dyspnea, a pale flabby tongue, and a deep weak pulse.

Key points: Soreness and weakness of the lower back and knees, deep and weak pulse, plus qi deficiency signs and symptoms.

Etiology and pathogenesis: This pattern usually develops as part of the process of aging, or arises due to congenital deficiency. Chronic illness and overstrain that impairs and consumes Kidney qi can also result in essence qi deficiency and manifest with hypofunction of the Kidney.

The Kidney stores essence, which is the fundamental nutritive material for replenishing the marrow supporting the bones, and maintaining normal *shén* activity. If the Kidney is deficient, it fails to store and secure, resulting in essence deficiency, which manifests as soreness and weakness of the lower back and knees, dizziness, poor memory, or physical and mental fatigue. The Kidney opens into the ear so if the Kidney is deficient then the ear loses nourishment, causing hearing loss or tinnitus.

The Kidney is a water organ, governs water metabolism, and controls the opening and closing of the Urinary Bladder. Thus Kidney deficiency causes disorders of water metabolism, resulting in water retention, edema, frequent or difficult urination, or even no urination. Additionally, panting and dyspnea can arise from Kidney qi deficiency, which fails to grasp qi. Impairment of the Kidney's qi transformation gives rise to a pale and flabby tongue, while the deficiency and lack of motive force results in a deep and weak pulse.

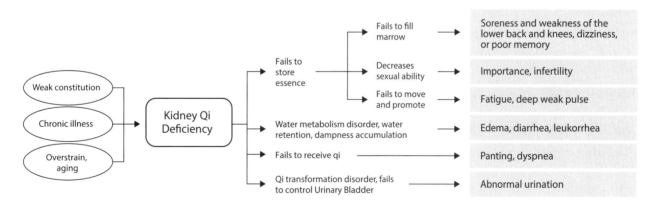

Chart 5.10 Etiology and pathogenesis of Kidney Qi Deficiency

TCM Disease	Western Disease	Herbal Formulas		Acupuncture	
Fatigue (虛勞)	Adrenal fatigue, CFS, Lyme disease, hypothyroidism, EBV, renal failure, fibromyalgia, malnutrition	Si Jun Zi Tang	Jin Gui Shen Qi Wan	ST-36, CV-6, BL-24, BL-26	BL-23, BL-52, CV-4, GV-4, KI-3
Impotence (陽痿)	Hormonal imbalances, sexual neurosis, MS, depression	Wu Zi Yan Zong Wan, Ban Long Wan		KI-1, KI-2, KI-10, KI-12, LR-8, GV-3, CV-1, CV-2, CV-6	
Urinary blockage (癃閉)	Enlarged prostate, chronic nephritis, uremia, urethral stricture	Ji Sheng Shen Qi Wan		KI-13, GV-4, GV-5	
Edema (水腫)	Chronic nephritis, chronic renal failure, malnutrition COPD, CHF	Zhen Wu Tang		SP-9, CV-7, CV-9, TB-5	
Diarrhea (泄瀉)	Colitis, IBS, Crohn's disease, inflammatory bowel disease, celiac disease	Si Shen Wan		KI-13, ST-25, ST-36, SP-5, BL-32, BL-37	
Tinnitus, deafness (耳聾耳鳴)	Aging related, Meniere's disease, TMJ disorders, acoustic neuroma, atherosclerosis, hypertension	Er Long Zuo Ci Wan		ST-1, SI-5, SI-16, SI-18, SI-19, SI-20, GB-2, GB-3, GB-10, GB-11, GB-20, GB-42, GB-43	
Lumbago (腰痛)	Sciatica, herniated disc, spinal stenosis, arthritis	Qing E Wan		Yaoyan, KI-4, KI-5, GV-9, BL-61	
Dizziness (眩暈)	Migraine, hypotension, hypertension, stroke, motion sickness, anemia	He Che Da Zao Wan		KI-1, KI-6, GV-11, GV-16, GV-20, Taiyang, Yintang	
Asthma (喘証)	Emphysema, COPD, cor pulmonale, CHF, pneumoconiosis, chronic bronchial asthma, chronic bronchitis	Qi Wei Du Qi Wan		KI-2, KI-4, KI-22, KI-23, KI-24, KI-25, KI-26, CV-17, CV-20, CV-22, Dingchuan	
Leukorrhea (帶下)	Bacterial vaginosis, yeast infection, vaginitis	Wan Dai Tang		KI-7, KI-12, BL-26	

Table 5.4 Diseases and treatments related to Kidney Qi Deficiency

2 Kidney Qi Failing to Secure Pattern | 腎氣不固 |

Definition: A group of signs and symptoms caused by the Kidney's failure to perform its securing or controlling functions. This pattern is also called 'jīng gate failing to secure' (精關不固 jīng guān bú gù) and 'Kidney essence failing to secure.'

Clinical manifestations: Sore, weak lower back region and knees, lassitude, listlessness, tinnitus, hearing loss, frequent copious urination, scanty or difficult urination, incontinence of urine, enuresis. In men: spermatorrhea, premature ejaculation. In women: continuous menstrual spotting, clear copious vaginal discharge, habitual miscarriage. Pale tongue. Weak pulse.

Key points: Frequent urination, dribbling after urination, incontinence, enuresis, spermatorrhea, premature ejaculation, clear copious vaginal discharge, habitual miscarriage, plus Kidney qi deficiency signs and symptoms.

Etiology and pathogenesis: This pattern is mostly caused by the decline of Kidney qi that accompanies aging. It may also arise from chronic illness or overstrain impairing Kidney qi, or due to constitution and congenital deficiency.

The Kidney is responsible for 'qi transformation' (氣化 qì huà), which controls the opening and closing of the Urinary Bladder. When deficient Kidney fails to transform qi, the Urinary Bladder fails to store and excrete, causing frequent urination, enuresis, oliguria, anuria, incontinence of urine, dribbling after urinating, or bedwetting.

The Kidney is in charge of the essence gate (精關 jīng guān), which opens and closes the anterior and posterior yin orifices (陰竅 yīn qiào). When Kidney qi is deficient, the essence gate fails to secure, resulting in seminal emission, impotence, premature ejaculation, copious clear vaginal discharge, infertility, and miscarriage.

Soreness, weakness, and aching of the lower back region and knees, loss of hearing, tinnitus, dizziness, pale tongue with thin white coating, a deep, thin, and weak pulse all arise from Kidney qi deficiency.`

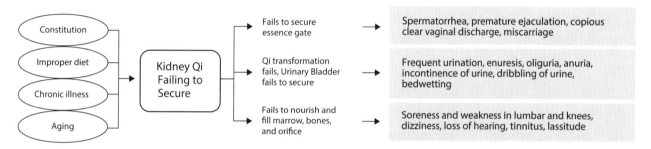

Chart 5.11 Etiology and pathogenesis of Kidney Qi Failing to Secure

TCM Disease	Western Disease	Herbal Formulas	Acupuncture
Fatigue (虛勞)	Adrenal fatigue, Lyme disease, hypothyroidism, CFS, EBV, malnutrition, anemia	Jin Gui Shen Qi Wan	CV-6, GV-4, BL-21
Spermatorrhea (遺精)	Spermatorrhea	Jin Suo Gu Jing Wan	KI-12, SP-6, CV-6
Urinary incontinence (小便失禁)	Urinary incontinence, overactive bladder, pelvic floor disorder	Bu Zhong Yi Qi Tang	BL-56
Enuresis (遺尿)	Enuresis	Suo Quan Wan	BL-28, CV-3, SP-6, LR-1
Turbid painful urinary dribbling (膏淋)	Diabetes, nephrotic syndrome, chronic prostatitis, pyelonephritis	You Gui Wan	KI-6, BL-28, CV-3, SP-9
Consumptive painful urinary dribbling (勞淋)	Chronic pyelonephritis, nephrotic syndrome, chronic UTI	Wu Bi Shan Yao Wan	CV-3, CV-6, BL-28, SP-9
Leukorrhea (帶下)	Bacterial vaginosis, yeast infection, vaginitis	Wan Dai Tang	KI-7, KI-12, BL-26
Irregular uterine bleeding (崩漏)	Functional uterine bleeding, uterus fibroids, polyps, adenomyosis	Gu Jing Wan	LR-1, LR-2, LR-3, KI-7, KI-8, KI-10, KI-13, KI-14, BL-56, CV-5, CV-6, CV-7
Habitual abortion (胎漏)	Habitual abortion, recurrent miscarriage	Bu Shen Gu Chong Wan	Zigong, LR-8, KI-6

(Sang Piao Xiao San; BL-23, BL-52, CV-4, KI-3, GV-20, ST-36)

Table 5.5 Diseases and treatments related to Kidney Qi Failing to Secure

Comparison: Kidney Qi Failing to Secure vs. Spleen Qi Sinking

Kidney qi failing to secure (腎氣不固 *shèn qì bú gù*) and Spleen qi sinking (脾氣下陷 *pí qì xià xiàn*) both contain qi deficiency signs and symptoms, such as listlessness, lassitude, low voice, pale complexion, pale tongue, and a weak pulse. And since failure to secure is the pathogenesis for both patterns, they also share similar leakage issues, such as urine or fecal incontinence.

The Spleen's securing function is responsible for holding up internal organs in their normal position and keeping blood circulation inside the vessels. The Spleen is also in charge of raising essential substances to the Lung for distribution to the entire body. Thus if the deficient Spleen qi fails to secure, the major clinical presentations are internal organ prolapse, bleeding, or chronic loose stools.

The Kidney's securing function is responsible for storing essence and controlling the opening and closing of the 'two yin orifices.' The Kidney also has the function of causing the clear to ascend and the turbid to descend. Thus if the deficient Kidney qi fails to secure, the major clinical presentations are of 'leakage', such as spermatorrhea, leukorrhea, miscarriage, menorrhagia, frequent urination, and loose stools.

The key points to distinguish these two patterns are as follows:
1) Leakage vs. prolapse
2) Kidney symptoms vs. Spleen symptoms

Pattern		Kidney Qi Failing to Secure	Spleen Qi Sinking
Pathogenesis		Deficient Kidney qi fails to control and secure the essence gate and yin orifices	Deficient Spleen qi fails to secure and hold
Symptoms	Common	Urine or fecal incontinence, chronic loose stools, listlessness, lassitude, pale complexion, low voice, pale tongue, weak pulse	
	Different	Urine, essence, Conception and Girdle vessels not secured, causing leakage: frequent urination, menorrhagia, spermatorrhea, leukorrhea, miscarriage	Internal organ prolapse: gastroptosis, renal ptosis, hepatoptosis, uterine prolapse, rectal prolapse
	Other	Soreness and weakness of the lower back and knees, tinnitus, dizziness, copious or difficult urination, infertility or sterility	Poor appetite, bloating and distention, or obesity
Tongue & pulse		Pale tongue; weak pulse	
Treatment strategy		Stabilize and tonify the Kidney, stop leakage	Tonify Spleen
Herbal formulas		Jin Suo Gu Jin Wan, Sang Piao Xiao San, Suo Quan Wan	Bu Zhong Yi Qi Tang

Table 5.6 Comparison of Kidney Qi Failing to Secure and Spleen Qi Sinking

3 Kidney Failing to Grasp Qi Pattern | 腎不納氣 |

Definition: A group of signs and symptoms involving respiratory issues caused by qi deficiency of the Kidney, which then fails to receive or grasp the qi.

Clinical manifestations: Chronic wheezing, rapid and weak breathing, cough, panting, difficult inhalation, shortness of breath, worse with exertion, feeble voice, spontaneous sweating, fatigue, and soreness and weakness of the lower back and knees. In severe cases: dyspnea, profuse cold sweating, cold limbs, dark complexion, and big pulse without root.

Key points: Chronic wheezing, dyspnea, cough, panting, difficult inhalation, worse with exertion, plus Kidney qi deficiency signs and symptoms.

Etiology and pathogenesis: This pattern usually develops from chronic cough or asthma, and impaired Lung qi weakening the Kidney. In addition, physical overstrain, congenital weakness with primary qi deficiency, and Kidney qi deficiency due to aging can all give rise to this pattern.

The Kidney receives clear qi inhaled by the Lung. It also regulates respiration to ensure deep breathing and to maintain normal gas exchange between inside and outside the body. When Kidney qi is deficient, it is unable to grasp the qi or maintain normal inspiration, thus causing shortness of breath, panting, and difficult inhalation. Since exertion consumes qi, the symptoms are worse with exertion.

Deficient qi fails at its functions to promote, push, and secure, resulting in feeble voice, spontaneous sweating, fatigue, and a deep and weak pulse. Severe yang qi deficiency can lead to yang qi collapse: dyspnea, profuse cold sweating, cold limbs, pale and dim complexion, and a big pulse without root.

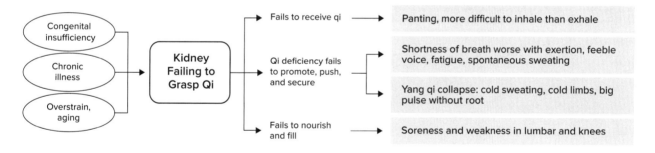

Chart 5.12 Pathogenesis of Kidney Failing to Grasp Qi

TCM Disease	Western Disease	Herbal Formulas		Acupuncture
Panting (喘証)	Emphysema, COPD, cor-pulmonale, CHF, chronic bronchitis pneumoconiosis, chronic bronchi-asthma	Jin Gui Shen Qi Wan, Du Qi Wan	Qi Wei Du Qi Wan, Shen Jie San	CV-16, CV-17, BL-13, BL-23, BL-43, BL-52, GV-12, LU-7, KI-3, KI-6, KI-7
Wheezing (哮証)				
Lung distention (肺脹)			Bu Fei Tang	
Cough (咳嗽)			Shen Jie San	

Table 5.7 Diseases and treatments related to Kidney Failing to Grasp Qi

Comparison: Kidney Failing to Grasp Qi vs. Lung Qi Deficiency

Kidney failing to grasp qi (腎不納氣 *shèn bù nà qì*) and Lung qi deficiency (肺氣虛 *fèi qì xū*) both involve respiratory dysfunction. Respiration involves the cooperation and coordination of the Lung and Kidney. The Lung governs the qi and is responsible for respiration, while the Kidney receives qi, anchors qi, and is the root of qi. Only when Kidney qi is vigorous can the Kidney maintain even and deep respiration by receiving the clear qi (清氣 *qīng qì*) inhaled from the environment and sent down by the Lung. Thus qi deficiency of either organ can result in panting, wheezing, dyspnea, shortness of breath, and abnormal respiration with symptoms that are worse with exertion.

When deficient Lung qi fails to descend, qi rebels upward causing panting, wheezing, and dyspnea characterized by shorter exhalation and longer inhalation. In contrast, when deficient Kidney qi fails to grasp qi, inhalation becomes shallow and difficult resulting in longer exhalation and shorter inhalation. Furthermore, Kidney failing to grasp qi will also present with soreness and weakness in the lower back and knees.

The key points to distinguish these two patterns are as follows:
1) Abnormal breathing pattern: harder to exhale than inhale indicates Lung qi deficiency pattern, while harder to inhale than exhale is caused by Kidney qi deficiency
2) Lung symptoms such as spontaneous sweating and cough vs. Kidney symptoms such as weakness in lumbar or knee pain

Pattern		Lung Qi Deficiency	Kidney Failing to Grasp Qi
Pathogenesis		Lung qi deficiency fails to descend, leads to short exhalation	Kidney qi deficiency fails to grab qi, leads to difficult inhalation
Symptoms	Common	Panting, wheezing, dyspnea, shortness of breath, feeble sound, fatigue, pale complexion	
	Different	Harder to exhale than inhale	Harder to inhale than exhale
	Other	Spontaneous sweating, catches cold frequently, cough	Soreness and weakness in the lower back and knees
Tongue & pulse		Pale and tender tongue; deep and weak pulse	
Treatment strategy		Tonify the Lung, augment qi, nourish yin	Tonify the Kidney to grasp qi
Herbal formulas		Sheng Mai San, Bu Fei Tang	Jin Gui Shen Qi Wan, Shen Ge San

Table 5.8 Comparison of Lung Qi Deficiency and Kidney Failing to Grasp Qi

4 Kidney Yang Deficiency Pattern | 腎陽虛証

Definition: A group of signs and symptoms caused by deficient Kidney yang, which fails to warm the body and limbs, lacks motive force to move and transform qi, and manifests as hypofunction of the body.

Clinical manifestations: Soreness and weakness of the lower back and knees with a cold sensation, intolerance of cold, cold limbs, early morning diarrhea, loose stools with undigested food, edema, frequent copious urination, frequent nocturnal urination, difficult urination, a pale flabby tongue, and a deep weak pulse. In men: impotence, spermatorrhea, and premature ejaculation. In women: menstruation disorder and infertility.

Key points: Disorder of sexual and reproductive function, general hypoactivity of physical function, plus deficiency cold signs and symptoms.

Etiology and pathogenesis: Kidney yang is the root of yang for the entire body. It promotes and warms the *zàng fǔ* and all tissues. When Kidney yang is intact, physical function is vigorous. Weak constitution, aging, chronic illness, physical and sexual overstrain, improper diet, and improper treatment can all damage yang, weaken its warming and promoting function, and result in Kidney yang deficiency pattern. Kidney yang deficiency pattern manifests as:

(1) Failure to warm: intolerance of cold, cold limbs, cold sensation in the lower back and knees, pale or dark complexion, dizziness and vertigo, and apathy.

(2) *Mìng mén* fire decline: reduced reproductive function. In men: impotence, premature ejaculation, spermatorrhea, oligospermia, azoospermia or even aspermia. In women: infertility, dysmenorrhea, amenorrhea, and low libido.

(3) Fire unable to warm earth, leading to Spleen dysfunction: early morning diarrhea, chronic loose stools, and watery stools with undigested food.

(4) Qi transformation (氣化 *qì huà*) failure: water metabolism disorder, which results in clear, copious, and frequent urination; frequent nocturnal urination; or difficult or no urination. There can be pitting edema that is worse in the lower body with scanty urine. If dampness or water attacks other organs there can be abdominal distention and bloating, palpitations, and panting.

(5) Pale tongue with a white coating. Deep and thin pulse, especially weak in proximal position.

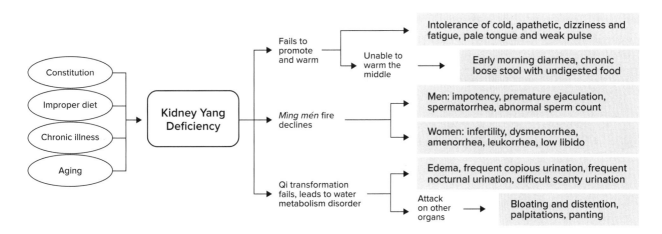

Chart 5.13 Etiology and pathogenesis of Kidney Yang Deficiency

TCM Disease	Western Disease	Herbal Formulas		Acupuncture	
Fatigue (虛勞)	Adrenal fatigue, hypothyroidism, CFS Lyme disease, EBV	Jin Gui Shen Qi Wan, Fu Gui Ba Wei Wan	You Gui Wan	BL-23, CV-4, GV-4, KI-3, ST-36	Moxa
Diarrhea (泄瀉)	Chronic enteritis, Crohn's disease, colitis, SIBO		Si Shen Wan		BL-20
Edema (水腫)	Chronic nephritis, malnutrition, CHF		Zhen Wu Tang		BL-20, CV-9, KI-7
Impotence (陽痿)	Sexual neurosis, hormonal imbalance		You Gui Wan		SP-6, CV-6, BL-28
Urinary blockage (癃閉)	Enlarged prostate		Ji Sheng Shen Qi Wan		BL-20, TB-4
Asthma (哮喘)	COPD, chronic asthma		Shen Jie San		BL-13, CV-6, CV-17
Infertility (不孕)	PCOS, hypothyroidism, LPD, POF		Yu Lin Zhu		CV-6, SP-6, KI-10
Lower back pain (腰痛)	Osteoarthritis, spinal stenosis, fibromyalgia		You Gui Wan		GV-3, BL-40, Yaoyan
Leukorrhea (帶下)	Bacterial vaginosis, yeast infection, vaginitis		Nei Bu Wan		SP-9, TB-5

Table 5.9 Diseases and treatments related to Kidney Yang Deficiency

Comparison: Kidney Qi Failing to Secure vs. Kidney Yang Deficiency

Kidney yang deficiency (腎陽虛 *shèn yáng xū*) and Kidney qi failing to secure (腎氣不固 *shèn qì bú gù*) both develop from Kidney qi deficiency and therefore manifest with the signs and symptoms of Kidney qi deficiency. Common signs and symptoms include a pale face, sore and weak lower back and knees, tinnitus, dizziness, copious or difficult urination, infertility, or sterility.

However, Kidney yang deficiency also presents with coldness due to yang failing to warm and promote, causing an intolerance of cold, cold limbs, edema below the waist, and loose stools. By contrast, Kidney qi failing to secure exhibits leakage due to Kidney failing to control and secure, causing frequent urination, menorrhagia, spermatorrhea, leukorrhea, or miscarriage.

The key points to distinguish these two patterns are:
1) Coldness: intolerance of cold
2) Leakage: frequent urination, menorrhagia, spermatorrhea, leukorrhea, miscarriage

Pattern		Kidney Yang Deficiency	Kidney Qi Failing to Secure
Pathogenesis	Common	Develops from Kidney qi deficiency	
	Different	Kidney yang fails to warm and transform qi, leading to coldness	Deficient Kidney qi fails to control and secure essence gate and yin orifices, leading to leakage
Symptoms	Common	Pale face, sore and weak lower back and knees, tinnitus, dizziness, copious urination, difficult urination, infertility or sterility	
	Different	Yang deficiency with cold: intolerance of cold, cold limbs, edema below the waist, loose stools	Urine, essence, Conception and Girdle vessels not secured, causing leakage: frequent urination, menorrhagia, spermatorrhea, leukorrhea, miscarriage, no obvious cold signs
Tongue & pulse		Pale flabby tongue with white coating; deep, feeble, weak or slow pulse	Pale tongue; weak pulse
Treatment strategy		Tonify and warm Kidney yang	Stabilize and tonify the Kidney, stop leakage
Herbal formulas		Jin Gui Shen Qi Wan, You Gui Yin	Jin Suo Gu Jin Wan, Sang Piao Xiao San, Suo Quan Wan

Table 5.10 Comparison of Kidney Yang Deficiency and Kidney Qi Failing to Secure

Comparison: Kidney Qi Deficiency vs. Kidney Yang Deficiency vs. Kidney Qi Failing to Secure vs. Kidney Failing to Grasp Qi

Kidney qi deficiency (腎氣虛 *shèn qì xū*), Kidney yang deficiency (腎陽虛 *shèn yáng xū*), Kidney qi failing to secure (腎氣不固 *shèn qì bù gù*), and Kidney failing to grasp qi (腎不納氣 *shèn bù nà qì*) all have similar presentations, including soreness and weakness of the lower back and knees, dizziness, tinnitus, fatigue, lassitude, a pale tongue, and a deep weak pulse. However, they are clinically different.

Kidney qi deficiency is a common and basic pattern of Kidney disease with a variety of causes including improper diet, aging, and chronic illness. With delayed or improper treatment, Kidney qi deficiency can develop into Kidney yang deficiency, which presents with coldness, such as intolerance of cold, cold pain in the lumbar area, and cold limbs.

Kidney failing to grasp qi and Kidney qi failing to secure are both subcategories of Kidney qi deficiency. The clinical manifestation of Kidney failing to grasp qi results from the dysfunction of the Kidney's relationship with the Lung, which presents with shallow and difficult breathing. In contrast, Kidney qi failing to secure involves leakage issues, such as essence and urine incontinence.

The key points to distinguish these four patterns are as follows:
- Chief complaints: soreness and weakness of the lower back and knees vs. leaking from two yin orifices vs. dyspnea vs. coldness

126 Part 1: Zang Organs

Pattern		Kidney Qi Deficiency	Kidney Qi Failing to Secure	Kidney Failing to Grasp Qi	Kidney Yang Deficiency
Pathogenesis		Kidney qi deficiency fails to store essence			
			Fails to secure the Girdle vessel and the two 'yin orifices'	Fails to receive qi	Fails to warm and promote
Symptoms	Common	Soreness and weakness of the lower back and knees, dizziness, tinnitus, fatigue, lassitude, pale tongue, and a deep weak pulse			
	Different		Frequent urination, nocturnal enuresis, spermatorrhea, premature ejaculation, clear copious vaginal discharge, habitual miscarriage, incontinence	Chronic panting, dyspnea, cough or asthma, exhale more than inhale, worse with exertion	Intolerance of cold, cold extremities, edema, pale complexion
Tongue & pulse		Pale tongue with white coating; deep and feeble or weak pulse			
				Or big pulse without root	Flabby tongue, greasy coating; slow pulse
Treatment strategy		Tonifies qi, strengthens the Kidney			
			Stabilize essence, stop seminal emission and spermatorrhea	Astringe Lung qi, relieve panting / cough	Warm and tonify Kidney yang
Herbal formulas		Jin Gui Shen Qi Wan	Sang Piao Xiao San	Du Qi Wan	Jin Gui Shen Qi Wan

Table 5.11 Comparison of Kidney Qi Deficiency, Kidney Qi Failing to Secure, Kidney Failing to Grasp Qi, and Kidney Yang Deficiency

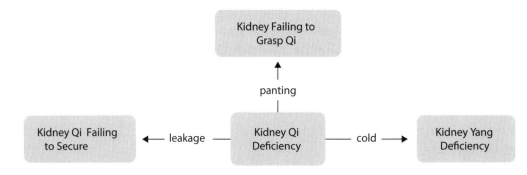

Chart 5.14   Kidney Qi Deficiency, Kidney Qi Failing to Secure, Kidney Failing to Grasp Qi, and Kidney Yang Deficiency

5 Kidney Yang Deficiency with Water Effusion |腎虛水泛|

Definition: A group of signs and symptoms caused by deficient Kidney yang, which fails to perform its qi transformation (氣化 qì huà) function, leading to water metabolism disorder and water retention.

Clinical manifestations: General pitting edema with greater severity in the lower extremities, abdominal distention, scanty urine, shortness of breath, cough and panting with sputum gurgling in the throat, palpitations, panting aggravated by exertion, intolerance of cold, cold extremities, a pale flabby tongue body with a thick or greasy white coating, and a deep, thin, and weak pulse.

Chapter 5 : Kidney Disease Patterns

Key points: Pitting edema worse in the lower extremities, scanty urination, intolerance of cold and cold limbs. In addition to the Kidney, this pattern must involve at least two other organs, such as the Heart, Lung, or Spleen.

Etiology and pathogenesis: This pattern may be caused by chronic illness, aging, improper diet, improper treatment, or a constitutional weakness that leads to Kidney yang deficiency. In most cases, this pattern develops from a Kidney yang deficiency pattern.

Kidney yang deficiency leads to a failure in qi transformation, resulting in water metabolism disorder and water retention. A decline of Kidney yang causes dysfunction of the Urinary Bladder, while water retention means less water is sent to the Urinary Bladder, causing scanty urination. General edema is due to water and fluids overflowing into the skin and muscles. Water upward-attacking the Spleen causes abdominal bloating and distention. If water and fluid overflow upward, they attack the Heart and Lung, causing palpitations and shortness of breath. Excess water and fluids transforms into phlegm, manifesting as cough and panting with sputum gurgling in the throat. Deficient yang fails to warm and nourish the extremities, causing intolerance of cold and cold extremities. A flabby tongue body, white tongue coating, and deep thin pulse are signs of yang deficiency causing an overflow of water and fluids.

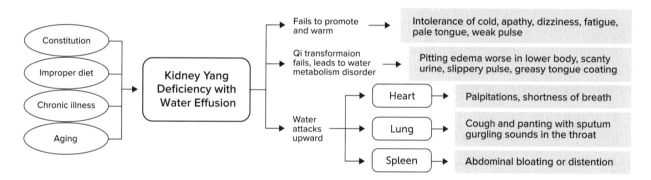

Chart 5.15 Etiology and pathogenesis of Kidney Yang Deficiency with Water Effusion

TCM Disease	Western Disease	Herbal Formulas		Acupuncture
Phlegm and thin mucus (痰飲証)	Ascites, gastroptosis, acute gastroenteritis, gastrectasis	Zhen Wu Tang	Wu Ling San with Jin Gui Shen Qi Wan	BL-20, BL-23, CV-4, CV-9, KI-7, ST-36
Edema (水腫)	Chronic nephritis, COPD, CHF, Chronic Kidney failure, malnutrition		Wu Pi Yin	
Lung distention (肺脹)	Emphysema, cor pulmonale, pulmonary edema		Bu Fei Tang, Ping Chuan Gu Ben Tang	

Table 5.12 Diseases and treatments related to Kidney Yang Deficiency with Water Effusion

Comparison: Kidney Yang Deficiency with Water Effusion vs. Cold-Water Shooting into the Lung vs. Water Qi Encroaching on the Heart

The major pathogenesis of Kidney yang deficiency with water effusion (腎虛水泛 *shèn xū shuǐ fàn*), cold-water shooting into the Lung (寒水射肺 *hán shuǐ shè fèi*), and water qi encroaching on the Heart (水氣凌心 *shuǐ qì líng xīn*) is Kidney yang deficiency failing to warm and transform, leading to excessive water accumulation. Thus they all present with edema, cold limbs, and a deep weak pulse.

Cold-water shooting into the Lung can be caused by exopathogenic cold combining with water, or exopathogenic cold invading and inciting pre-existing phlegm-thin mucus caused by Kidney and Spleen yang deficiency. This phlegm-thin mucus obstructs the Lung qi, which fails to descend and disperse, resulting in cough with profuse white foamy sputum, dyspnea, and an inability to lie down flat. On the other hand, water qi encroaching on the Heart is due to water-thin mucus obstructing the Heart yang, which leads to palpitations and oppression or tightness in the chest.

The above two patterns are different clinical manifestations of Kidney yang deficiency with water effusion. When this water effusion upwardly attacks the Heart, it leads to the pattern of water qi encroaching on the Heart. When it upwardly attacks the Lung, it leads to the pattern of cold-water shooting into the Lung. These three patterns may appear together in the same disease.

The key points to distinguishing these three patterns are as follows:
1) Area of edema: upper body vs. lower body
2) Major symptoms: difficult urination vs. cough with profuse white foamy sputum vs palpitations

Pattern		Kidney Yang Deficiency with Water Effusion	Cold-Water Shooting into the Lung	Water Qi Encroaching on the Heart
Pathogenesis	Common	Kidney yang deficiency fails to warm and transform qi, leads to water accumulation, generates phlegm-thin mucus		
	Different		Exopathogenic cold invades with water or exopathogenic cold inciting pre-existing phlegm-thin mucus	Spleen and Kidney yang deficiency leads to water accumulation that upward obstructs Heart yang
Symptoms	Common	Edema, cold limbs, pale face, pale flabby tongue with slippery coating, weak and slippery pulse		
	Different	Pitting edema, worse in lower extremities, difficult or scanty urination	Cough with profuse white foamy sputum, facial edema, dyspnea, inability to lie down flat	Palpitations, oppression or pain in the chest, shortness of breath, facial edema, inability to lie down flat
Tongue & pulse		Pale flabby tongue with white coating; deep, thin, and weak pulse	White greasy tongue coating; soft and slow, slippery, or wiry pulse	Pale flabby tongue with white coating; deep thread and weak, or knotted pulse
Treatment strategy		Warm Kidney, promote diuresis to drain water-dampness	Release the exterior, transform phlegm-thin mucus, warm the Lung, cause rebellious Lung qi to descend	Unblock Heart yang, benefit yin, calm *shén*, eliminate irritability
Herbal formulas		Zhen Wu Tang	Xiao Qing Long Tang	Gui Zhi Gan Cao Long Gu Mu Li Tang

Table 5.13 Comparison of Kidney Yang Deficiency with Water Effusion, Cold-Water Shooting into the Lung, and Water Qi Encroaching on the Heart

6 Kidney Yin Deficiency Pattern | 腎陰虛証 |

Definition: A group of signs and symptoms caused by a deficiency in Kidney yin, which fails to nourish the body, producing deficiency fire. It is also called Kidney water deficiency (腎水虧虛 *shèn shuǐ kuī xū*) and original or true yin deficiency (真陰虧虛 *zhēn yīn kuī xū*).

Clinical manifestations: Soreness and weakness of the lower back and knees, dizziness, vertigo, tinnitus, insomnia, low-grade fever in the afternoon or evening, malar flush, night sweats, hot flashes, five-center heat, steaming bone disorder, dry mouth and throat, poor memory, emaciation, a red tongue with scanty coating, and a thin and rapid pulse. In men: premature ejaculation, inhibited ejaculation, excessive sexual desire, or nocturnal emissions. In women: scanty menses, amenorrhea, dysmenorrhea, or heavy menses.

Key points: Soreness and weakness of the lower back and knees, dizziness, vertigo, tinnitus, nocturnal emissions in men, and abnormal menses in women, plus deficiency heat signs and symptoms.

Etiology and pathogenesis: This pattern may be caused by chronic illness consuming yin fluids; later stages of febrile disease; aging; weak constitution; physical or sexual overstrain; or excessive consumption of warm and dry food, alcohol, herbs, or medication.

Yin deficiency produces internal heat, thus symptoms such as low-grade fever, malar flush, hot flashes, five-center heat, and night sweats arise. Additionally, there may be menorrhagia for women and premature ejaculation or nocturnal emissions for men. Yin deficiency also leads to deficient body fluids, manifesting as dry mouth and throat. Consumption of Kidney yin fails to nourish the bones, causing soreness and weakness of the lower back and knees, as well as hair loss and loosening of teeth. Yin deficiency also leads to a failure of the Kidney to produce marrow to fill the brain, which causes dizziness, vertigo, poor memory, and insomnia. Deficient yin is unable to nourish the upper orifices, resulting in tinnitus and deafness. Kidney yin deficiency also leads to Kidney essence deficiency, which fails to fill the Penetrating and Conception vessels, causing scanty menses or amenorrhea. This yin deficiency will present with a red cracked tongue with scanty or no coating, and a thin rapid pulse.

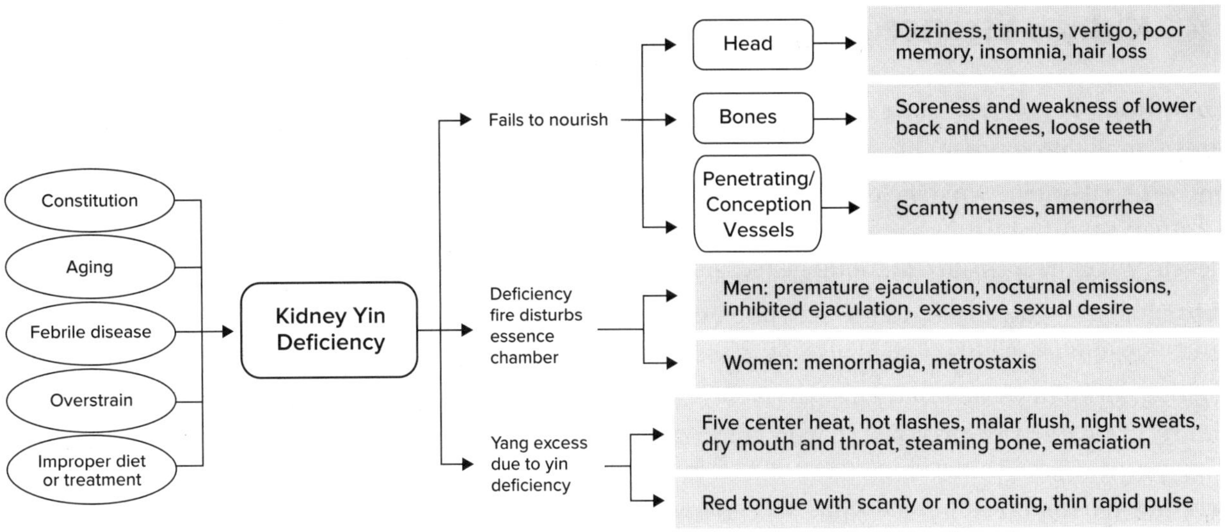

TCM Disease	Western Disease	Herbal Formulas		Acupuncture	
Insomnia (失眠)	Menopause syndrome, anxiety, depression	Liu Wei Di Huang Wan	Huang Lian E Jiao Tang, Tian Wang Bu Xin Dan	BL-23, KI-3, KI-6	BL-23, HT-7, SP-6, Anmian
Fatigue (虛勞)	Anemia, diabetes, CFS, Lyme disease TB		Zuo Gui Wan		ST-36, BL-43
Turbid painful urinary dribbling (膏淋)	Diabetes, UTI, cystitis, Kidney stone, bladder infection		Zhi Bai Di Huang Wan		BL-28, CV-3, SP-9
Bloody painful urinary dribbling (血淋)	UTI, kidney or bladder, infections, diabetes, kidney stone, cancer		Zhi Bai Di Huang Wan		BL-28, CV-3, SP-6, SP-9, SP-10
Nocturnal emission (夢遺)	Nocturnal emission		Zhi Bai Di Huang, Jin Suo Gu Jing Wan		HT-7, BL-15, BL-52
Wasting and thirsting disorder (消渴)	Diabetes mellitus		Zhi Bai Di Huang Wan		BL-13, SP-10, Yishuxue, BL-20
Dizziness vertigo (眩暈)	Hypertension, Meniere's disease, labyrinthitis		Zuo Gui Wan		BL-18, BL-20, LR-2
Painful obstruction of throat (喉痹)	Pharyngitis, laryngitis		Bai He Gu Jin Wan		LU-7, LU-10, CV-23, LI-18
Sudden blindness (暴盲)	Retinal detachment, central retinal vein thrombosis		Qi Ju Di Huang Wan, Ming Mu Di Huang Wan		BL-1, BL-18, BL-20, Qiuhou, GB-39, LR-3
Amenorrhea (閉經)	Hyper- or hypothyroidism, eating disorder, hormone imbalance, premature ovarian failure (POF)		Zuo Gui Wan		SP-6, CV-6, SP-10
Irregular uterine bleeding (崩漏)	Premature menopause, hormone imbalance		Qing Hai Wan		SP-6, SP-10, CV-6, ST-36

Table 5.14 Diseases and treatments related to Kidney Yin Deficiency

7 Kidney Essence Deficiency Pattern | 腎精不足

Definition: A group of signs and symptoms caused by the deficiency of Kidney essence, which retards growth and development or causes senility.

Clinical manifestations: Sore and weak lower back and knees. In children: poor physical and mental development, late closure of fontanels, small and short body, 'five types of developmental delay,' and 'five types of flaccidity.' In adults: senility, prematurely gray hair, loss of hair and teeth, tinnitus, dizziness, poor memory, absentmindedness, mental developmental delay, weak legs and feet, sexual dysfunction, sterility or infertility, or premature aging. A pale tongue and a deep, weak, thin pulse.

Key points: Growth developmental delay in children; sterility, infertility, or premature aging in adults without apparent heat or cold signs and symptoms.

Etiology and pathogenesis: This pattern is mostly caused by prenatal deficiency, but also can be caused by postnatal malnutrition, failure to replenish primary qi, chronic illness, or sexual hyperactivity consuming Kidney essence.

Kidney essence is the basic substance for physical growth and development. If essence is deficient in children, it fails to fill marrows (brain, spinal, and bone marrow) and transform into blood. This delays growth and development, resulting in late closure of fontanel, small and short body, weak bones, 'five types of developmental delay,' and 'five types of flaccidity.' Essence is the basic material of physical and mental activities. Failure of essence to fill brain marrow can cause poor memory, absentmindedness, mental slowness, or developmental delay. Kidney manifests on the hair, and governs the bones; teeth are a surplus of bone. Thus Kidney essence deficiency leads to premature gray hair, thin hair, and loss of teeth.

Tiān kúi is part of congenital essence and is the major component of reproductive essence. It is responsible for puberty, development of secondary sexual characteristics, menarche, sperm production, maturation of sexual instinct, and healthy sexual capacity. Thus Kidney essence deficiency gives rise to sexual dysfunction, sterility, or infertility. A pale tongue and a thin weak pulse are also signs that Kidney essence is failing to nourish and fill.

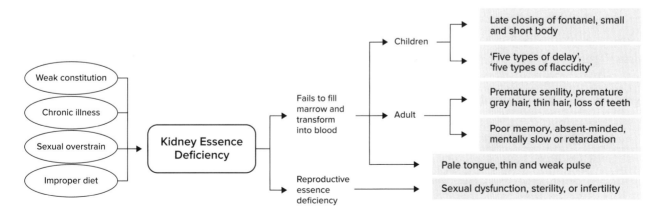

Chart 5.17 Etiology and pathogenesis of Kidney Essence Deficiency

TCM Disease	Western Disease	Herbal Formulas	Acupuncture
Impotence (陽痿)	Hormonal imbalances, sexual neurosis, MS, depression	Wu Zi Yan Zong Wan, Zan Yu Dan	SP-6, CV-6, BL-28
Premature ejaculation (早泄)			
Infertility (不孕)	Hypothyroidism, small uterus, LPD, PCOS, POF	Wu Zi Yan Zong Wan, He Che Da Zao Wan	CV-6, SP-6, KI-10
Amenorrhea (閉經)	Hypothyroidism, Kallmann syndrome, craniopharyngioma	You Gui Wan, He Che Da Zao Wan	SP-6, CV-6, SP-10
Fatigue (虛勞)	Hypothyroidism, anemia, malnutrition, depression, fibromyalgia symptoms	You Gui Wan	Moxa ST-36
Tinnitus, deafness (耳聾，耳鳴)	Tinnitus, deafness	Er Long Zuo Ci Wan	TB-3, TB-17, GB-2, GB-43
Dizziness, vertigo (眩暈)	Hypotension, anemia, Meniere's disease, hypoglycemia, neurasthenia	You Gui Wan	GB-20, BL-18, LR-2
Atrophy disorder (痿証)	Acute transverse myelitis, polyneuritis, PMA, MG, muscular dystrophy, ALS	Hu Qian Wan	ST-30, ST-34, ST-41, GB-30, GB-39, SP-10
Five types of developmental delay (五遲)	Achondroplasia, congenital hypothyroidism, malnutrition	Liu Wei Di Huang with Bu Zhong Yi Qi Tang	ST-36
Five types of flaccidity (五軟)			

You Gui Yin, He Che Da Zao Wan (spanning Herbal Formulas column)
BL-23, CV-4, GV-4, KI-3 (spanning Acupuncture column)

Table 5.15 Diseases and treatments related to Kidney Essence Deficiency

Comparison: Kidney Yin Deficiency vs. Kidney Essence Deficiency

Kidney essence is an aspect of Kidney yin; both produce marrow, transform blood, and nourish bones. Thus Kidney yin deficiency (腎陰虛 shèn yīn xū) and Kidney essence deficiency (腎精不足 shèn jīng bù zú) share many symptoms, including soreness and weakness in the lower back and knees, poor memory, low libido, reproductive dysfunction, and a thin pulse.

However, Kidney essence is the basic material for growth and development, and is the fundamental substance for reproduction. Thus the major presentation of Kidney essence deficiency involves issues with growth, development, and reproductive function. In children this presents as poor or delayed growth, late closure of fontanels, and a small and short body. In adults this presents as premature senility, infertility, and sterility. In contrast, the major presentation for Kidney yin deficiency is its failure to nourish, which generates yin deficiency heat, five-center heat, hot flashes, night sweats, steaming bone disorder, low-grade fever in the afternoon and evenings, and emaciation.

The key points to distinguish these two patterns are as follows:
1) Deficiency heat vs. no heat
2) Delayed growth and development, premature senility, infertility or sterility
3) Tongue and pulse

Pattern		Kidney Yin Deficiency	Kidney Essence Deficiency
Pathogenesis	Common	Deficiency	
	Different	Deficient Kidney yin fails to nourish, generates heat	Deficient Kidney essence fails to fill marrow, transform blood, and nourish *shén*
Symptoms	Common	Soreness and weakness of the lower back and knees, poor memory, low libido, reproductive disorders, thin pulse	
	Different	Deficiency heat: low-grade fever in the afternoon or evening, five center heat, hot flashes, night sweats, steaming bone disorder, emaciation	No heat signs Children: poor and delayed growth, late closure of fontanels, small and short body Adults: premature senility, infertility, sterility
Tongue & pulse		Red tongue with scanty coating; rapid pulse	Pale tongue; deep, weak pulse (especially at *chi* position)
Treatment strategy		Nourish and tonify Kidney yin	Replenish essence
Herbal formulas		Liu Wei Di Huang Wan, Zuo Gui Wan	Wu Zi Yan Zhong Wan, He Che Da Zao Wan

Table 5.16 Comparison of Kidney Yin Deficiency and Kidney Essence Deficiency

Kidney disease patterns relationship and development

Kidney disease patterns are mostly caused by chronic illness or congenital weakness, and generally develop from Kidney qi deficiency. For instance, the sub-patterns Kidney qi failing to secure and Kidney failing to grasp qi are essentially different clinical manifestations of Kidney qi deficiency. Furthermore, Kidney qi deficiency can develop into Kidney yin deficiency or Kidney yang deficiency, depending on individual constitutions and etiologies. When Kidney yang deficiency leads to water retention due to the failure of qi transformation, the resulting pattern is Kidney yang deficiency with water effusion.

Kidney essence deficiency is usually caused by congenital insufficiency, but it can also develop from Kidney qi deficiency. Conversely, Kidney qi deficiency can develop from Kidney essence deficiency. These two patterns commonly co-exist.

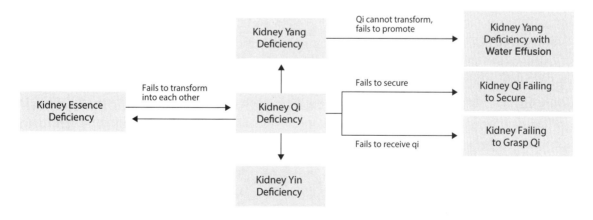

Chart 5.18 Kidney disease pattern relationship and development

Summary of Kidney Disease Patterns

Key points: soreness and weakness of the lower back and knees; growth, development, and reproductive disorders; water metabolism disorders: edema, difficult or frequent urination; respiratory disorders: panting or asthma, shortness of breath; symptoms related to the brain, marrow, bone, hair, ears, or the two yin orifices affecting bowel movements and urination		

Patterns	Clinical manifestations	
	Common	Different
Kidney Qi Deficiency	Soreness and weakness in the lower back and knees, dizziness, tinnitus, fatigue, lassitude, and deep weak pulse	
Kidney Qi Failing to Secure		Leakage due to Urinary Bladder or Kidney failing to secure, frequent urination, enuresis, spermatorrhea, premature ejaculation, clear copious vaginal discharge, habitual miscarriage, pale tongue with a thin white coating
Kidney Failing to Grasp Qi		Kidney fails to receive qi, chronic panting, dyspnea, cough or asthma, difficult inhalation, worse with exertion, pale tongue with a thin white coating
Kidney Yang Deficiency		Cold symptoms, edema, intolerance of cold, cold limbs, edema, nocturnal urination, early morning diarrhea, pale complexion, pale flabby tongue with white glossy coating, weak and slow pulse
Kidney Yang Deficiency with Water Effusion		Edema in the lower extremities, pitting edema worse in the lower extremities, cold symptoms, scanty urine, cough with sputum, palpitations
Kidney Yin Deficiency		Yin deficiency fails to balance, leads to deficiency heat, hot flashes, malar flush, five center heat, night sweats, thirst, red cracked tongue with scanty or no coating, thin and rapid pulse
Kidney Essence Deficiency		Essence fails to be filled. Children: poor physical and mental development. Adults: senility, premature graying of hair, sexual dysfunction, sterility or infertility

Table 5.17 Summary of Kidney disease patterns

Part 2

FU ORGANS

Fǔ (腑) organs include the Stomach, Small Intestine, Large Intestine, Urinary Bladder, Gallbladder, and Triple Burner.* These yang organs are mainly responsible for digesting food and transmitting nutrients to the entire body. *Fǔ* organs are typically hollow organs with empty cavities. Based on the physiological functions and anatomical structures of *fǔ* organs, their pathological changes are more likely to result in excess patterns such as obstruction and stagnation.

CONTENTS

CHAPTER 6: STOMACH DISEASE PATTERNS, 136

CHAPTER 7: SMALL INTESTINE DISEASE PATTERNS, 156

CHAPTER 8: LARGE INTESTINE DISEASE PATTERNS, 165

CHAPTER 9: GALLBLADDER DISEASE PATTERNS, 183

CHAPTER 10: URINARY BLADDER DISEASE PATTERNS, 196

---

*Functionally, the Triple Burner is regarded as a *fǔ* organ, but one that does not match up with any specific organ. (One theory suggests that the Triple Burner is the space between the other organs). It has two major functions. It serves as a passageway for water metabolism: its qi transforming (氣化) function converts water into body fluids and discharges water waste. It also provides a passageway for primal qi (元氣) to course freely throughout the body. When the Triple Burner is obstructed, it leads to qi stagnation, and to water metabolism disorder, manifested as difficult urination, edema, abdominal bloating and distention.

Although it lacks a specific organ of its own, its functions are inseparable from the operations of the Lung, Spleen, Kidney and Urinary Bladder. Thus pathological changes associated with dysfunction of the Triple Burner are reflected in the patterns of other organs such as Urinary Bladder damp-heat, heat congesting the Lung, cold invading the Lung, Spleen qi deficiency or dampness encumbering the Spleen, or Kidney qi deficiency. But there is no Triple Burner pattern as such.

Chapter 6
Stomach Disease Patterns

Physiological characteristics and functions of the Stomach

The Stomach is one of the most important *fǔ* organs. Along with the Spleen, it is called the 'root of post-natal qi' (後天之本 *hòu tiān zhī běn*) because it is the origin of qi and blood produced after birth. The Stomach is also called the 'sea of water and grains' (水谷之海 *shuǐ gǔ zhī hǎi*), the 'great granary' (太倉 *tài cāng*), and the Minister of Granary (倉廩之官 *cāng lín zhī guān*).

The Stomach channel begins at the lateral side of the ala nasi, encircles the face, travels down the neck, enters the supraclavicular fossa, and passes through the diaphragm. It then enters the Stomach and connects with the Spleen. The straight portion of the channel descends from the supraclavicular fossa, travels along the abdomen and down the anterior thigh and leg, and ends at the lateral tip of the second toe.

The Spleen and Stomach are located in the middle burner and are interconnected by channels and membranes, forming an interior-exterior relationship. They are related to the Earth phase. One is *zàng* and ascending, the other is *fǔ* and descending. They coordinate and cooperate to maintain normal digestive function. The Spleen and Stomach are the pivot of the body's qi circulation. The Stomach favors moisture and disfavors dryness, whereas the Spleen favors dryness and disfavors dampness. Together, they transform and transport water and dampness, maintaining normal water metabolism.

The physiological characteristic of the Stomach is that it has an abundance of qi and blood because it is the source of qi and blood. Thus Stomach patterns are usually excessive in nature and rarely deficient. According to one ancient text, "excess patterns belong to *yáng míng* and deficient patterns belong to *tài yín*," which, in the case of middle burner dysfunction, means that the Stomach is more prone to excess patterns and the Spleen more to deficiency. However, this is only a general rule. Even though the Spleen and Stomach are closely related and affect each other, they have unique physiological functions and pathological characteristics. As a result, both of them can have excess and deficient aspects.

1 | Receiving food and drink

The Stomach is in charge of receiving, containing, and fermenting food and drink. Thus the Stomach is called the 'sea of grain and water.'

2 | Decomposition of food and drink

Decomposition or 'rotting and ripening' (腐熟 *fǔ shú*) is the process of granulating, grinding, and fermenting food into chyme, which enables the Spleen to extract the refined essence from food.

3 | Governs descending

The Stomach sends the decomposed food down to the Small Intestine for further extraction of the essence and separation of the waste.

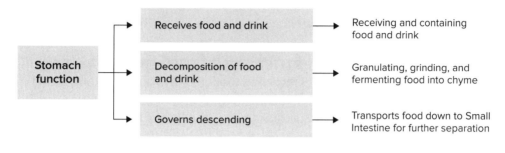

Chart 6.1 Stomach function summary

Common etiological factors in Stomach patterns

Improper diet is one of the most common causes of Stomach dysfunction. However, exopathogens, emotional stress, or chronic illness can all lead to pathological changes in the Stomach. The following are common etiological factors for Stomach disease patterns:
  (1) Exopathogenic cold, heat, dampness or dryness invasion
  (2) Improper diet: overeating; undereating; excessive consumption of raw, cold, greasy, hot, spicy, or dry food; excessive intake of alcohol or caffeine
  (3) Improper treatment: overuse of medication; herbs that are too hot, too dry, too cold, or too greasy
  (4) Emotional stress: excessive worry, anger, thinking, or anxiety
  (5) Chronic illness with Spleen deficiency
  (6) Constitution, aging

Pathological changes and major clinical manifestations of the Stomach

The pathological changes of the Stomach are usually related to Stomach qi failing to descend, which can lead to rebellious Stomach qi, Stomach failing to decompose, and Stomach failing to receive food and drink.

1 | Vomiting, nausea, belching, hiccups, and acid regurgitation

Definition: Vomiting, nausea, belching, hiccups and acid regurgitation are all signs and symptoms related to Stomach qi rebellion.
  (1) Vomiting or emesis is the forceful expulsion of Stomach contents through the mouth.
  (2) Nausea is a sensation of unease and discomfort in the epigastrium with an involuntary urge to vomit.

(3) Hiccups are reflexive spasms of the diaphragm accompanied by a rapid closure of the glottis, producing an audible sound.
(4) Belching, also known as eructation, burping, or ructus, is a normal process to relieve distention from air accumulation in the Stomach.
(5) Acid regurgitation involves Stomach acid flowing back into the esophagus and up to the mouth, leaving a sour, bitter taste in the mouth.

Etiology and pathomechanisms: Stomach qi rebellion is the pathogenesis of this group of symptoms. The physiological function of the Stomach is receiving food and drink and sending it downward to the Small Intestine. When Stomach qi is impaired, it will fail to receive or send food downward, resulting in Stomach qi rebellion and causing vomiting, nausea, belching, hiccups, and acid regurgitation.

There are two pathomechanisms for Stomach qi rebellion:
(1) Qi, phlegm, or dampness stagnation or obstruction; improper diet such as overconsumption of raw, cold, greasy, hot, spicy, or dry foods, and overconsumption of alcohol or caffeine; exopathogen invasion such as cold, dampness, dryness or heat; excessive emotional stress; or improper treatment such as overuse of medications or herbs that are too hot, dry, cold or greasy.
(5) Stomach's lack of power to send food downward due to chronic illness, aging, malnutrition, or a weak constitution.

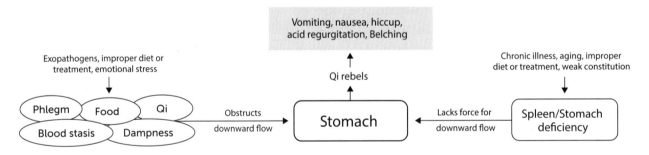

Chart 6.2 Etiology and pathomechanism of vomiting, nausea, hiccups, belching, and acid regurgitation

2 | Aversion to food

Definition: Characteristics of food aversion due to Stomach dysfunction include a loss of appetite, no desire to eat, or abdominal and epigastric discomfort or pain after eating.

Etiology and pathomechanisms: An aversion to food may result from either a slowing down of the Stomach's decomposition process or an impairment of the Stomach's descending function. These two conditions are the underlying pathomechanisms to food aversion or loss of appetite.

There are three possible causes for the process of slowed decomposition: (1) *Cold*: yang qi is the motive force for the decomposition process and can become deficient due to exopathogenic cold invasion, an improper diet of overeating cold raw or greasy food, improper treatments overusing cold herbs or medications, or chronic illness and aging. (2) *Stagnation*: overeating can lead to food stagnation in the Stomach. (3) *Lack of moisture*: normal Stomach function requires nourishment from yin fluids, which can be impaired by chronic illness, aging, an improper diet of overeating spicy, acrid foods, alcohol, or improper treatments using overly stimulating medications.

Descending and ascending is the basic movement for qi circulation and there are three possible ways this movement can be disrupted: (1) *Stagnation*: dampness or phlegm resulting from exopathogenic dampness invasion, an improper diet of overeating cold, raw or greasy food, food stagnation due to overeating, or qi stagnation resulting from emotional stress. (2) *Lack of moisture or lack of motive force*: yin deficiency and yang deficiency due to chronic illness, aging, or constitution can result in the Stomach lacking nourishment and power to perform its descending function. (3) *Qi movement disorder*: chronic illness, improper diet, and emotional stress, such as worry, sorrow, and fear, can impair the Spleen's ascending function, which in turn will adversely affect the Stomach's descending function.

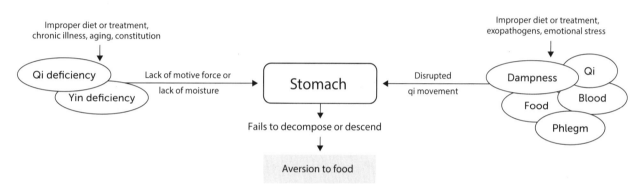

Chart 6.3 Etiology and pathomechanism of aversion to food

3 | Epigastric bloating, distention, and discomfort

Definition: A sensation of bloating and/or distention in the epigastrium and abdomen. In severe cases there is an enlargement of the abdomen.
  (1) Bloating (滿 *mǎn*) is a subjective sensation of fullness that is only felt by the patient.
  (2) Distention (痞 *pǐ*) means bloating that is both a subjective and objective sign that may be seen or felt by both the patient and the practitioner.
  (3) Epigastric discomfort (嘈雜 *cáo zá*): an uncomfortable feeling, neither pain nor nausea, it is emptiness, a burning and uneasy sensation in the epigastric region.

Etiology and pathomechanisms: Any disorder in the circulation of qi in the epigastric area, such as qi obstruction or qi deficiency, can cause qi accumulation that leads to bloating, distention, and pain. Etiological factors that lead to qi obstruction include the invasion of exopathogenic dampness, improper diet resulting in food stagnation, and emotional stress causing organ dysfunctions that produce phlegm or blood stasis. Meanwhile, a weak constitution, improper diet or treatment, long-term medications, surgery, and chronic illness can all lead to qi deficiency, which fails to move and release accumulation and stagnation. Additionally, the pathogenesis of epigastric discomfort (嘈雜 *cáo zá*) can result from Stomach qi or yin deficiency, which causes Stomach dysfunction due to a lack of nourishment.

140 Part 2: Fu Organs

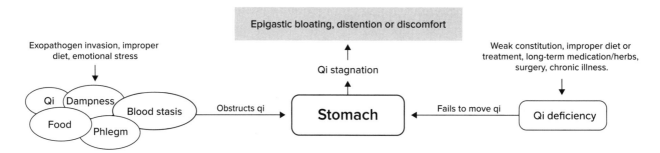

Chart 6.4 Etiology and pathomechanisms of epigastric bloating, distention, and discomfort

4 | Other signs and symptoms related to the Stomach

The following signs and symptoms can also appear in Stomach patterns: excessive appetite, bad breath, severe thirst, swollen or bleeding gums.

Physiological Function	Pathological Change	Clinical Manifestation
Controls receiving	Fails to receive	Aversion to food, poor appetite
Decomposes food and drink	Fails to rot and ripen; then Spleen is unable to extract refined essence from the food and fails to transform and transport; food stays inside stomach longer, causing blockage	Poor appetite, bloating and distension, epigastric discomfort
Governs descending	Fails to descend, leads to rebellious qi	Nausea, vomiting, belching, hiccups, acid regurgitation

Table 6.1 Physiological functions, pathological changes, and clinical manifestations of the Stomach

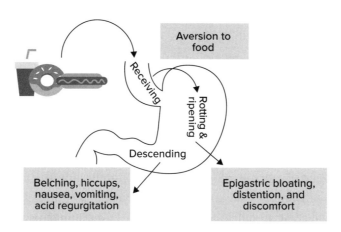

Chart 6.5 Summary of Stomach pathology

Common patterns in Stomach disease

As the postnatal root of qi and blood, the Stomach is the organ with abundant qi and blood. Thus the Stomach is prone to patterns of excess.

There are six Stomach patterns commonly seen in the clinic. According to their pathogenesis and clinical manifestation, these patterns can be divided into two groups: deficiency patterns and excess patterns. Deficiency patterns include Stomach yin deficiency and Stomach deficiency cold. Excess patterns include Stomach fire, cold invading the Stomach, blood stagnation in the Stomach, and food stagnation in the Stomach.

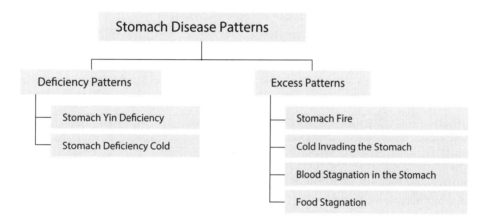

Chart 6.6   Common Stomach disease patterns

	Etiology	Patterns
Deficiency	Improper diet, improper treatment, emotional stress, chronic illness, constitution, aging	Stomach Yin Deficiency, Stomach Deficiency Cold
Excess	Exopathogens invasion, improper diet, improper treatment, emotional stress	Stomach Fire, Cold Invading the Stomach, Blood Stagnation in the Stomach, Food Stagnation

Table 6.2 Classification of common Stomach patterns

1 Stomach Yin Deficiency Pattern | 胃陰虛 |

Definition: A group of signs and symptoms involving Stomach yin deficiency that leads to the lack of nourishment and poor lubrication of the Stomach, resulting in Stomach qi rebellion.

Clinical manifestations: Epigastric pain with a burning sensation, hunger but no desire to eat, epigastric discomfort, dry mouth and throat, nausea, hiccups, acid regurgitation, dry stools, a red tongue with a scanty dry coating, and a thin, rapid pulse.

Key points: Hunger but no desire to eat, rebellious Stomach qi symptoms, plus yin deficiency signs and symptoms.

Etiology and pathogenesis: There are several causes of Stomach yin deficiency: high fevers in febrile diseases can erode the Stomach yin, in which case yin deficiency symptoms manifest during the later stages of the disease; emotional stress; qi stagnation generating heat that consumes Stomach yin; severe vomiting or diarrhea; overconsumption of spicy, aromatic, dry and pungent food or alcohol; or overuse of warm and dry herbs, which can damage Stomach yin.

The Stomach favors moisture and disfavors dryness. If Stomach yin fails to nourish, Stomach qi rebels, which causes nausea and hiccups. Without sufficient nourishment, the Stomach cramps, resulting in epigastric pain and a burning sensation from deficiency heat. When the Stomach lacks nourishment, it gives rise to a feeling of discomfort, which is neither pain, nor nausea, but an emptiness, burning, and uneasy sensation.

Deficiency heat decomposes food and causes the patient to experience the sensation of hunger. However, the deficient yin cannot nourish the Stomach, which is then unable to receive more food. Thus, despite hunger there is no desire to eat. The deficiency heat will also cause a dry mouth, dry stools, a red tongue with a scanty or peeled coating, and a thin rapid pulse.

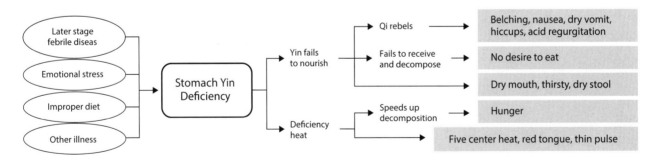

Chart 6.7 Etiology and pathogenesis of Stomach Yin Deficiency

TCM Disease	Western Disease	Herbal Formulas		Acupuncture
Epigastric pain (胃痛)	Atrophic gastritis, gastric neurosis, Peptic ulcer, GERD, gastric carcinoma	Sha Shen Mai Men Dong Tang, Yi Wei Tang	Yi Wei Tang	CV-12, ST-36, SP-6	CV-4, CV-6, PC-6, KI-3, ST-44
Wasting and thirsting disorder (消渴)	Diabetes, hyperthyroidism		Yu Nu Jian	ST-44, KI-3, BL-20, BL-21
Hiccups (嗝嗝)	GERD, alcoholism, diabetes, stroke, MS, tumors, steroid or tranquilizer use		Ju Pi Zhu Ru Tang	BL-17, CV-17

Table 6.3 Diseases and treatments related to Stomach Yin Deficiency

Comparison: Stomach Yin Deficiency vs. Spleen Yin Deficiency

Stomach yin deficiency (胃陰虛 *wèi yīn xū*) and Spleen yin deficiency (脾陰虛 *pí yīn xū*) share many symptoms, including epigastric discomfort, nausea, vomiting, dry belching, abdominal bloating, and distention.

Stomach yin deficiency is relatively acute and usually occurs in the later stage of febrile diseases, after severe vomiting, diarrhea, or major surgery with massive blood loss, or due to diet. Hunger but no desire to eat is the hallmark symptom for Stomach yin deficiency.

Spleen yin deficiency is a chronic condition. It does not have a single momentous cause in the clinic. It is usually caused by long-term mental or physical overstrain, chronic illness with deficiency of internal organs, or a weak constitution. Chapped lips with no hunger and no desire to eat are the distinguishing symptoms of Stomach yin deficiency.

The key points to distinguish these two patterns are as follows:
1) Nature and course of disease: acute and short course vs. chronic and long course
2) Etiology: severe illness or improper diet vs. long-term chronic overstrain or weak constitution
3) Hunger but no desire to eat vs. no hunger and no desire to eat with dry chapped lips

Pattern	Stomach Yin deficiency	Spleen Yin Deficiency
Etiology	High fever, severe vomiting, diarrhea, sweating, or following a major surgery, too much spicy pungent food or alcohol	Long-term mental or physical overstrain, chronic illness, or weak constitution
Pathogenesis	Yin deficiency fails to nourish the Stomach, disrupting its receiving, decomposing, and transporting function	Yin deficiency fails to nourish the Spleen that then fails to transport and transform
Characteristics	Relatively acute, exogenous disease, course develops quicker, easier to treat	Chronic, endogenous disease, course develops slowly, difficult to treat
Symptoms — Common	Epigastric discomfort, nausea, vomiting, dry belching, distention and bloating, yellow urine, dry stools, five center heat, red tongue with scanty or peeled coat, rapid and thin pulse	
Symptoms — Different	Hunger but no desire to eat, hiccups, belching	No hunger, no desire to eat, discomfort after eating, dry chapped lips
Treatment strategy	Nourish yin, tonify the Stomach	Tonify the Spleen, harmonize the middle
Herbal formulas	Sha Shen Mai Men Dong Tang, Yi Wei Tang, Yu Nu Jian	Ma Zi Ren Wan, Zhong He Li Yin Tang

Table 6.4 Comparison of Stomach Yin Deficiency and Spleen Yin Deficiency

Comparison: Stomach Yin Deficiency vs. Large Intestine Dryness

Stomach yin deficiency (胃陰虛 wèi yīn xū) and Large Intestine dryness (大腸液虧 dà cháng yè kuī) both appear with constipation and dry stools. However, they have different clinical manifestations because of their difference in location, etiology, and pathogenesis.

Stomach yin deficiency is more acute and severe, usually occurring after febrile diseases, major surgery, or severe vomiting and diarrhea. Improper diet and alcohol use can also damage Stomach yin. Its key symptoms are dull stomachache, hunger with no desire to eat, epigastric discomfort, belching, and nausea. Constipation with dry stools is not the primary symptom.

Large Intestine dryness is caused by insufficient body fluids that fail to nourish and moisten the Large Intestine. It usually occurs in older patients and those with chronic illness. Constipation with dry stools is the primary symptom.

The key points to distinguish these two patterns are as follows:
1) Acute vs. chronic
2) Main symptoms: hunger but no desire to eat vs. constipation with dry stools

Pattern	Stomach Yin Deficiency	Large Intestine Dryness
Etiology	High fever, severe vomiting or diarrhea, major surgery, excessive spicy and pungent food or alcohol	Aging, chronic illness
Pathogenesis	Insufficient Stomach yin fails to nourish and moisten the Stomach, leading to rebellious qi	Insufficient body fluid fails to nourish and moisten the Large Intestine, slowing transportation
Nature	More acute, severe	Chronic, mild
Symptoms — Common	Dry mouth and throat, dry stool, difficulty defecating, bad breath, red tongue with dry coating	
Symptoms — Different	Dull stomachache, hunger with no desire to eat, epigastric discomfort, fullness, dry belching	Constipation, no bowel movements for days
Tongue & pulse	Red tongue with little or no coating; thread and rapid pulse	Red tongue with dry yellow coating; rapid or choppy pulse
Treatment strategy	Nourish yin, clear heat from the Stomach	Generate fluids, moisten dryness, unblock the bowels
Herbal formulas	Sha Shen Mai Men Dong Tang, Yi Wei Tang, Yu Nu Jian	Qing Ye Tang, Qing Ao Run Chang Tang, Wu Ren Wan

Table 6.5 Comparison of Stomach Yin Deficiency and Large Intestine Dryness

2 Stomach Deficiency Cold Pattern | 胃中虛寒 |

Definition: A group of signs and symptoms involving digestive system hypofunction where deficient Stomach yang fails to warm, leading to deficiency cold and resulting in rebellion of Stomach qi. This pattern is also called Stomach yang deficiency and is commonly combined with Spleen yang deficiency.

Clinical manifestations: Discomfort or dull pain in the epigastrium that improves after eating and is better with pressure and warmth, no appetite, preference for warm drinks and foods, vomiting of clear fluid, absence of thirst, cold and weak limbs, tiredness, pale complexion. Pale and moist tongue. Deep, weak, and slow pulse.

Key points: Dull, vague, cold pain in epigastrium that is relieved by warmth, pressure and by eating, plus yang deficiency signs and symptoms.

Etiology and pathogenesis: The Stomach is the organ with abundant qi and blood, so Stomach qi or yang deficiency is very rare. However, long-term improper diet, such as overeating raw and cold foods, improper treatment, overuse of herbs or medications, aging, chronic deficiency illness, especially related with Spleen and Kidney yang deficiency, or severe vomiting and diarrhea can impair Stomach qi and yang.

The nature of cold is to congeal and stagnate, thus cold may cause contraction and obstruction within the channels and collaterals. This blocks qi and blood circulation, causing pain that is aggravated by cold and relieved by warmth. Since the cold is generated by yang deficiency, the pain is relieved by pressure and eating. Stomach yang deficiency fails to descend and receive, so there is epigastric and abdominal distention, bloating, and no appetite.

Yang qi has the function of warming the body; when there is not enough power to warm the body, there is intolerance of cold, cold limbs, preference for warm food and drink but no particular thirst, a pale tender tongue, and a slow pulse.

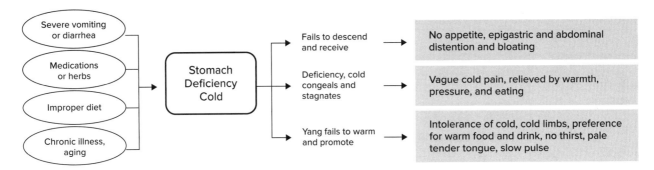

Chart 6.8 Etiology and pathogenesis of Stomach Deficiency Cold

TCM Disease	Western Disease	Herbal Formulas		Acupuncture	
Epigastric pain (胃痛)	Atrophic gastritis, gastric neurosis, peptic ulcer, GERD, gastric carcinoma		Xiao Jian Zhong Tang		ST-25, SP-4, CV-14
Epigastric discomfort (嘈雜)	GERD, ulcer, gastritis, esophagitis, hernia, SIBO		Yi Gong San		ST-10
Hiccups (呃逆)	GERD, stroke, MS, diabetes, kidney failure	Huang Qi Jian Zhong Tang, Xiao Jian Zhong Tang, Liang Fu Wan	Liu Jun Zi Tang	ST-36, CV-6, CV-12, BL-20, BL-21, PC-6	BL-17
Belching (噯氣)	GERD, lactose intolerance, IBS, aerophagia		Xuan Fu Dai Zhe Tang		TB-6, CV-10, ST-44
Vomiting (嘔吐)	Motion sickness, gastroenteritis, pregnancy, stomach flu		Li Zhong Wan		SP-6, LI-4
Fatigue (虛勞)	Adrenal fatigue, hypothyroidism, CFS Lyme disease, EBV		Si Jun Zi Tang		CV-4, GV-4, BL-23, BL-24, BL-26
Morning sickness (妊娠惡阻)	GERD, alcoholism, diabetes, stroke, MS, tumors, steroid or tranquilizer use		Xiang Sha Liu Jun Zi Tang		PC-6

Table 6.6 Diseases and treatments related to Stomach Deficiency Cold

Comparison: Stomach Deficiency Cold vs. Spleen Yang Deficiency

Stomach deficiency cold (胃中虛寒 *wèi zhōng xū hán*) and Spleen yang deficiency (脾陽虛 *pí yáng xū*) share many clinical symptoms, treatment strategies, and herbal formulas. The Spleen governs transformation and transportation, and the Stomach governs receiving and decomposing. Physiologically, they cooperate and coordinate food digestion, assimilation, and distribution. Therefore, pathologically, they are also closely connected. When there is a yang deficiency in one organ, it usually involves both and manifests as Spleen and Stomach yang deficiency. However, in the early stages of illness, the patterns may appear separately.

The key point to distinguish these two patterns is Stomach yang deficiency includes vomiting clear fluids, while Spleen yang deficiency has loose stools and dampness-related symptoms such as edema, copious vaginal discharge, and phlegm.

Pattern		Stomach Deficiency Cold	Spleen Yang Deficiency
Etiology		Improper diet, improper treatment, pathogenic cold attack, or chronic illness	
		Severe vomiting or diarrhea	Aging
Pathogenesis		Yang deficient Stomach fails to descend and decompose, manifesting as rebellious qi	Yang deficient Spleen fails to transport and transform, disrupting water metabolism, causing dampness and phlegm
Characteristics		Interior, deficiency, cold	
		Rare	More common
Symptoms	Common	Vague cold pain in epigastrium that is relieved by warmth and pressure, epigastric and abdominal bloating and distention, pale complexion, cold and weak limbs, pale tender tongue with white, thin, glossy coating, and weak and slow pulse	
	Different	Epigastric pain relieved by eating, vomiting with clear fluids	Edema with scanty urine, loose stools, symptoms of dampness like copious vaginal discharge and phlegm
Treatment strategy		Tonify and warm the middle, expel cold, relieve pain	Tonify and warm the middle, expel cold, stop diarrhea
Herbal formulas		Xiao Jian Zhong Tang, Huang Qi Jian Zhong Tang	Li Zhong Wan

Table 6.7 Comparison of Stomach Deficiency Cold and Spleen Yang Deficiency

3 Stomach Fire Pattern | 胃熱熾盛 |

Definition: A group of signs and symptoms caused by exuberant fire disrupting Stomach function. This pattern is also known as excess heat in the Stomach.

Clinical manifestations: Epigastric burning pain that resists pressure, thirst with desire to drink cold water, excessive appetite, insatiable hunger, bad breath, painful, swollen, bleeding gums, sores in the mouth, vomit with sour or bitter taste, acid regurgitation, constipation with dry stools, scanty yellow urine, a red tongue with yellow coating, and a slippery and rapid pulse.

Key points: Burning epigastric pain, excessive appetite, plus interior excess heat signs and symptoms.

Etiology and pathogenesis: An improper diet, such as overconsumption of pungent, spicy, warm, and dry foods, alcohol, caffeine, and medications, may transform into heat and fire. Emotional stress can lead to qi stagnation that generates fire and attacks the Stomach. Pathogenic heat can also directly invade the Stomach.

Heat and fire gathers and stagnates in the Stomach, which burns up the body fluids, causing thirst with a desire to drink cold water. Excess heat speeds Stomach decomposition and transportation, increasing peristalsis, which results in the patient eating a lot but still feeling hungry. When heat scorches inside the Stomach, it causes epigastric burning pain. When heat flares up along the Stomach channel, it putrefies flesh and impairs the blood vessels, which causes painful, swollen, bleeding gums, sores in the mouth, and bad breath. Constipation with dry stools, scanty yellow urine, a red tongue with yellow coating, and a slippery rapid pulse are all signs and symptoms of excess heat.

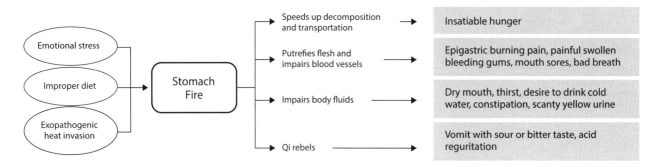

Chart 6.9 Etiology and pathogenesis of Stomach Fire

TCM Disease	Western Disease	Herbal Formulas		Acupuncture
Epigastric pain (胃痛)	Atrophic gastritis, gastric neurosis, peptic ulcer, GERD, gastric carcinoma	Xiao Xian Xiong Tang	Qing Wei San	ST-36, ST-45, PC-6, TB-6, GB-34, LR-2
Wasting and thirsting disorder (消渴)	Diabetes, hyperthyroidism	Yu Nu Jian, Xiao Ke Fang		ST-44, KI-3, BL-20, BL-21
Swollen gums (牙齦腫痛)	Periodontitis, ulcerations of oral cavity	Qing Wei San		LI-4, ST-6, ST-7
Vomiting (嘔吐)	Food poisoning, gastroenteritis, stomach flu, pregnancy, cholecystitis, ear infection, GERD	Ju Pi Zhu Ru Yin		BL-17, CV-17

Acupuncture column also includes: ST-34, ST-44, CV-12, CV-13, LI-4, LI-11, SP-15, CV-15

Table 6.8 Diseases and treatments related to Stomach Fire

Comparison: Stomach Fire vs. Stomach Yin Deficiency

Stomach fire (胃熱熾盛 *wèi rè chì shèng*) and Stomach yin deficiency (胃陰虛 *wèi yīn xū*) have the same pathological location and etiological factor of heat in the Stomach, and therefore share many symptoms including hunger, thirst, burning epigastric pain, dry stools, a red tongue, and a rapid pulse.

However, the pathogeneses of these two patterns are different. Stomach fire involves excess heat, which may have invaded from the exterior, transformed from other pathogenic factors, or resulted from an imbalanced diet, emotional stress, or improper lifestyle (smoking, drinking, drug abuse, caffeine). Excess heat speeds up the Stomach's decomposition and transformation function, and damages body fluids. It is an acute and excess syndrome with severe symptoms. Stomach yin deficiency, on the other hand, reflects damaged yin fluids, usually caused by febrile disease, major surgery, severe vomiting and diarrhea, improper diet, or improper treatment. The resulting yin-yang imbalance generates deficiency heat. It is a more chronic, deficient, and mild condition.

The key points to distinguish these two patterns are as follows:
(1) Hunger and food intake: excess intake, but still hungry vs. hunger but no desire to eat
(2) Thirst: thirst and desire to drink cold water vs. thirst with preference for warm or room temperature water
(3) Tongue and pulse

Pattern		Stomach Fire	Stomach Yin Deficiency
Etiology and pathogenesis		Exopathogens transfer inside or improper diet, excess heat speeds up Stomach decomposition and transformation function, damages body fluids	Febrile disease, bleeding, vomiting, diarrhea, or improper diet impairs or consumes yin, yin-yang imbalance generates deficiency heat
Characteristics		Excess heat, acute, short course, usually appears in early stage of febrile disease	Deficiency heat, chronic, long course, usually appears in later stage of febrile disease
Symptoms	Common	Hunger, thirst, burning pain in epigastrium, dry stool, red tongue, rapid pulse	
	Different	Overeats but still feels hungry, thirst and desire for cold drinks, severe pain that resists pressure, fever, bad breath, bleeding or swollen gums	Hungry but no desire to eat, thirst and preference for warm drinks, dull and vague pain improved with pressure, low-grade fever, dry belching, hiccups
Tongue		Red tongue with yellow coating	Red tongue with little or no coating
Pulse		Rapid, excess	Thin, rapid, deficient
Treatment strategy		Drain Stomach fire, and nourish the yin	Nourish yin, clear heat from the Stomach
Herbal formula		Qing Wei San	Sha Shen Mai Men Dong Tang, Yi Wei Tang, Yu Nu Jian

Table 6.9 Comparison of Stomach Fire and Stomach Yin Deficiency

4 Cold Invading the Stomach Pattern | 寒邪犯胃 |

Definition: A group of signs and symptoms involving the failure of Stomach qi to descend due to pathogenic cold invading the Stomach.

Clinical manifestations: Acute severe colicky epigastric and abdominal pain that is aggravated by cold and relieved by warmth, nausea, vomiting, epigastric pain relieved by vomiting or warmth, diarrhea with some undigested food, no thirst, profuse clear saliva, pale complexion, cold limbs, a pale tongue with moist white coating, and a wiry or deep tight pulse.

Key points: Epigastric cold pain, plus interior excess cold signs and symptoms.

Etiology and pathogenesis: This pattern usually arises due to excessive intake of raw, cold food and drink, or due to exopathogenic cold directly invading the Stomach.

Cold is a yin pathogen and easily damages yang qi, impairing its warming function, which causes cold limbs, pale complexion, a pale tongue, and a slow pulse. The nature of cold is congealing and stagnating. It blocks and obstructs the flow of qi and blood, resulting in pain that is relieved by warmth. When cold disrupts the Stomach's descending function, it stagnates qi, causing pain that worsens in response to cold or eating and improves after vomiting. Cold also slows down the Stomach's decomposition and descending function, resulting in undigested food accumulation in the Stomach that leads to diarrhea with some undigested food.

When yin excess causes a relative yang deficiency, the body is unable to warm and transform water and fluid, which causes accumulation of cold-dampness and leads to vomiting with clear fluid and a white moist tongue coating. When yang qi is deficient, the force behind blood circulation is weak, resulting in a slow pulse. Cold causes constriction and spasms, so the pulse may also be tight.

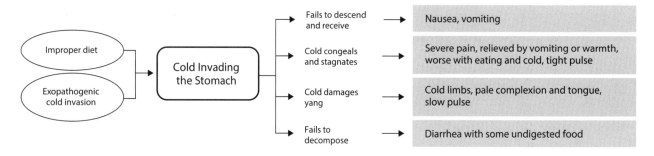

Chart 6.10 Etiology and pathogenesis of Cold Invading the Stomach

TCM Disease	Western Disease	Herbal Formulas		Acupuncture	
Epigastric pain (胃痛)	Acute or chronic gastritis, gastric and duodenal ulcer, gastric carcinoma, gastroneurosis, pyloric obstruction	Liang Fu Wan	Liang Fu Wan	ST-21, ST-34, SP-4, CV-13	CV-12, ST-36, PC-6
Vomiting (嘔吐)	Food poisoning, gastroenteritis, stomach flu, pregnancy		Hou Po Wen Zhong Tang		PC-6, ST-36, CV-17
Diarrhea (泄瀉)	Food poisoning, gastroenteritis, stomach flu		Huo Xiang Zheng Qi San With Wen Zhong Tang		ST-25, ST-36, CV-6, BL-25

Table 6.10 Diseases and treatments related to Cold Invading the Stomach

Comparison: Cold Invading the Stomach vs. Stomach Deficiency Cold

Cold invading the Stomach (寒邪犯胃 *hán xié fàn wèi*) and Stomach deficiency cold (胃中虛寒 *wèi zhōng xū hán*) have the same pathological location and etiological factor of cold in the Stomach, and therefore share many symptoms including cold epigastric pain that is relieved by warmth, pale complexion, pale tongue, and a slow pulse.

However, the pathogeneses for these two patterns are different. Cold invading the Stomach is caused by exopathogenic cold invasion that is acute and severe, making it an excess pattern. Stomach deficiency cold is caused by Stomach yang deficiency generating interior cold that is chronic and mild, making it a deficiency pattern.

The key points to distinguish these patterns are as follows:
(1) Nature of illness: acute and severe vs. chronic and mild
(2) Characteristics of the pain:
- Aggravated by pressure vs. relieved by pressure
- Colicky, excruciating pain vs. dull, vague pain

(3) Tongue and pulse

Pattern		Cold Invading the Stomach	Stomach Deficiency Cold
Etiology and pathogenesis		Excessive intake of raw cold food and drink, direct exopathogenic cold attack, Stomach yang impaired by cold, fails to descend and decompose	Long-term improper diet or chronic illness, Stomach yang deficiency then generates deficiency cold, fails to descend
Characteristics		Acute, severe, short course, excess	Chronic, mild, long course, deficiency
Symptoms	Common	Epigastric cold pain relieved by warmth, pale complexion and tongue, slow pulse	
	Different	Severe colicky pain that is resistant to pressure and worse after eating, pain relieved by warmth and after vomiting	Dull vague pain that is relieved by warmth and pressure and reduced after eating
	Other	Cold sensation in epigastric area, feels like an ice pack	Pale complexion, mental and physical fatigue, cold limbs, intolerance of cold
Tongue		Pale tongue, white glossy coating	Pale flabby tongue, thin white and moist coating
Pulse		Wiry or tight	Deep and weak
Treatment strategy		Dispel cold, warm middle burner, regulate Stomach, relieve pain	Tonify and warm Stomach, expel cold, relieve pain
Herbal formulas		Liang Fu Wan, Da Jiang Zhong Tang	Xiao Jiang Zhong Tang, Huang Qi Jiang Zhong Tang

Table 6.11 Comparison of Cold Invading the Stomach and Stomach Deficiency Cold

Comparison: Cold Invading the Stomach vs. Cold-Dampness Encumbering the Spleen

Cold invading the Stomach (寒邪犯胃 *hán xié fàn wèi*) and cold-dampness encumbering the Spleen (寒濕困脾 *hán shī kùn pí*) share the same pathogen and location: cold in the middle burner. Thus both patterns present with epigastric and abdominal pain that is relieved by warmth, nausea or vomiting, poor appetite, pale complexion, and cold limbs.

However, the pathogeneses of these two patterns are different. Cold invading the Stomach is caused by exopathogenic cold invasion that results in an acute onset, severe symptoms, and a short course. On the other hand, cold-dampness encumbering the Spleen is usually related to eating habits or living and working environments, which generate cold and dampness in the middle burner that impairs the Spleen yang, resulting in symptoms that are mild and longer course.

The key points to distinguish these two patterns are as follows:
   (1) Nature of illness: acute and severe vs. sub-acute or chronic and mild
   (2) Characteristics of the pain: colicky, excruciating pain vs. dull, distending pain
   (3) Tongue and pulse

Pattern		Cold Invading the Stomach	Cold-Dampness Encumbering the Spleen
Etiology and pathogenesis		Excessive intake of raw, cold food and drink or direct exopathogenic cold attack, Stomach yang impaired by cold fails to descend and decompose	Long-term improper diet consuming cold or raw food, or sweet and greasy food, living or working in cold damp environments, impairs the Spleen yang
Characteristics		Acute, severe, short course, excess	Sub-acute, chronic, mild, long course, excess
Symptoms	Common	Epigastric and abdominal cold pain relieved by warmth, nausea or vomiting, poor appetite, pale complexion, cold limbs	
Symptoms	Different	Severe colicky epigastric pain that is resistant to pressure and worse after eating, pain relieved by warmth or vomiting	Fullness, distention, and dull pain in the epigastrium and abdomen that is relieved by warmth
Symptoms	Others	Cold sensation in the epigastrium that feels like an ice pack	Yin jaundice, heaviness of the whole body, edema with scanty urine, bland but slimy taste in the mouth
Tongue		Pale tongue with white glossy coating	Flabby tongue with greasy coating
Pulse		Wiry or tight	Slow, moderate, slippery, or deep thin
Treatment strategy		Dispel cold, warm the middle, regulate the Stomach to relieve pain	Strengthen the Spleen, dry dampness
Herbal formulas		Liang Fu Wan, Da Jiang Zhong Tang	Liu Jun Zi Tang, Ping Wei San, Wu Ling San

Table 6.12 Comparison of Cold Invading the Stomach and Cold-Dampness Encumbering the Spleen

5 Food Stagnation Pattern | 食滯腸胃 |

Definition: A group of signs and symptoms caused by improper food intake that leads to food being retained in the Stomach.

Clinical manifestations: Epigastric and abdominal distention pain that resists pressure, rotten belching, acid regurgitation, aversion to food, sour vomiting, pain usually relieved after vomiting, diarrhea with sticky foul-smelling stools or constipation, a thick greasy tongue coating, and a slippery or deep excess pulse.

Key points: Epigastric and abdominal pain and distention, sour vomiting, sticky foul diarrhea, or acid regurgitation.

Etiology and pathogenesis: Improper diet, such as eating foods that are unhygienic or difficult to digest, overeating, overdrinking, and a weak constitution with Spleen and Stomach qi deficiency, can all lead to food stagnation.

The Stomach is a *fǔ* organ, empty and open, preferring to descend and be unobstructed. Improper diet, overeating, or food intake that surpasses the Stomach's rotting and ripening capability leads to undigested food remaining in the Stomach longer than is healthy. This affects the Stomach's descending function and results in qi stagnation, which manifests as distention, bloating, distress and fullness in the epigastrium, or even pain. Rebellious qi brings up undigested food, acid regurgitation or sour and rotten vomit, nausea, and bad breath. When inadequately processed food is transported downward, the intestines becomes overtaxed, causing aversion to food, frequent flatulence, or diarrhea with foul stools. Heat steams up stagnated rotten food, which condenses on the tongue's surface as a thick coating.

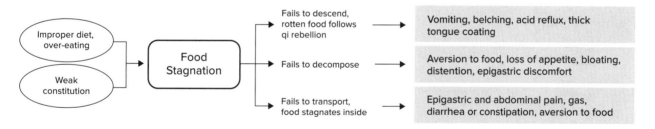

Chart 6.11 Etiology and pathogenesis of Food Stagnation

TCM Disease	Western Disease	Herbal Formulas	Acupuncture	
Epigastric pain (胃痛)	Atrophic gastritis, gastric neurosis, Peptic ulcer, GERD, gastric carcinoma	Bao He Wan, Zhi Shi Dao Zhi Wan	CV-10, CV-12, CV-13, ST-21, ST-44, SP-4, PC-6	LR-13, ST-36, LI-10, LI-13, ST-20, ST-25
Vomiting (嘔吐)	Food poisoning, gastroenteritis, stomach flu, pregnancy			CV-17, ST-36
Diarrhea (泄瀉)	Food poisoning, gastroenteritis, stomach flu, food allergy			ST-25, ST-36, CV-6, BL-25

Table 6.13 Diseases and treatments related to Food Stagnation

6 Blood Stagnation in the Stomach Pattern | 血瘀胃脘 |

Definition: A group of signs and symptoms that is marked by stabbing epigastric pain due to blood stagnation.

Clinical manifestations: Severe stabbing epigastric pain that may be worse at night or after eating and worse with pressure, nausea, vomiting, possibly vomiting blood, black tar-like stool, dull complexion and lips, a tongue that is purple or has purplish spotting, and a wiry or choppy pulse.

Key points: Stabbing epigastric pain, purple tongue, and choppy pulse.

Etiology and pathogenesis: Improper diet, toxic foods or herbs, overconsumption of alcohol, or long-term emotional stress usually cause this pattern. It can also be constitutional.

Blood stasis obstructs qi movement. Blood and qi fail to nourish the Stomach muscle and tissues, resulting in stabbing, piercing pain in a fixed location that is worse with pressure. Since blood stagnation accumulates more at night, pain is worse at that time. Food intake increases obstruction, so pain worsens after eating.

Blood stasis means blood cannot perform its normal functions. As a result, the Stomach qi is not nourished and fails to descend. Rebellious Stomach qi causes nausea and vomiting. If blood stagnation also causes bleeding, then symptoms of vomiting of blood or black stools arise. If blood stasis obstructs the vessels, it will appear as distended veins. The choppy and irregular pulse arises from impaired blood circulation.

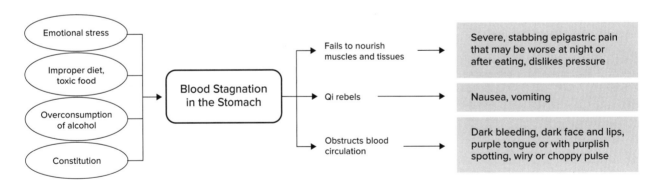

Chart 6.12   Etiology and pathogenesis of Blood Stagnation in the Stomach

TCM Disease	Western Disease	Herbal Formulas	Acupuncture
Epigastrium pain (胃痛)	Carcinoma of the stomach, gastric and duodenal ulcer, pyloric obstruction	Ge Xia Zhu Yu Tang, Shi Xiao San, Dan Shen Yin	ST-19, ST-21, ST-34, ST-40, KI-21, TB-6, PC-6, SP-4, SP-10, GB-34, CV-11, CV-12, BL-17, LI-4
Abdominal pain (腹痛)			
Hematochezia (便血)			
Hematemesis (吐血)			

Table 6.14   Diseases and treatments related to Blood Stagnation in the Stomach

Summary of Stomach Disease Patterns

Key points: nausea, vomiting, belching, hiccups, poor appetite, acid regurgitation, distention and bloating, epigastric discomfort or pain

	Patterns	Clinical manifestations	
		Common	Different
Deficiency	Stomach Yin Deficiency	Epigastric and abdominal pain with burning sensation, hunger but no desire to eat, dry mouth and throat, nausea, hiccups, dry stool, red tongue with a scanty dry coating, thin and rapid pulse	
	Stomach Deficiency Cold	Epigastric cold pain relieved by warmth, pale complexion and tongue, slow pulse	Dull vague pain relieved by pressure and reduced after eating, pale flabby tongue with a thin, white, and moist coating, deep and weak pulse
Excess	Cold Invading the Stomach		Severe colicky pain that resists pressure and is worse after eating, pain relieved after vomiting, tongue is pale with a white glossy coating, pulse is wiry or tight
	Stomach Fire	Epigastric and abdominal pain that resists pressure, bad breath, red tongue with a yellow coating, slippery and rapid pulse	Thirst and desire to drink cold water, excessive appetite, insatiable hunger, swelling and bleeding of the gums, constipation with dry stool
	Food Stagnation		Rotten belching, acid regurgitation, aversion to food, sour vomiting, pain usually relieved after vomiting or diarrhea, stool with sticky foul odor, constipation
	Blood Stagnation in the Stomach	Severe, stabbing epigastric pain that may be worse at night or after eating or with pressure, nausea, vomiting, possibly vomiting of blood, black tar-like stool, dull complexion and lips, purple tongue, wiry or choppy pulse	

Table 6.15 Summary of Stomach disease patterns

Chapter 7
Small Intestine Disease Patterns

Physiological characteristics and functions of the Small Intestine

The Small Intestine is located in the lower abdomen and is connected above to the Stomach through the pylorus and connected below to the Large Intestine. It is about a 20-feet long, hollow tubular organ with a tortuous, looped-back, and piled-up form. The Small Intestine channel starts at the ulnar side of the tip of the little finger and courses up the medial side of the arm to the posterior aspect of the shoulder. From the supraclavicular fossa, a branch connects with the Heart, Stomach, and Small Intestine. It is internally-externally connected with the Heart.

Known as the Minister of Reception (受盛之官 *shōu shèng zhī guān*), the Small Intestine receives partially digested food from the Stomach and further refines it, separating the clear from the turbid or the 'pure from the impure,' assimilating the purified nutrients, and moving the impure wastes onwards to the Large Intestine and Urinary Bladder for elimination.

1 | Receives and transforms

Receiving (受盛 *shòu shèng*) means accepting and storing, while transforming (化物 *huà wù*) means changing, digesting, compounding, and absorbing. Food in the Stomach is granulated, ground, and fermented into chyme that is then transported downward to the Small Intestine, where it will stay for a period of time to be further digested and absorbed. After the preliminary digestion by the Stomach, the Small Intestine conducts further digestion and absorption, extracting food and water essence to be used by the body as nutrients.

2 | Separates and secretes the clear and turbid

To separate the clear (分清 *fēn qīng*) means to absorb the food and water essence parts of the food received from the Stomach. With the assistance of the Spleen's ascending and transporting function, the food and water essence is sent up to the Lung and Heart to be distributed to the entire body.

To secrete the turbid (别浊 *bié zhuó*) involves two processes: one is moving solid food waste onward to the Large Intestine for elimination as stool; second is assisting the Kidney's qi transformation function by sending water waste to the Urinary Bladder for elimination as urine. Since the Small Intestine involves the body's water metabolism, it is said that the "Small Intestine governs *yè*-fluids" (小肠主液 *xiǎo cháng zhǔ yè*).

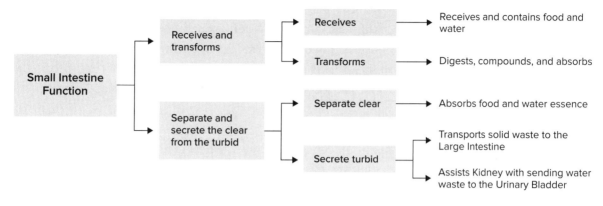

Chart 7.1 Small Intestine function summary

Common etiological factors in Small Intestine patterns

Small Intestine dysfunction can be the result of several factors including emotional stress, chronic illness, aging, improper lifestyle, and constitution. But the most common causes of Small Intestine dysfunction are improper diet and the direct invasion of exopathogens. The following are common etiological factors for Small Intestine disease patterns:

(1) Exopathogenic cold or damp-heat invasion
(2) Improper diet: overconsumption of cold, raw, spicy and hot, or greasy food, or the intake of unhygienic food or water
(3) Emotional stress
(4) Improper treatment, such as the overuse of cold, diaphoretic, or greasy herbs, or the lack of proper care after chronic illness
(5) Chronic illness that impairs Small Intestine function
(6) Constitution and aging

Pathological changes and major clinical manifestations of Small Intestine disease

Pathological changes in the Small Intestine are mostly caused by the Small Intestine failing to receive and transform, and failing to separate and secrete the clear and turbid. The major symptoms include abnormal urination and loose stools or diarrhea.

1 | Abnormal urination

Definition: Abnormal urination includes changes in quantity, such as copious or scanty urination; frequency, such as frequent, nocturnal, or reduced urination; color, such as yellow or clear urination; or changes in elimination, such as burning pain, dripping, or difficult urination. However, abnormal urination due to Small Intestine dysfunction mostly manifests in changes in quantity and frequency.

Etiology and pathomechanisms: The quantity and frequency of urination is based on the amount of fluid sent to the Urinary Bladder from the Small Intestine. When exopathogenic cold invades the Small Intestine, such as from improper diet of overeating cold foods, improper treatments, or yang deficiency resulting from chronic illness, the Small Intestine is unable to perform its function of transforming and separating the clear from the turbid, leading to excess fluid pouring into the Urinary Bladder and causing frequent and copious urination.

If pathogenic heat invades or accumulates in the Small Intestine, the heat consumes fluids, leading to less fluid being sent to the Urinary Bladder, resulting in scanty and short urination.

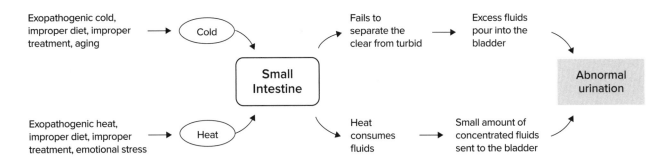

Chart 7.2 Etiology and pathomechanism of abnormal urination

2 | Loose stools or diarrhea

Definition: Frequent passing of watery or shapeless feces.

Etiology and pathomechanisms: Exopathogenic cold invasion, improper diet or treatment, chronic illness, and aging can all impair the function of the Small Intestine in transforming and absorbing fluids as well as in separating the clear from the turbid. This excess of fluids and unseparated food and water along with waste then pours down to the Large Intestine, increasing intestinal peristalsis and leading to diarrhea or loose stools.

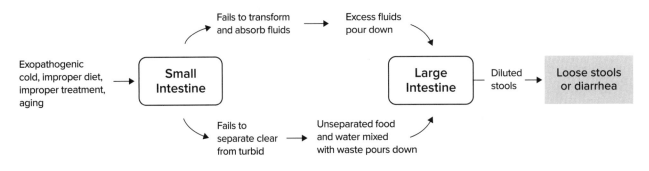

Chart 7.3 Etiology and pathomechanism of loose stools or diarrhea

3 | Other signs and symptoms related to the Small Intestine

Other signs and symptoms related to the Small Intestine include abdominal pain, abdominal distention, or borborygmus.

Physiological Function		Pathological Change	Clinical Manifestation
Receive and transform	Digestion and absorption	Fails to transform, unable to digest and absorb, causes unseparated food and water mixed with waste to pour down into the Large Intestine	Diarrhea or loose stools
	Reception and transportation	Fails to receive or transport, causes stagnation	Abdominal distention or pain
Separate and secrete the clear and turbid	Separate clear from turbid	Fails at reabsorption or ascending clear fluids, causes excess fluids to be sent to Bladder	Copious urination
	Secrete solid waste	Unabsorbed fluids pour down to the Large Intestine and dilute the stool	Diarrhea or loose stools, scanty urine

Table: 7.1 Physiological functions, pathological changes, and clinical manifestations of the Small Intestine

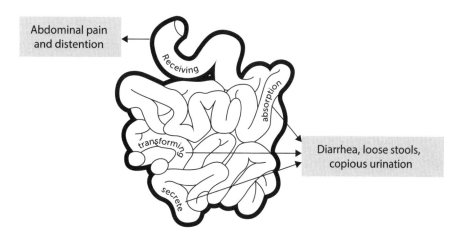

Chart 7.4 Small Intestine function and pathological symptoms

Common patterns in Small Intestine disease

Small Intestine Excess Fire, Small Intestine Qi Stagnation, and Small Intestine Deficiency Cold are the three most common patterns seen in the clinic. Small Intestine disease also includes some other patterns such as Small Intestine Qi Tied (小腸氣結 *xiǎo cháng qì jié*), infestation of worms in the Small Intestine, blood stagnation in the Small Intestine, damp-heat in the Small Intestine, and heat and cold combined in the Small Intestine. However, these patterns are either rarely seen in the clinic or not commonly recognized.

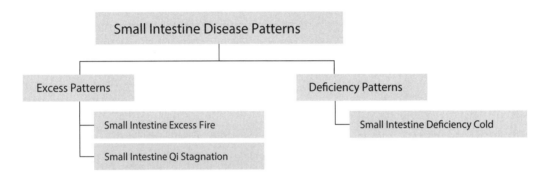

Chart 7.5 Common Small Intestine disease patterns

	Etiology	Patterns
Deficiency	Improper diet, chronic illness, physical overstrain, constitution, aging	Small Intestine Deficiency Cold
Excess	Exopathogens invasion, improper diet, emotional stress	Small Intestine Excess fire, Small Intestine Qi Stagnation

Table 7.2 Classification of common Small Intestine patterns

1 Small Intestine Deficiency Cold Pattern | 小腸虛寒 |

Definition: A group of signs and symptoms caused by Small Intestine yang deficiency failing to warm, manifesting in hypoactivity.

Clinical manifestations: Dull pain in the lower abdomen that is relieved by pressure and warmth, borborygmus, loose stools, frequent or clear and copious urination, intolerance of cold, cold limbs, low energy, a pale tongue with a thin white coating, and a deep, weak, or slow pulse.

Key points: Dull pain in the lower abdomen that is relieved by pressure and warmth, loose stools, and frequent or clear and copious urination, plus yang deficiency signs and symptoms.

Etiology and pathogenesis: This pattern can be caused by improper diet, overconsumption of cold food or cold drink impairing yang qi, exopathogenic cold invasion, or physical overstrain impairing yang qi. Chronic illness or weak constitution with Spleen and Stomach deficiency can also develop into this pattern.

The Small Intestine controls receiving and transforming as well as the reabsorption of fluids. It receives digested food from the Stomach and separates the clear from the turbid by reabsorbing and sending food and water essence up to the Lung with assistance from the Spleen and transporting the turbid into the Large Intestine to be excreted as stool. It also transports water waste to the Urinary Bladder to be excreted as urine. When yang qi is deficient, the Small Intestine lacks the motive force to reabsorb fluid, leading to excess fluid accumulation, diluting the stools in the Large Intestine, resulting in watery stools. When excess fluids pour down to the Urinary Bladder, there is frequent, clear and copious urination.

Yang qi has the function of warming the body. When the yang is insufficient, there is not enough power to warm the body. This gives rise to an intolerance of cold, cold limbs, and a preference for warm food and drink. The nature of cold is to congeal, constrict, and stagnate, thus cold may cause contraction and obstruction that blocks qi and blood circulation, which leads to pain that is aggravated by cold and relieved by warmth and pressure. A pale tender tongue and a slow feeble pulse all indicate yang deficiency.

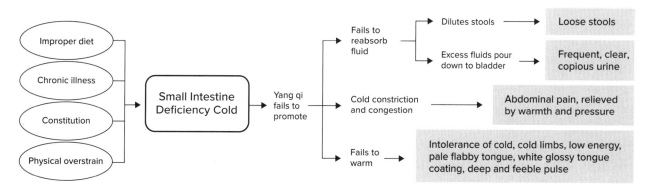

Chart 7.6 Etiology and pathogenesis of Small Intestine Deficiency Cold

TCM Disease	Western Disease	Herbal Formulas		Acupuncture	
Loose stools or diarrhea (泄瀉)	Chronic enteritis, Crohn's disease, chronic colitis, IBS, celiac disease, food allergies, SIBO	Wu Zhu Yu Tang	Shen Ling Bai Zhu San, Li Zhong Wan	ST-25, ST-36, ST-39, CV-4	BL-25, ST-37, SP-9
Abdominal pain (腹痛)	Diverticulitis, Crohn's disease, lead poisoning, celiac disease, IBS, lactose intolerance, food allergies		Fu Zi Li Zhong Wan		CV-12, SP-3, PC-6
Frequent urination (尿頻)	Overactive bladder, anxiety disorders, cystocele, benign prostatic hyperplasia, bladder stones, diabetes insipidus, diuretics, interstitial cystitis, pyelonephritis		Sang Piao Xiao San, Suo Quan Wan, Bu Zhong Yi Qi Tang		BL-28, BL-32, KI-3

Table 7.3 Diseases and treatments related to Small Intestine Deficiency Cold

2 Small Intestine Excess Fire Pattern | 小腸實火 |

Definition: A group of signs and symptoms caused by excessive heat accumulating inside the Small Intestine, presenting with burning painful urination as a major clinical manifestation.

Clinical manifestations: Frequent urination with painful, urgent, and burning sensation, scanty dark yellow urine or bloody urine, irritability, thirst with desire to drink cold water, sore throat, canker sores, tongue ulcers, a red tongue with yellow coating, and a rapid pulse. There may also be early stage exterior symptoms such as fever and chills and a superficial pulse.

Key points: Frequent urination with painful, burning, and urgent sensation or bloody urine, plus interior excess heat signs and symptoms.

Etiology and pathogenesis: This pattern can be caused by exopathogen invasion; improper diet, such as overconsumption of greasy, fatty, hot, and spicy foods, hot-natured herbs, or alcohol; and emotional strain, such as anxiety and excessive stress.

The Small Intestine governs yè-fluids (主液 zhǔ yè) and is responsible for separating the clear from the turbid. Thus if there is excess heat in the Small Intestine, the clear fluids fail to be separated and reabsorbed, resulting in excessive fluids combined with heat pouring down into the Urinary Bladder, disrupting the Urinary Bladder's qi transformation function, causing frequent urination with a burning, urgent, and painful sensation. If heat injures the blood vessels, then hematuria may result.

When pathogenic heat flares up, disturbing the *shén*, it may cause irritability or insomnia. If the pathogenic heat follows the Heart channel and flares upward, it may decompose the tissues and flesh of the mouth and tongue, leading to a red tongue, sore throat, and canker or tongue sores. When heat impairs the body fluids, there are signs and symptoms of thirst with a desire to drink cold water as well as yellow and scanty urination. If this pattern developed from exopathogen invasion, then chills and fever would appear in the early stages of the illness. This internal excess heat would also present a red tongue with yellow coating and a surging rapid pulse.

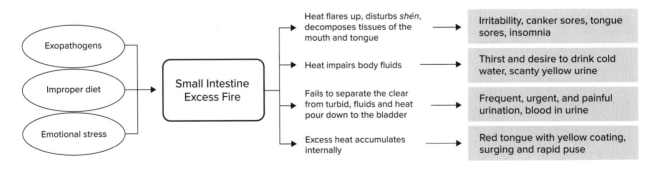

Chart 7.7 Etiology and pathogenesis of Small Intestine Excess Fire

TCM Disease	Western Disease	Herbal Formulas		Acupuncture	
Hot painful urinary dribbling (熱淋)	Cystitis, bladder infection, kidney infection, pyelonephritis, urethritis, interstitial cystitis, prostatitis	Dao Chi San, Zhu Ling Tang	Ba Zheng San	SI-2, SI-5, HT-5, HT-8, ST-39	LI-11, BL-28, BL-48
Hematuria (血淋)	UTI, pyelonephritis, prostatitis, glomerulonephritis, vasculitis, kidney or bladder stone or cancer		Xiao Ji Yin Zi		BL-22, BL-23, BL-27, PC-7, PC-8

Table 7.4 Diseases and treatments related to Small Intestine Excess Fire

3 Small Intestine Qi Stagnation Pattern | 小腸氣滯 |

Definition: A group of signs and symptoms caused by qi stagnation in the Small Intestine with twisting colicky pain in the lower abdomen as a major clinical manifestation. This pattern is also known as Small Intestine Qi Pain (小腸氣痛 *xiǎo cháng qì tòng*).

Clinical manifestations: Lower abdominal twisting colicky pain, which may extend to the scrotum area, abdominal distention, dislike of pressure on the abdomen, borborygmus, flatulence, and abdominal pain relieved by passing gas, a normal tongue with a white coating, and a deep wiry pulse.

Key points: Lower abdominal twisting pain, borborygmus, and pain relieved by passing gas.

Etiology and pathogenesis: Mostly caused by exopathogenic cold invasion, this pattern may result from improper diet such as overconsumption of cold or raw food, or due to cold climate and unsuitable attire. This pattern can also develop from excessive emotions, especially from anger and wailing.

When exopathogenic cold invades the Small Intestine, it congeals and constricts, leading to qi stagnation in the area that causes distention and pain. Since passing gas will reduce the local tension, the pain will be relieved after passing gas and worsen with pressure. If qi stagnation pushes down the Small Intestine, trapping it in the scrotum, there will be colicky or twisting pain in the lower abdomen, radiating to the scrotum and testicle area.

When qi and dampness lodge in the Small Intestine and there is a stalemate, borborygmus may result. Colicky pain pushes blood outward, increasing tension of the vessels, so there is a wiry pulse. Since the pathological changes are located in the lower part of the body, the pulse will also be deep.

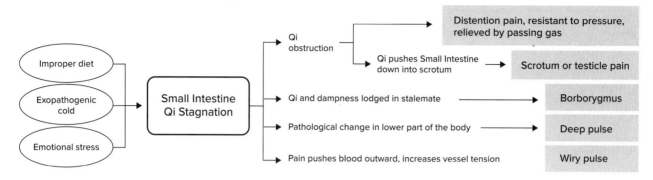

Chart 7.8 Etiology and pathogenesis of Small Intestine Qi Stagnation

TCM Disease	Western Disease	Herbal Formulas		Acupuncture	
Cold hernia (寒疝)	Inguinal hernia, umbilical hernia, femoral hernia	Mu Xiang Shun Qi Wan, Wu Yao Wan, Ju He Wan	Nuan Gan Jian	CV-12, CV-6, ST-36, TB-6, LR-1	CV-3, CV-6, SP-6
Qi hernia (氣疝)	Inguinal hernia, umbilical hernia, femoral hernia		Tian Tai Wu Yao San		
Abdominal pain (腹痛)	Diverticulitis, Crohn's disease, lead poisoning, celiac disease, IBS, lactose intolerance, food allergies, SIBO		Wu Zhu Yu Tang plus Shao Yao Gan Cao Tang		SP-6, LR-3, LI-4, ST-25

Table 7.5 Diseases and treatments related to Small Intestine Qi Stagnation

Summary of Small Intestine Disease Patterns

	Patterns	Clinical manifestations
Deficiency	Small Intestine Deficiency Cold	Dull pain in lower abdomen, which is relieved by pressure and warmth, borborygmus, loose stool, frequent or clear and copious urination. A pale tongue with a thin white coating, and a deep weak or slow pulse.
Excess	Small Intestine Excess Fire	Frequent urination with painful, urgent, and burning sensation. Scanty dark yellow or bloody urine. Irritability, thirst, and desire to drink cold water, sore throat, canker sores or tongue ulcers. Red tongue with yellow coating and a rapid pulse.
Excess	Small Intestine Qi Stagnation	Lower abdominal twisting (colicky) pain, which may extend to scrotum area, abdominal distention, dislike of pressure on abdomen, borborygmi, flatulence, abdominal pain relieved by passing gas. A normal tongue with a white coating, and a deep and wiry pulse.

Key points: abnormal urination (frequent and/or copious urination, scanty and short urination), loose stools or diarrhea

Table 7.6 Summary of Small Intestine disease patterns

Chapter 8
Large Intestine Disease Patterns

Physiological characteristics and functions of the Large Intestine

The Large Intestine is connected to the Small Intestine above and the anus below. The Large Intestine channel begins at the radial side of the tip of the index finger and continues proximally along the radial edge of the arm to the elbow, up to the lateral aspect of the arm to the shoulder. It descends internally, connecting first to the Lung and then the Large Intestine. Thus the Large Intestine and the Lung are internally-externally related and they are both associated with the phase of metal and the emotion of grief.

The Large Intestine is called the Minister of Transportation (傳導之官 *chuán dǎo zhī guān*). The physiological function of the Large Intestine is mainly to receive food waste sent down from the Small Intestine. After reabsorbing any remaining food and water essences, the Large Intestine transports the waste and transforms it into stool for excretion through the anus, all of which are accomplished by the propelling function of the Large Intestine qi.

1 | Transportation

The Large Intestine receives the food waste sent down from the Small Intestine and transports it downward to the anus for excretion.

2 | Reabsorption

The Large Intestine reabsorbs any remaining food and water essences from the food waste. This food and water essence, with the assistance of the Spleen's ascending function, will be sent upward to the Lung for distribution. The Large Intestine reabsorbs water essence and transforms desiccated food waste into stool, playing an important part in the body's water metabolism. Thus it is said that the Large Intestine governs *jīn*-fluids (大腸主津 *dà cháng zhǔ jīn*).

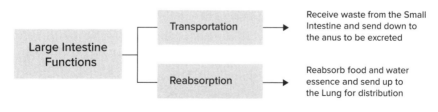

Chart 8.1 Large Intestine function summary

Common etiological factors in Large Intestine patterns

Exopathogenic factors invasion and improper diet are the two major etiological factors for Large Intestine disease. But aging and chronic illness may also result in a Large Intestine pattern. The following are common etiological factors for Large Intestine disease patterns:

(1) Exopathogenic cold-dampness or damp-heat invasion
(2) Improper diet: overconsumption of cold, raw, greasy, or hot and spicy food; or intake of unhygienic food or water
(3) Improper treatment: overuse of cold or hot herbs, diaphoretics, or greasy herbs; or lack of proper care after chronic illness
(4) Chronic illness impairs Large Intestine function
(5) Constitution and aging

Pathological changes and major clinical manifestations of Large Intestine disease

Pathological changes of the Large Intestine are usually caused by disorder of the Large Intestine transmitting and transporting function, as well as the organ's failure to reabsorb fluids. The most common clinical manifestation of Large Intestine disorder are diarrhea or loose stools, and constipation.

1 | Diarrhea or loose stools

Definition: Frequent passing of watery or shapeless feces.

Etiology and pathomechanisms: Diarrhea or loose stools are usually caused by excess fluids or dampness accumulating in the Large Intestine with increased intestinal peristalsis.

Dampness can arise from the exterior invasion of exopathogenic damp-heat, cold-dampness, or improper diet, such as eating unhygienic food. In these cases, the diarrhea and loose stools may also be accompanied by exterior signs and symptoms such as fever, chills, and a superficial pulse.

Chronic illness, aging, improper diet or treatment, and emotional stress can all cause *zàng fǔ* organ dysfunction, giving rise to internal dampness, especially of the Spleen, Kidney, Lung, Small Intestine, Large Intestine, and Triple Burner. If the Spleen fails to transport and transform, the Kidney fails to transform qi, the Lung fails to descend and disperse, the Triple Burner fails in the passage of water, and the Small Intestine and Large Intestine fail to reabsorb fluids and dessicate food waste, then dampness and water accumulation will pour downward to the Large Intestine and dilute stools, leading to diarrhea or loose stools.

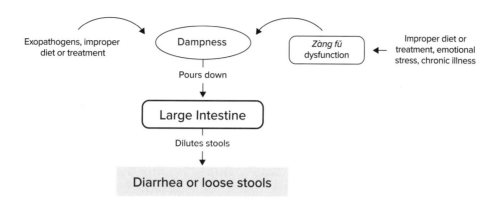

Chart 8.2 Etiology and pathomechanism of diarrhea or loose stools

2 | Constipation

Definition: Difficulty in passing stools, prolonged intervals between stools, or a desire to defecate without the ability to do so, either partially or completely.

Etiology and pathomechanisms: Constipation is associated with the dysfunction of the Large Intestine's ability to transport. The cause of this dysfunction can be divided into three pathways of disease development:

(1) The Large Intestine lacks moisture. This may be due to pathogenic heat in the Large Intestine and Stomach, which consumes body fluids, or to yin or blood deficiency arising from a chronic illness, aging, profuse sweating, bleeding, or improper treatment.

(2) The Large Intestine loses its motive force and power of transportation. This may be caused by qi stagnation arising from emotional stress, or by qi and yang deficiency as a result of aging or chronic illness.

(3) The Large Intestine is obstructed by a pathological accumulation such as food, blood, or phlegm stagnation. This may result from improper diet, emotional stress, or dysfunction of a *zàng fǔ* organ.

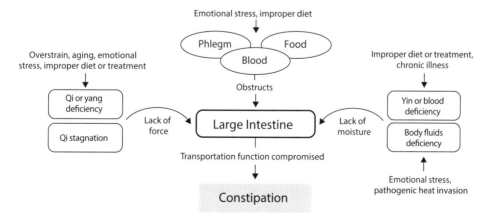

Chart 8.3 Etiology and pathomechanism of constipation

3 | Other signs and symptoms related to the Large Intestine

The following signs and symptoms can also appear in Large Intestine patterns: abdominal distention, bloating, and borborygmus.

	Etiology	Patterns
Deficiency	Improper diet, improper treatment, chronic illness, constitution, aging	Large Intestine Deficiency Cold, Large Intestine Dryness
Excess	Exopathogen invasion, improper diet, improper treatment	Large Intestine Cold-Dampness, Large Intestine Damp-Heat, Large Intestine Heat Accumulation

Table 8.1 Classification of common Large Intestine patterns

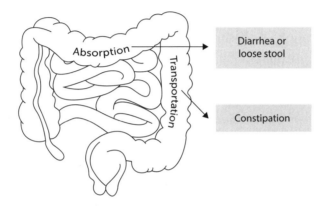

Chart 8.4 Large Intestine function and pathological symptoms

Common patterns in Large Intestine disease

There are five common Large Intestine disease patterns seen in the clinic. Based on the clinical manifestations, Large Intestine patterns are either excess or deficient. Depending on the nature of the pathogens, excess patterns can be divided into two groups: heat and cold. Excess heat patterns includes Large Intestine Damp-Heat and Large Intestine Heat Accumulation, while excess cold patterns include Large Intestine Cold-Dampness. Deficiency patterns include Large Intestine Deficiency Cold and Large Intestine Dryness.

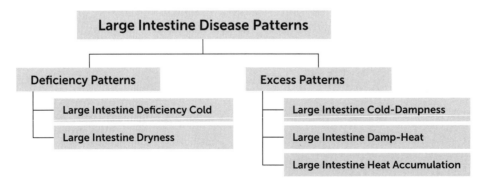

Chart 8.5 Common Large Intestine disease patterns

	Etiology	Patterns
Deficiency	Improper diet, improper treatment, chronic illness, constitution, aging	Large Intestine Deficiency Cold, Large Intestine Dryness
Excess	Exopathogen invasion, improper diet, improper treatment	Large Intestine Cold-Dampness, Large Intestine Damp-Heat, Large Intestine Heat Accumulation

Table 8.2 Classification of common Large Intestine patterns

1 Large Intestine Deficiency Cold Pattern | 大腸虛寒 |

Definition: A group of signs and symptoms arising from yang qi deficiency of the Large Intestine that causes a failure to transport and leads to abnormal bowel movements.

Clinical manifestations: Chronic loose stools or constipation, borborygmus, fecal incontinence, anal prolapse, dull abdominal pain with a preference for warmth and pressure, intolerance of cold, cold limbs, clear copious urine, a pale tongue with white coating, and a deep, slow, feeble pulse.

Key points: Abnormal bowel movements, diarrhea or constipation, plus yang deficiency cold signs and symptoms.

Etiology and pathogenesis: This pattern can be caused by improper diet, overconsumption of cold foods, and prolonged diarrhea and dysentery impairing yang qi. Aging and a weak constitution with yang deficiency can also develop into this pattern.

The Large Intestine controls the transportation and reabsorption of fluids. It receives digested food from the Small Intestine, reabsorbs fluids, and then dessicates and transforms the food waste into stool to be sent down for elimination through the anus. When yang qi is deficient, the Large Intestine lacks the motive force to reabsorb fluids, leading to excess fluid accumulation that dilutes the stools, resulting in watery stools. Since yang qi is the motive force for intestinal peristalsis, a deficiency can also slow down peristalsis, leading to constipation.

Yang qi has the function of warming the body. When it is deficient, there is insufficient power to warm the body, giving rise to an intolerance of cold, cold limbs, and a preference for warm food and drink. The nature of cold is to congeal and stagnate, which causes obstruction of qi and blood circulation, leading to pain that is aggravated by cold and relieved by warmth and pressure. The tongue will be pale and tender and the pulse will be slow and feeble.

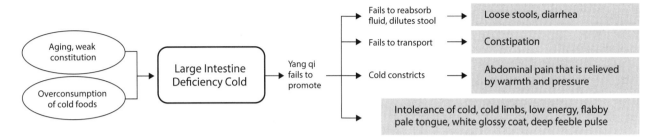

Chart 8.6 Etiology and pathogenesis of Large Intestine Deficiency Cold

TCM Disease	Western Disease	Herbal Formulas	Acupuncture
Abdominal pain (腹痛)	Chronic dysentery, chronic enteritis, ulcerative colitis, Crohn's disease, SIBO, IBS, parasites	Liang Fu Wan, Fu Zi Li Zhong Wan	ST-25, ST-36, ST-37, CV-6, BL-20, BL-25
Chronic dysentery (慢性痢疾)			
Diarrhea (泄瀉)			
Constipation (便秘)	Habitual constipation, hypothyroid, SIBO, IBS		ST-25, ST-36, ST-44, SP-6, CV-4, KI-3, TB-6

Table 8.3 Diseases and treatments related to Large Intestine Deficiency Cold

Comparison: Large Intestine Deficiency Cold vs. Spleen Yang Deficiency vs. Kidney Yang Deficiency

Large Intestine deficiency cold (大腸虛寒 *dà cháng xū hán*), Spleen yang deficiency (脾陽虛 *pí yáng xū*), and Kidney yang deficiency (腎陽虛 *shèn yáng xū*) all share the major pathogenesis of yang qi deficiency, and therefore they all manifest with chronic diarrhea, loose stools, dull abdominal pain with a preference for warmth and pressure, a pale flabby tongue, a deep feeble pulse, and other yang deficiency signs and symptoms. However, the major organs undergoing pathological change are different in each pattern.

The location of the Large Intestine is in the lower burner where its function is to receive digested food from the Small Intestine, absorb fluids, and excrete stools. Thus Large Intestine yang deficiency diarrhea involves the dysfunction of fluid absorption, which results in excess fluid causing borborygmus and diluted stools that resemble duck droppings.

In Spleen yang deficiency, the location of pathological change is in the middle burner. The Spleen's failure to transform and transport generates dampness that floods into the Large Intestine and dilutes stools. This leads to intermittent soft and loose stools, which are worse after eating greasy and cold foods. Spleen yang deficiency will also present with poor appetite, distention, and discomfort after the intake of food.

The Kidney is in the lower burner, but its yang qi provides motive force for the entire body. Therefore, when Kidney yang is deficient, there is not enough power for the rotting and ripening of food, leading to water metabolism dysfunction and diarrhea with undigested food. Early morning or 'cockcrow' diarrhea occurs because deficient Kidney yang cannot lift Spleen yang during the early morning, which is the coldest time of the day. As a result, Spleen yang descends and causes abdominal pain and diarrhea. Since pathogenic coldness is expelled through defecation, abdominal pain will be relieved after the diarrhea passes.

The key points to distinguish these three patterns are as follows:
1)   Shape of the stool
2)   Time of the diarrhea
3)   Accompanying symptoms

Pattern		Large Intestine Deficiency Cold	Spleen Yang Deficiency	Kidney Yang Deficiency
Etiology		Chronic illness, improper diet, weak constitution, aging		
Pathogenesis		Yang deficiency lack of power to reabsorb fluids	Failure to transport and transform	Failure to provide yang qi for digestion and absorption
Characteristics		Chronic, deficiency, cold		
Symptoms	Common	Chronic diarrhea, loose stool, dull abdominal pain, pale flabby tongue with white moist coating, deep and slow, or deep and feeble pulse		
	Different	Loose stools like duck droppings, light color without strong odor, borborygmus	Intermittent soft and loose stools, worse with intake of greasy or cold foods	Early morning diarrhea with undigested food, abdominal cramps relieved after bowel movement
	Other	Borborygmus	Poor appetite, distention and discomfort after eating	Cold limbs and body, impotence, irregular menses
Treatment strategy		Tonify and warm Large Intestine	Tonify Spleen, warm yang, stop diarrhea	Warm and tonify Kidney, stop diarrhea
Herbal formulas		Liang Fu Wan	Shen Ling Bai Zhu San	Si Shen Wan

Table 8.4 Comparison of Large Intestine Deficiency Cold, Spleen Yang Deficiency, and Kidney Yang Deficiency

Comparison: Large Intestine Deficiency Cold vs. Small Intestine Deficiency Cold

Large Intestine deficiency cold (大腸虛寒 *dà cháng xū hán*) and Small Intestine deficiency cold (小腸虛寒 *xiǎo cháng xū hán*) have similar etiology and pathogenesis with almost identical symptoms, including dull pain in the lower abdomen that is relieved by pressure and warmth, borborygmus, loose stools or diarrhea, clear copious urine, cold limbs, a pale tongue with a thin white coating, and a deep weak or slow pulse. Their treatment strategies are also the same, and therefore in clinic we refer to these two patterns as 'deficiency cold in the lower burner.'

Since the Small Intestine is located above the Large Intestine, when the Small Intestine fails to separate the clear from the turbid and fails to absorb the food and water essences, the Large Intestine can substitute with its reabsorption function, reducing the amount of food and water essences that would otherwise have been eliminated. Thus loose stools or diarrhea caused by Small Intestine deficiency cold is mild and the stool shape is soft. In contrast, the Large Intestine directly connects with the anus and when Large Intestine deficiency cold causes failure to reabsorb fluids, that excess fluid dilutes the contents of the Large Intestine, resulting in watery, muddy, or shapeless stools resembling duck droppings. Furthermore, Large Intestine deficiency cold may also manifest with constipation, fecal incontinence, or rectal prolapse.

The Small Intestine 'governs *yè*-fluids', separates and secretes, and is involved in water metabolism. When Small Intestine yang qi is deficient, it fails to reabsorb fluids, leading to excess fluids pouring down to the Urinary Bladder. Thus the main symptom for Small Intestine deficiency cold is clear copious urination.

The key points to distinguish these two patterns are as follows:
1) Stool shape: soft stool vs. stool resembling duck droppings
2) Presence of fecal incontinence or rectal prolapse
3) Main symptom: abnormal urination vs. abnormal stools

Pattern		Small Intestine Deficiency Cold	Large Intestine Deficiency Cold
Etiology		\multicolumn{2}{c}{Improper diet, chronic illness, and constitution}	
Pathogenesis		Failure to separate clear from turbid, leads to extra fluids pouring down	Failure to reabsorb fluids, dilutes stool
Characteristics		Chronic, deficiency, cold	
Symptoms	Common	Dull pain in the lower abdomen, relieved by pressure and warmth, borborygmus, loose stools or diarrhea, clear copious urine, cold limbs, a pale tongue with thin white coating, and a deep weak or slow pulse	
	Main	Clear copious urine	Diarrhea or loose stools
	Stool	Soft	Watery, muddy, or like duck drops
	Other		Fecal incontinence, rectal prolapse
Treatment strategy		Warm and tonify the Intestines	
Herbal formulas		Wu Zhu Yu Tang, Fu Zi Li Zhong Wan, Liang Fu Wan	

Table 8.5 Comparison of Small Intestine Deficiency Cold and Large Intestine Deficiency Cold

2 Large Intestine Dryness Pattern | 大腸液虧 |

Definition: A group of signs and symptoms involving a deficiency of yin fluids in the Large Intestine that causes a failure to transport and results in dry stools or difficult defecation.

Clinical manifestations: Dry stools, difficult defecation, no bowel movements for days, thirst, dry mouth, red tongue with a dry, scanty coating, and a thin or thin and rapid pulse.

Key points: Constipation, dry stools, plus body fluids deficiency signs and symptoms.

Etiology and pathogenesis: This pattern is usually associated with a yin deficiency constitution or yin and blood deficiency that arises from aging. Diarrhea, vomiting, and chronic illness can also contribute to this condition. Additionally, it can occur in the later stages of febrile diseases when body fluids are impaired or after prolonged bleeding or postpartum bleeding that damages blood and body fluids.

When body fluids are insufficient, the Large Intestine will lack nourishment and moisture. This impairs its transportation function and slows down peristalsis. The intestinal waste dries up and is delayed from elimination, leading to dry stools and difficult defecation. This lack of body fluids will be accompanied by dry mouth, thirst, scanty urine, a dry tongue coating, and a thin pulse. If dryness turns into heat, there will be a red tongue and a rapid pulse.

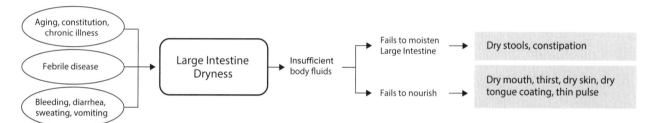

Chart 8.7 Etiology and pathogenesis of Large Intestine Dryness

TCM Disease	Western Disease	Herbal Formulas	Acupuncture
Constipation (便秘)	Postpartum constipation, habitual constipation, hemorrhoids, IBS, aphthous ulcers, hyperthyroid, chronic pancreatitis, or side effect associated with radiation therapy	Run Chang Wan, Ma Zi Ren Wan, Zeng Ye Cheng Qi Tang	ST-25, ST-36, ST-44, SP-6, CV-4, KI-3, KI-6, LI-11, TB-6

Table 8.6 Diseases and treatments related to Large Intestine Dryness

3 Large Intestine Cold-Dampness Pattern | 大腸寒濕 |

Definition: A group of signs and symptoms caused by cold-dampness accumulation inside the Large Intestine, impairing its transforming and reabsorbing functions.

Clinical manifestations: Borborygmus, paroxysmal cold pain of the umbilicus and abdomen, watery diarrhea, a white and glossy or thick tongue coating, and a slippery or wiry tight pulse. There may be accompanying exterior symptoms such as chills and fever, headache, and a superficial pulse.

Key points: Watery diarrhea with borborygmus and pain in the umbilicus and abdominal region, plus cold-dampness signs and symptoms.

Etiology and pathogenesis: This pattern arises from exopathogenic cold-dampness invasion or improper diet, such as overconsumption of cold, raw, and greasy food, or due to the intake of unhygienic food, resulting in accumulation of cold-dampness diluting the stools and disrupting the Large Intestine's transporting function.

Dampness pours down and dilutes stools, forming clear, diluted, and even watery stools with an acute onset. Cold causes contraction and stagnation of qi, thus leading to paroxysmal abdominal pain. When qi and dampness attack each other, intestinal sounds ensue. When the qi is stronger than the dampness, the sound is loud. Cold causes constriction, so the pulse is tight or wiry. Dampness is viscous and sticky, so the pulse can also be slippery and the tongue has a thick and greasy coating.

If this pattern is caused by exopathogenic cold-dampness invasion, protective qi will rise up against the pathogen. This process may weaken or impair the protective qi's warming function and therefore the patient feels an aversion to cold. Meanwhile, the struggle between the protective qi and the exopathogens will create heat and lead to an increase in body temperature, resulting in chills and fever. When yang qi rises up against exopathogens, the result is a superficial pulse.

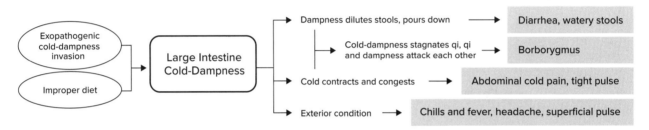

Chart 8.8 Etiology and pathogenesis of Large Intestine Cold-Dampness

TCM Disease	Western Disease	Herbal Formulas	Acupuncture
Abdominal pain (腹痛)	Acute enteritis, ulcerative colitis, Crohn's disease, food poisoning, viral gastroenteritis	Wei Ling Tang, Huo Xiang Zheng Qi San	ST-25, ST-36, CV-6, CV-12
Dysentery (痢疾)			
Diarrhea (泄瀉)			

Table 8.7 Diseases and treatments related to Large Intestine Cold-Dampness

Comparison: Large Intestine Cold-Dampness vs. Large Intestine Deficiency Cold

Large Intestine deficiency cold (大腸虛寒 dà cháng xū hán) and Large Intestine cold-dampness (大腸寒濕 dà cháng hán shī) share the same etiological factors and pathological location, and thus clinical manifestations are similar, including diarrhea, loose or watery stools, abdominal cold pain, and a pale tongue with a white glossy coating.

However, the nature and pathogenesis of these two patterns are different. Large Intestine deficiency cold is a deficiency condition that is mostly caused by endopathogenic factors. Yang qi deficiency fails to promote the Large Intestine's function of reabsorbing fluids and transporting food wastes, leading to cold-dampness accumulation in the Large Intestine that can cause loose stools or constipation. On the other hand, Large Intestine cold-dampness is a condition of excess that is usually caused by exopathogenic factors. Cold and dampness lodge in the Large Intestine, disrupting its function.

The key points to distinguish these two patterns are as follows:
1) Acute, short course, severe vs. chronic, long course, mild
2) Whether there is preference for pressure
3) Forceful pulse or feeble pulse

Pattern		Large Intestine Deficiency Cold	Large Intestine Cold-Dampness
Etiology and pathogenesis		Weak constitution or improper diet impairs yang qi, failure to reabsorb fluids dilutes stools	Exopathogenic cold invasion or improper diet causes cold-dampness accumulation, disrupts reabsorption function
Characteristics		Chronic, deficiency, mild	Acute onset, short course, excess, more severe
Symptoms	Common	Diarrhea, loose or watery stools, cold, pale tongue with white glossy coating, deep pulse	
	Different	Dull abdominal pain, preference for warmth and pressure, intolerance of cold, cold limbs, a flabby tongue, a slow feeble pulse	Severe watery stool with borborygmus, cold pain of the umbilicus and abdomen, pulse may be wiry or tight
	Stools	Loose stools or constipation	Watery stools, diarrhea
Treatment strategy		Warm and tonify the Large Intestine, stop diarrhea	Warm the interior, eliminate dampness, stop diarrhea
Herbal formulas		Liang Fu Wan	Wei Ling Tang, Huo Xiang Zheng Qi San

Table 8.8 Comparison of Large Intestine Deficiency Cold and Large Intestine Cold-Dampness

4 Large Intestine Damp-Heat Pattern | 大腸濕熱 |

Definition: A group of signs and symptoms caused by damp-heat accumulation in the Large Intestine that inhibits its ability to transport and reabsorb, leading to diarrhea or dysentery.

Clinical manifestations: Abdominal pain, diarrhea with pus and blood, tenesmus, loose stools with discomfort or burning sensation of the anus, yellow sticky stools with strong foul odor, possibly fever, thirst, scanty yellow urine, a red tongue with a yellow greasy coating, and a slippery and rapid pulse. There may also be accompanying exterior symptoms such as chills and fever, headache, and a superficial pulse.

Key points: Dysentery or diarrhea, plus damp-heat signs and symptoms.

Etiology and pathogenesis: This pattern mostly happens between summer and fall and is often caused by exopathogenic summer-heat invading the intestines or from eating unhygienic food, causing damp-heat and turbidity to accumulate inside the Large Intestine.

Damp-heat invading the Large Intestine disrupts its transporting and reabsorbing function, thus damp-heat pours down and results in diarrhea. Damp-heat accumulation in the Large Intestine putrefies flesh and injures blood vessels, producing blood and pus. Damp-heat obstructs qi flow in the intestines causing a qi and dampness stalemate that results in tenesmus. Heat leads to rotting and decay, so the stool is sticky with a foul odor. Fever, thirst, a red tongue with a yellow coating, and a rapid pulse are all caused by heat, while a greasy tongue coating and a slippery pulse are caused by dampness.

If this pattern is caused by exopathogenic damp-heat invasion, protective qi will rise up against the pathogen. This process may weaken or impair the protective qi's warming function, causing the patient to feel an aversion to cold. Meanwhile, the struggle between the protective qi and exopathogen will create heat, leading to an increase in body temperature. Thus there may be chills and fever. The pulse will also be superficial as a result of yang qi rising up against the exopathogen.

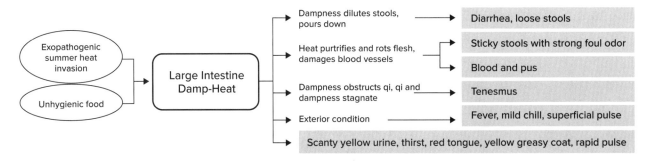

Chart 8.9 Etiology and pathogenesis of Large Intestine Damp-Heat

TCM Disease	Western Disease	Herbal Formulas		Acupuncture	
Abdominal pain (腹痛)	Crohn's disease, diverticulitis, appendicitis, IBD	Ge Gen Qin Lian Tang, Tao He Cheng Qi Tang	Shao Yao Tang	ST-25, ST-36, ST-44, SP-9	SP-3, PC-6
Dysentery (痢疾)	Acute bacillary dysentery, amebic dysentery, Crohn's disease		Bai Tou Weng Tang		ST-37, CV-12, LI-11
Diarrhea (泄瀉)	Acute enteritis, ulcerative colitis, IBS, IBD, dysentery, gastroenteritis		Ge Gen Qin Lian Tang		BL-25, ST-37
Intestinal abscess (腸癰)	Intestinal abscess, appendicitis, diverticulitis, ulcerative colitis		Da Huang Mu Dan Tang		Lan Wei Xue, LI-11
Hemorrhoid (痔瘡)	Hemorrhoid		Huai Jiao Wan		GV-1, BL-35, BL-57, Er Bai

Table 8.9 Diseases and treatments related to Large Intestine Damp-Heat

Comparison: Large Intestine Damp-Heat vs. Large Intestine Cold-Dampness

Large Intestine damp-heat (大腸濕熱 *dà cháng shī rè*) and Large Intestine cold-dampness (大腸寒濕 *dà cháng hán shī*) both involve accumulation of dampness in the Large Intestine as one of the major pathogeneses. They are both acute onset, short course, excess conditions usually caused by improper diet and intake of unhygienic food or drink. They present with abdominal pain, diarrhea, chills and fever, headache, a superficial pulse, and other exterior signs and symptoms. However, one pattern involves dampness with heat while the other involves dampness with cold, and therefore the clinical manifestation is different.

The key points to distinguish these two patterns are as follows:
1) Stool color, odor, and shape
2) Abdominal pain: cold vs. burning pain
3) Accompanying signs and symptoms: borborygmus vs. burning sensation of the anus
4) Tongue and pulse

Pattern		Large Intestine Damp-Heat	Large Intestine Cold-Dampness
Etiology	Common	Exopathogenic factors invasion, improper diet, intake of unhygienic food and water	
	Different	Damp-heat	Cold-dampness
Characteristics		Acute onset, short course, excess, may be exterior combined with interior	
		Heat	Cold
Symptoms	Common	Diarrhea, abdominal pain, thick tongue coating, slippery pulse, may have chills and fever, superficial pulse	
	Stools	Muddy, sticky yellow stool with pus and blood, strong foul odor	Watery diarrhea, light color, less odor
	Other	Tenesmus, discomfort or burning sensation of the anus	Borborygmus, paroxysmal cold pain
	Exterior	Thirst, yellow urine, may have fever and mild chills	May have chills and mild fever
Tongue		Red with yellow thick coating	Pale with white thick coating
Pulse		Rapid and slippery	Slow and slippery, or superficial and tight
Treatment strategy		Expel dampness, clear heat, stop diarrhea	Warm the interior, expel dampness, stop diarrhea
Herbal formulas		Ge Gen Qin Lian Tang, Bai Tou Weng Tang	Wei Ling Tang, Huo Xiang Zheng Qi San

Table 8.10 Comparison of Large Intestine Damp-Heat and Large Intestine Cold-Dampness

Comparison: Large Intestine Damp-Heat vs. Damp-Heat Encumbering the Spleen

Damp-heat encumbering the Spleen (濕熱睏脾 shī rè kùn pí) and Large Intestine damp-heat (大腸濕熱 dà cháng shī rè) share many symptoms including fever, diarrhea or sticky loose stools, yellow urine, a red tongue with a greasy yellow coating, and a slippery and rapid pulse. Both are characterized as excess heat conditions. However, the pathological location is different (middle burner vs. the lower burner), and therefore the clinical manifestations are different.

Besides diarrhea, damp-heat encumbering the Spleen will present with signs and symptoms related to Spleen dysfunction such as nausea, poor appetite, or abdominal distention and bloating. It is usually sub-acute or chronic, mild, and has a long course. In contrast, in Large Intestine damp-heat, diarrhea will be the only complaint and it is acute, has a short course, and may be very severe with blood or pus in the stool. Damp-heat encumbering the Spleen may also present with jaundice, edema, or scanty urine.

The key points to distinguish these two patterns are as follows:
1) Severity and nature of onset: sub-acute or chronic onset vs. acute, long course vs. short course, mild diarrhea vs. severe diarrhea with pus and blood
2) Location: middle burner vs. lower burner
    Spleen (middle burner) symptoms: abdominal fullness, distention, poor appetite, and nausea or vomiting
    Large Intestine (lower burner) symptoms: diarrhea with blood and pus

Pattern	Damp-Heat Encumbering the Spleen	Large Intestine Damp-Heat
Pathogenesis	Damp-heat disrupts Spleen and Stomach function	Damp-heat disrupts Large Intestine's transportation function
Characteristics	Sub-acute or chronic, long course, mild, excess, heat	Acute, short course, severe, excess, heat
Symptoms — Common	Fever, diarrhea, or sticky loose stools, yellow urine, a red tongue with yellow greasy coating, a slippery and rapid pulse	
Symptoms — Main	Abdominal fullness and distention, poor appetite, nausea, vomiting, jaundice, edema, or scanty urine	Abdominal pain, with severe diarrhea or with pus and blood in the stool
Symptoms — Location	Middle burner	Lower burner
Tongue & pulse	Red tongue with yellow greasy coating; slippery and rapid pulse	
Treatment strategy	Clear heat, transform dampness, regulate qi, harmonize the middle burner	Clear heat, transform dampness, stop diarrhea
Herbal formulas	Lian Po Yin, Zhong Man Fei Xiao Wan, Yin Chen Hao Tang	Ge Gen Qin Lian Tang, Bai Tou Weng Tang, Shao Yao Tang

Table 8.11 Comparison of Damp-Heat Encumbering the Spleen and Large Intestine Damp-Heat

5 Large Intestine Heat Accumulation Pattern ｜大腸熱結｜

Definition: An interior excess heat pattern involving the retention of dry feces in the intestines due to a mixture of excess pathogenic heat with waste materials in the intestines, manifesting with high fever, abdominal pain, and severe constipation. It is also known as the *yáng míng* organ (*fǔ*) pattern in six-channel pattern identification.

Clinical manifestations: Tidal fever or high fever that peaks at 3 p.m., abdominal pain and distention that resists touch or pressure, severe constipation, thirst with a desire to drink cold water, diarrhea with dark greenish watery stools and strong foul odor, coma, delirium, mania, irritability, insomnia, a thorny tongue with a thick, dry, yellow, or dark brown coating, and a deep, forceful pulse.

Key points: Severe abdominal pain that is resistant to pressure, distention, bloating, constipation with dry stools, plus interior excess heat signs and symptoms.

Etiology and pathogenesis: This pattern usually arises from excess heat invasion, which may be due to improper diet, such as overconsumption of hot, spicy, or greasy food, alcohol, or unhygienic food; or from profuse sweating that impairs body fluids. It can also result from improper treatments, such as overusing diaphoretic herbs, leading to body fluids leakage. Additionally, Large Intestine dryness can also increase internal heat leading to the development of this pattern.

Pathogenic heat consumes body fluids and dries up the intestinal tract. Dry stools and impeded qi movement leads to abdominal fullness and pain with no defecation. When dry stools form, it is bound with heat accumulation in the intestines, creating more heat and strongly scorching heat. The body temperature increases and worsens around 3 p.m. to 5 p.m. since Large Intestine yang qi reaches its peak at this time.

When pathogenic heat rises, it disturbs and harasses the Heart *shén*. Thus there is vexation, restlessness, insomnia, and irritability. In severe cases, there may be coma, delirious speech, and mania.

Heat clumps and dries stools, obstructing the contents of the Large Intestine. Meanwhile, the patient drinks a lot of water due to excessive thirst, which produces water waste. The water waste then passes around the intestinal obstructions and is expelled outside the body as diarrhea. Since the water waste has to pass by the obstruction of dry stools and is consumed by pathogenic heat, it becomes viscous and turbid. This is called "heat clumping with circumfluence" (熱結旁流 *rè jié páng liú*) and produces a type of diarrhea that is foul-smelling, dark green, and watery.

Excessive heat and dry stools obstructing the intestinal tract, steams up the turbid from the intestines, giving the tongue a thick, dry, yellow, or brown coating. The dry stools obstruct internally in the lower part of the body, therefore the pulse is deep, but forceful.

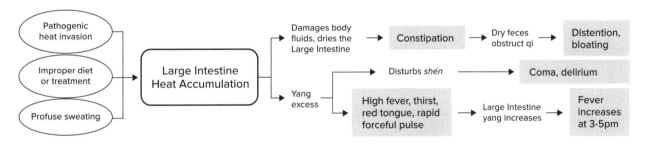

Chart 8.10   Etiology and pathogenesis of Large Intestine Heat Accumulation

TCM Disease	Western Disease	Herbal Formulas	Acupuncture	
Abdominal pain (腹痛)	Acute appendicitis, acute cholecystitis, acute pancreatitis, intestinal obstruction, postoperative constipation, intestinal adhesion	Da Cheng Qi Tang, Xiao Cheng Qi Tang, Tiao Wei Cheng Qi Tang, Tao He Cheng Qi Tang, Da Chai Hu Tang	ST-4, ST-5, LI-1, LI-4, LI-11, SP-5, TB-6	ST-25, CV-12
Constipation (便秘)				ST-25, ST-44, BL-25
yáng míng organ (*fǔ*) pattern (陽明腑實証)				ST-25, BL-25
Warm disease (溫病)	Dysentery, cholera, campylobacteriosis, stomach flu	Ge Gen Tang add Huang Qin, Sang Bai Pi, Gua Lou		ST-37

Table 8.12   Diseases and treatments related to Large Intestine Heat Accumulation

Comparison: Large Intestine Heat Accumulation vs. Large Intestine Dryness

Large Intestine dryness (大腸液虧 *dà cháng yè kuī*) and Large Intestine Heat Accumulation (大腸熱結 *dà cháng rè jié*) both present with constipation, dry stools, dry mouth, and thirst with bad breath. However, the pathogenesis and nature of these two patterns are different. Large Intestine dryness is a condition of deficiency that develops from an insufficiency of body fluids to nourish the Large Intestine, which leads to intestinal tract dryness and failure to move and expel stool.

In contrast, Large Intestine heat accumulation is a condition of excess that is usually caused by exopathogenic heat invasion or improper diet. The pathogenesis involves excess heat clumping with dry feces that obstruct the intestines. Thus, besides constipation, dry stools, severe abdominal pain with distention and bloating, which are the main symptoms of this pattern, there are also obvious excess heat signs such as high fever, a red face, a red tongue with dark yellow coating, and a rapid forceful pulse.

The key points to distinguish these two patterns are as follows: Large Intestine heat accumulation is usually severe, acute, and an emergency situation, combined with fever and severe abdominal pain, while Large Intestine dryness is mild and chronic.

Pattern		Large Intestine Dryness	Large Intestine Heat Accumulation
Etiology		Constitution, aging, diarrhea, bleeding, vomiting, chronic illness	Exopathogenic heat invasion, improper diet, improper treatment
Pathogenesis		Deficiency in blood and body fluids fails to nourish the intestines	Excess heat clumps with dry feces and obstructs the intestines
Characteristics		Deficiency, chronic, mild	Excess, acute, severe
Symptoms	Common	Constipation, dry stools, dry mouth, thirst, bad breath, red tongue, dry yellow coating, scanty urine	
Symptoms	Different	Pale complexion if developed from blood deficiency, dizziness, thin pulse	High fever, severe abdominal pain, distention, and bloating, resistant to pressure, red tongue, thick, dark brown coating, deep forceful pulse
Treatment strategy		Nourish and replenish fluids in the Large Intestine, laxative to relieve constipation	Purgative, clear heat, remove clumps
Herbal formulas		Run Chang Wan	Da Cheng Qi Tang

Table 8.13 Comparison of Large Intestine Dryness and Large Intestine Heat Accumulation

Comparison: Large Intestine Heat Accumulation vs. Large Intestine Damp-Heat

Large Intestine heat accumulation (大腸熱結 *dà cháng rè jié*) and Large Intestine damp-heat (大腸濕熱 *dà cháng shī rè*) are both excess heat conditions exhibiting symptoms of fever, thirst with desire to drink cold water, abdominal pain, yellow urine, a red tongue with yellow greasy coating, and a rapid slippery pulse. However, the etiological factors and pathogenesis are different and therefore they have distinct clinical manifestations.

The pathogenesis of Large Intestine heat accumulation involves pathogenic heat consuming body fluids and drying up the intestinal tract, which leads to dry stools bound with heat that accumulates inside and scorches the Large Intestine. This results in constipation, abdominal pain that is resistant to pressure, and greenish watery diarrhea. There may also be *shén* disturbance, such as irritability, restlessness, coma, or manic behavior. In contrast, Large Intestine damp-heat involves dampness and heat accumulation in the Large Intestine that disrupts its reabsorption and transportation function, allowing damp-heat to pour down and cause diarrhea.

The key points to distinguish these two patterns are as follows:
1) Constipation vs. diarrhea
2) Diarrhea:
    - Stools with pus and blood vs. greenish yellowish watery stools
    - Abdominal pain relieved after diarrhea vs. not relieved
3) Presence of *shén* disturbance

Pattern		Large Intestine Heat Accumulation	Large Intestine Damp-Heat
Pathogenesis		Excess heat damages body fluids, dried Large Intestine tract, leading to heat and dry feces clumping together, blocks qi, disrupts Large Intestine transmitting and transport function	Damp-heat accumulates in the Large Intestine, putrefying and rotting flesh, damages blood vessels, dilutes and pours down stool, qi and dampness stagnate
Characteristics		Acute onset, short course, interior excess heat	
Symptoms	Main	Constipation or diarrhea	Diarrhea
Symptoms	Common	Fever, thirst and desire to drink cold water, abdominal pain, yellow urine, red tongue with yellow greasy coating, rapid and slippery pulse	
Symptoms	Different	Fever increases around 3-5pm, distention and bloating, severely dry stools or greenish watery stools with foul odor, abdominal pain not relieved after bowel movement	Tenesmus, watery stools with pus and blood, stools with foul odor and discomfort or burning sensation of the anus, abdominal pain relieved after bowel movement
Symptoms	Shén	Irritability, restlessness, agitation, coma, delirium, manic behavior	
Treatment strategy		Purge clumped heat, promote bowel movement	Clear heat, resolve dampness, stop diarrhea
Herbal formulas		Da Cheng Qi Tang, Xiao Cheng Qi Tang, Tiao Wei Cheng Qi Tang	Ge Gen Qin Lian Tang, Bai Tou Weng Tang

Table 8.14 Comparison of Large Intestine Heat Accumulation and Large Intestine Damp-Heat

Summary of Large Intestine Disease Patterns

	Patterns	Clinical Manifestations	
		Common	Different
	Key points: diarrhea, loose stools, or constipation		
Deficiency	Large Intestine Deficiency Cold	Chronic loose stools, borborygmus, fecal incontinence, rectal prolapse, dull abdominal pain, preference for warmth and pressure, intolerance of cold, cold limbs, clear copious urine, possibly constipation, a pale tongue with white coating, and a deep, slow, feeble pulse	
	Large Intestine Dryness	Constipation, dry stools, dry mouth and thirst, bad breath, red tongue, dry yellow coating, scanty urine	Scanty tongue coat, thin pulse
Excess	Large Intestine Heat Accumulation		High fever, severe abdominal pain, distention and bloating, resistance to pressure, dark green foul-smelling diarrhea, red tongue, thick, dark brown coating, deep and forceful pulse
	Large Intestine Damp-Heat	Diarrhea, abdominal pain, thick tongue coating, and slippery pulse. There may be chills and fever, and superficial pulse	Muddy sticky yellow stool with pus and blood and strong foul odor, tenesmus, discomfort or burning sensation of the anus, thirst, yellow urine, may have fever and mild chills, red tongue with thick yellow coating, a rapid and slippery pulse
	Large Intestine Cold-Dampness		Watery diarrhea, light colored, less odor, borborygmus, paroxysmal cold pain, pale tongue with white greasy coating, a slow slippery or superficial tight pulse

Table 8.15 Summary of Large Intestine disease patterns

Chapter 9
Gallbladder Disease Patterns

Physiological characteristics and functions of the Gallbladder

The Gallbladder is located in the right hypochondriac region, on the inferior surface of the Liver between the quadrate and right lobes. The Gallbladder channel begins near the outer corner of the eye and descends down the side of the body along the rib margin, and down the lateral leg, ending on the lateral side of the fourth toe. Its internal branches connect with the Stomach and the Small Intestine channels, and joins the Liver and Gallbladder organs.

The Gallbladder is a hollow capsule-shaped organ that contains bile. The bile comes from the Liver and is the accumulation of the surplus part of Liver qi. The bile is a pure and refined essence, which is greenish in color and bitter in taste, playing an important role in assisting the absorption of food. The bile is called the 'essence juice' (精汁 *jīng zhī*) or 'lucid juice.' That is why the Gallbladder is called 'the *fǔ* organ of essence juice' (中精之腑 *zhōng jīng zhī fǔ*) or 'the *fǔ* organ of lucid juice' (中清之腑 *zhōng qīng zhī fǔ*) in *Spiritual Pivot,* Chapter 8.

Although functionally the Gallbladder resembles a *zàng* organ because it only stores bile and does not receive, transform, or transport digested waste products, its anatomical shape is more similar to a *fǔ* organ. For this reason, the Gallbladder is included in the six *fǔ* organs and is also categorized as an 'extraordinary organ.'

There are two physiological characteristics of the Gallbladder. The first is that the Gallbladder qi governs ascending. The Gallbladder is a *shào yáng* or yang within yang organ that is located east, belongs to the wood phase, and governs early spring when the time of life is full of vitality, growth, and development. Secondly, the Gallbladder is an organ that favors peace, calm, and quiet and disfavors being harassed and bothered.

1 | Storing and secreting bile, aiding digestion

The Gallbladder itself is empty. After bile is produced by the Liver, it is condensed and stored in the Gallbladder. Directed by the coursing and dispersing functions of the Liver, bile is secreted by the Gallbladder into the Small Intestine to participate in the process of food digestion and absorption, assisting the Small Intestine in separating the clear from the turbid.

2 | Governing decision-making and judgment

The Gallbladder is called the Minister of Justice (中正之官 *zhōng zhèng zhī guān*). In the process of spiritual activities, awareness, and consciousness, the Gallbladder is in charge of making judgments and decisions. This function plays an important role in preventing and eliminating the adverse effects of certain mental stimulations such as shock, fear, or fright, in order to maintain and control the normal qi and blood circulation and to ensure harmonious relationships among the *zàng fǔ* organs. *Simple Questions*, Chapter 8 states: "The Gallbladder is an upright official who is in charge of judgment and decision."

The Gallbladder assists the Liver to course and discharge, regulating mental and emotional activities. The Liver controls planning and strategizing, while the Gallbladder governs judgment and decision-making. When the Gallbladder and Liver are harmonized, there is mental balance and stability; even severe mental stimulation has little effect and one can recover faster from such stimulation. Thus only when the Liver and Gallbladder work in coordination can mental and emotional activities, such as careful thinking, good judgment, and decisiveness, be well maintained.

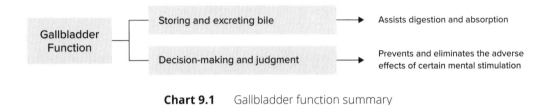

Chart 9.1 Gallbladder function summary

Common etiological factors in Gallbladder patterns

Gallbladder disease develops similarly to Liver disease with the major causes being emotional stress, exopathogens, diet, and lifestyle. The following are common etiological factors of Gallbladder disease patterns:

(1) Exopathogenic wind, cold, heat, dryness, dampness, summer-heat, or pestilential qi
(2) Emotional stress: anger, depression, worry, fear, sadness, and fright
(3) Improper diet: overconsumption of hot spicy or pungent food, alcohol, or medications
(4) Congenital defects
(5) Chronic illness

Pathological changes and major clinical manifestations of the Gallbladder

The Gallbladder's failure to store bile, causing bile to steam upward and outward, its failure to secrete bile, and its failure at decision-making and good judgment are the major pathological changes in Gallbladder disease and results in the following signs and symptoms.

1 | Bitter taste in the mouth

Definition: Bitter taste in the mouth.

Etiology and pathomechanism: The physiological function of the Gallbladder is to store and secrete bile. Bile is a greenish fluid with a bitter taste that aids digestion and is produced by the Liver and stored in the

Gallbladder. When there is excess heat accumulation in the Gallbladder, bile steams upward to the mouth, resulting in a bitter taste. Pathogenic heat can come from exopathogenic heat invasion or from emotional stress, causing qi stagnation that generates heat, or from overconsumption of alcohol and hot spicy foods.

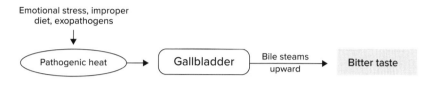

Chart 9.2 Etiology and pathomechanism of bitter taste in the mouth

2 | Jaundice

Definition: Yellow staining of the skin and sclera by abnormally high blood levels of the bile pigment bilirubin.

Etiology and pathomechanism: Bile is a greenish fluid that aids digestion and is secreted by the Liver and stored in the Gallbladder. The yellow-orange pigment in bile that forms from the breakdown of red blood cells is called bilirubin. There are two major causes for high levels of bilirubin in the blood that lead to jaundice: first is pathogenic heat that steams the bile outward; and second is an obstruction of the Gallbladder duct where the bile generated by the Liver cannot enter the Gallbladder for storage and is instead pushed outward.

Pathogenic heat can be caused by improper diet, such as overconsumption of hot, spicy, or greasy foods, and overconsumption of alcohol. It may also be due to exopathogenic heat invasion or emotional stress. The Gallbladder duct can be blocked by phlegm, blood stasis, and stones, which all belong to secondary pathogens caused by chronic illness, improper diet, exopathogen invasion, or emotional stress.

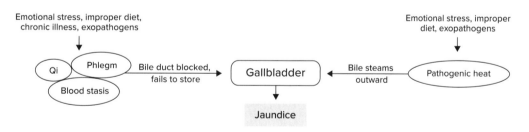

Chart 9.3 Etiology and pathomechanism of jaundice

3 | Timidity and paranoia

Definition: Lack of courage, startles easily, suspicious of others, doubtful, and skeptical.

Etiology and pathomechanism: Gallbladder qi deficiency can come from a weak constitution or chronic illness, especially Spleen and Stomach deficiency, or long-term emotional stress. The Gallbladder is in charge of judgment and decision-making and assists the Liver to course and discharge, regulating emotional activities. If Gallbladder qi is deficient, it will fail to be activated and motivated, resulting in indecisiveness, poor judgment, a lack of courage, and being easily startled.

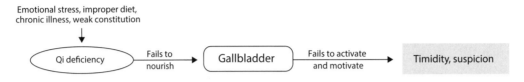

Chart 9.4 Etiology and pathomechanism of timidity and paranoia

4 | Other signs and symptoms related to Gallbladder

The following signs and symptoms may also appear in Gallbladder disease patterns: indigestion, hypochondriac pain, headache, dizziness, tinnitus, ear pain, and blurry vision.

Physiological Function	Pathological Change	Clinical Manifestation
Storage and excretion of bile	Bile steams upward	Bitter taste in the mouth
	Bile flows outward	Jaundice
Judgment, decision-making	Gallbladder qi deficiency	Frightened, timid, insomnia

Table 9.1 Physiological functions, pathological changes, and clinical manifestations of the Gallbladder

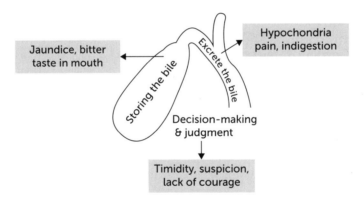

Chart 9.5 Gallbladder function and pathological symptoms

Common patterns in Gallbladder disease

Gallbladder disease can be divided into two groups: excess and deficiency. Based on the nature and characteristics of the Gallbladder, its disease patterns tend to be more excessive than deficient. However, a weak constitution and chronic illness may lead to deficiency patterns. Common excess patterns include Gallbladder Heat and Gallbladder Stagnation with Phlegm Disturbance, while the most common deficiency pattern is Gallbladder Qi Deficiency

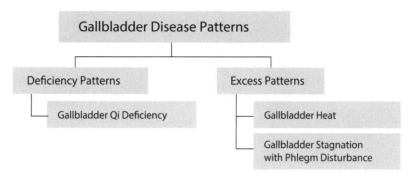

Chart 9.6   Common Gallbladder disease patterns

	Etiology	Patterns
Deficiency	Chronic illness, constitution	Gallbladder Qi Deficiency
Excess	Exopathogens invasion, emotional stress	Gallbladder Heat, Gallbladder Stagnation with Phlegm Disturbance

Table 9.2 Classification of common Gallbladder patterns

1 Gallbladder Qi Deficiency Pattern | 膽氣虛証 |

Definition: A group of signs and symptoms caused by Gallbladder qi insufficiency that leads to indecisiveness and poor judgment.

Clinical manifestations: Dizziness, blurry vision, nervousness, timidity, startles easily, paranoia, lack of courage and initiative, indecisiveness, insomnia, dream-disturbed sleep, shortness of breath, a pale tongue, and a thin and wiry or weak pulse.

Key points: Timidity, startles easily, paranoia, lack of courage, plus qi deficiency signs and symptoms.

Etiology and pathogenesis: This pattern is mostly due to constitution. It can also develop from chronic illness, especially Spleen and Stomach deficiency not generating enough qi to nourish the Gallbladder. It can also result from long-term emotional stress due to fear, worry, sadness, or anger.

Gallbladder qi deficiency leads to poor judgment and decision-making. It causes nervousness, timidity, propensity towards being easily startled, paranoia, lack of courage and initiative, and difficulty making decisions. Qi deficiency fails to nourish and motivate, resulting in dizziness, shortness of breath, pale tongue and weak pulse. If Gallbladder qi deficiency disrupts the Heart and Liver, there will also be insomnia, dream-disturbed sleep, and a wiry pulse.

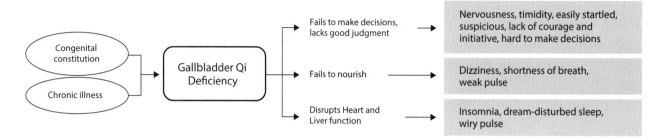

Chart 9.7 Etiology and pathogenesis of Gallbladder Qi Deficiency

TCM Disease	Western Disease	Herbal Formulas		Acupuncture	
Fright (驚悸)	Anxiety, panic attack, paranoia, PTSD, schizophrenia, dementia, Alzheimer's		Wen Dan Tang		PC-6, HT-7, CV-17, GV-20, Yintang
Depression (鬱証)	Depression, postpartum depression, neurosis, menopause syndrome, ADD/ADHD	Ding Zhi Wan	Yue Ju Wan	GB-40, LR-8, ST-36, SP-6, CV-4, BL-18, BL-47	BL-15, BL-20, HT-7, GV-14, CV-17
Mania, psychosis (癲狂)	Hysteria, neurosis, schizophrenia, OCD, PTSD, ADD/ADHD, anxiety attack, psychosis, mania		Wen Dan Tang add Ci Shi, Long Gu, Mu Li		GV-14, GV-16, GV-26, PC-6, HT-7
Insomnia (不寐)	Anxiety, neurosis, ADD/ADHD, menopausal syndrome, depression		An Shen Ding Zhi Wan		HT-7, Anmian, Yintang
Collapse (厥証)	Vasovagal syncope, hypotension, cardiac syncope, bradycardia		Ding Zhi Wan		GV-20, GV-26

Table 9.3 Diseases and treatments related to Gallbladder Qi Deficiency

2 Gallbladder Heat Pattern | 膽熱証 |

Definition: A group of signs and symptoms that arises from heat accumulation and stagnation inside the Gallbladder with a clinical manifestation of bitter taste in the mouth, alternating chills and fever, and a wiry and rapid pulse. This pattern is also called heat congestion in the Gallbladder.

Clinical manifestations: Irritability, short temper, tinnitus or ear pain, headache, insomnia or dream-disturbed sleep, hypochondriac distention pain, anorexia, bitter taste in the mouth, dry mouth and thirst, red face, nausea and vomiting, constipation, scanty dark yellow urine, alternating chills and fever, yellow sclera and skin, a red tongue with yellow coating, and a rapid wiry pulse.

Key points: Bitter taste in the mouth, dry throat, dizziness and tinnitus. Or alternating chills and fever with jaundice, plus interior heat signs and symptoms.

Etiology and pathogenesis: This pattern occurs when exopathogens or emotional stress leads to qi stagnation that transforms into heat.

The Gallbladder stores bile, but when pathogenic heat harasses inside, the bile is steamed upward and overflows, leading to a bitter taste in the mouth, dry mouth, and thirst. The Gallbladder is the organ of justice (中正之官 zhōng zhèng zhī guān). It governs ascending and prefers peace, calm, and quiet. When pathogenic heat harasses inside, it disrupts the Gallbladder, ascends upward, and disturbs the Heart *shén* and the Liver *hún*, resulting in irritability, insomnia, or dream-disturbed sleep.

The Gallbladder channel runs along the side of the body and acts as a pivot. When pathogenic heat congests in the Gallbladder, this affects yang qi's ability to exit and enter, which can manifest with alternating chills and fever. If heat congests in the Gallbladder channel and disrupts other organs, it will cause headache, dizziness, ear pain, tinnitus, hypochondriac distention pain, nausea or vomiting, or anorexia. Dry mouth and thirst, constipation, dark yellow and scanty urine, a red face and tongue, and a rapid pulse are all caused by heat steaming inside, consuming body fluids.

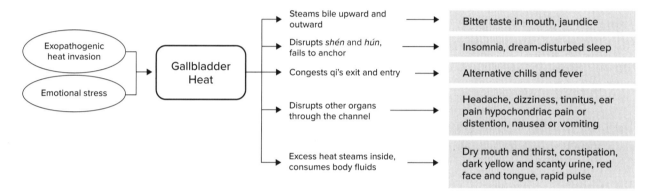

Chart 9.8 Etiology and pathogenesis of Gallbladder Heat

TCM Disease	Western Disease	Herbal Formulas		Acupuncture	
Dizziness and vertigo (眩暈)	Hypertension, hypotension, BPPV, Parkinson's disease, SCA, Meniere's syndrome, anxiety	Da Chai Hu Tang, Xiao Chai Hu Tang	Long Dan Xie Gan Tang	GB-43, GB-34, BL-19, BL-18, LI-11, LR-4, LI-4	GB-20, GV-20, LR-2, SP-6
Hypochondriac pain (脇痛)	Hypochondriasis, costochondritis, pleurisy, arthritis, osteoporosis, intercostal neuralgia		Jin Ling Zi San		GB-24, LR-13, LR-14,
Jaundice (黃疸)	Acute cholecystitis, baby jaundice, Gilbert's syndrome, obstruction or inflammation of the bile duct		Yin Chen Hao Tang		SP-9, CV-12, GV-9
Insomnia (不寐)	Anxiety, neurosis, ADD/ADHD, menopausal syndrome, depression		Wen Dan Tang		HT-7, Anmian, Yintang

Table 9.4 Diseases and treatments related to Gallbladder Heat

Comparison: Gallbladder Heat vs. Liver Fire Blazing

Gallbladder heat (膽熱 *dǎn rè*) and Liver fire blazing (肝火上炎 *gān huǒ shàng yán*) are both caused by qi stagnation generating heat as a result of emotional stress or improper diet. The Liver and Gallbladder have a close relationship as internally-externally paired organs, so they share many clinical signs and symptoms such as headache, dizziness, bitter taste in the mouth, tinnitus, red eyes, irritability, insomnia, dream-disturbed sleep, hypochondriac pain, a red tongue with yellow coating, and a rapid wiry pulse. Both of them can be treated with Long Dan Xie Gan Tang, so many books identify them as the same pattern. However, their channels pass through different parts of the body and thus they have some differences in clinical manifestation.

Liver fire blazing involves excess fire flaring up through the Liver channel, disrupting the clear orifice (清竅 qīng qiào), which causes severe headache, dizziness, vertigo, and tinnitus. Liver fire also disrupts the Heart *shén*, leading to irritability, anger, or mania. And, since the eyes are the orifice of the Liver, another major symptom is red eyes.

In comparison, the main symptoms of Gallbladder heat rising upward and disrupting the clear orifice are a bitter taste in the mouth, dry throat, dizziness, tinnitus, and headache. Red eyes are mild and not the chief complaint. Since the Gallbladder directly secretes bile into the Stomach, Gallbladder heat will disrupt the Stomach's descending function, resulting in nausea or vomiting. Other differentiating symptoms for Gallbladder dysfunction are jaundice and alternating chills and fever.

The Liver governs anger, while the Gallbladder is in charge of decision-making. Thus Liver fire blazing usually leads to a quick temper, while Gallbladder heat mostly causes frequent sighing.

The key points to distinguish these two patterns are as follows:
1) Chief complaints: bitter taste in the mouth vs. red eyes and headache
2) Presence of jaundice
3) *Shén* disturbance: mild vs. severe
4) Alternating chills and fever vs. fever only

Pattern		Gallbladder Heat	Liver Fire Blazing
Etiology		Emotional stress, improper diet, exopathogenic heat invasion	
Pathogenesis		Excess heat accumulation inside that steams upward	
		Fails to store bile	Fails to course and discharge
Characteristics		Acute or sub-acute, excess, heat	
Symptoms	Common	Headache, dizziness, bitter taste in the mouth, tinnitus, red eyes, red tongue with yellow coating, and a rapid and wiry pulse	
	Main	Bitter taste in the mouth, dry throat, tinnitus	Headache, red eyes, dizziness
	Different	Mild headache and red eyes	Severe headache
		Jaundice, alternating chills and fever	Fever
Emotions		Frequent sighing	Short temper, irritable
Treatment strategy		Clear heat from Gallbladder	Purge fire
Herbal formulas		Wen Dan Tang	Jia Wei Xiao Yao San

Table 9.5 Comparison of Gallbladder Heat and Liver Fire Blazing

3 Gallbladder Stagnation with Phlegm Disturbance | 膽鬱痰擾証 |

Definition: A group of signs and symptoms that refers to phlegm-heat disturbing the Gallbladder, resulting in its dysfunction. It has also been translated as heat-phlegm in the Gallbladder or depressed Gallbladder with phlegm harassing.

Clinical manifestations: Fright, timidity, susceptibility, easily startled, panic attacks, paranoia, irritability, restlessness, dizziness, tinnitus, nausea, bitter taste in the mouth, chest distress, hypochondriac distention, insomnia, dream-disturbed sleep, palpitations, a red tongue with thick yellow greasy coating, and a slippery and wiry pulse. Patient often has a history of mental illness.

Key points: Fright, easily startled, panic attacks, paranoia, insomnia, dizziness, chest distress, hypochondriac distention, bitter taste in the mouth, plus heat-phlegm signs and symptoms.

Etiology and pathogenesis: This pattern is derived mainly from emotional stress. Emotional stimuli causes qi stagnation, qi stagnation generates phlegm, and phlegm accumulation produces fire, resulting in the coalescence of heat and phlegm that disrupts the Gallbladder.

The Gallbladder is the organ for justice (中正之官). It favors peace, calm, and quiet. Pathogenic heat harassing inside will disrupt the Gallbladder, leading to timidity and susceptibility to fright and being easily startled. If the heat disrupts the *shén* and *hún*, it causes insomnia and dream-disturbed sleep. Phlegm-heat disrupts clear yang, resulting in dizziness and vertigo while phlegm-heat obstructs qi in the Gallbladder channel, leading to tinnitus, ear pain, chest distress, or hypochondriac distention.

The Gallbladder pertains to wood while the Heart pertains to fire. Wood generates fire, thus, Gallbladder phlegm-heat accumulation may lead to Heart fire excess, which manifests with palpitations, irritability, restlessness, and insomnia. A red tongue with thick yellow greasy coating and slippery and wiry pulse indicate phlegm accumulation with heat.

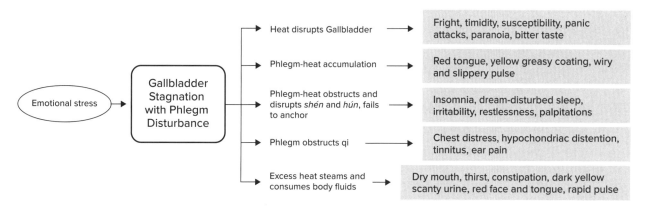

Chart 9.9 Etiology and pathogenesis of Gallbladder Stagnation with Phlegm Disturbance

TCM Disease	Western Disease	Herbal Formulas		Acupuncture
Dizziness and vertigo (眩暈)	Parkinson's disease, SCA, hypertension, Meniere's syndrome, anxiety	Huang Lian Wen Dan Tang	Tian Ma, Gou Teng	GB-34, GB-24, ST-40, LI-11, TB-6, CV-12	LR-2, GB-20, GV-20
Insomnia (失眠)	Anxiety, panic attack, menopause syndrome, ADD/ADHD		Huang Lian, Yuan Zhi, Bai Zi Ren		Anmian, HT-5, HT-6, HT-7
Qi constraint (氣鬱)	Plum-pit syndrome or globus hystericus (Mei He Qi)		Ban Xia Hou Po Tang, Yue Ju Wan		CV-17, CV-22, CV-23, LR-2, LR-3, PC-6, ST-36, ST-40, SP-9

Table 9.6 Diseases and treatments related to Gallbladder Stagnation with Phlegm Disturbance

Comparison: Gallbladder Stagnation with Phlegm Disturbance vs. Gallbladder Heat

Gallbladder stagnation with phlegm disturbance (膽鬱痰擾 *dǎn yù tán rǎo*) and Gallbladder heat (膽熱 *dǎn rè*) both involve heat in the Gallbladder that causes irritability, short temper, tinnitus or ear pain, dry mouth, bitter taste in the mouth, hypochondriac distention or pain, red face, nausea or vomiting, constipation, scanty dark yellow urine, insomnia or dream-disturbed sleep, a red tongue with yellow coating, and a rapid pulse.

Gallbladder stagnation with phlegm disturbance mostly develops from emotional stress. Since phlegm is one of the major etiological factors, it is chronic, longer course, and involves recurrent attacks. Clinically, it also manifests with phlegm characteristics such as dizziness, greasy tongue coating, and slippery pulse. Patients mostly have a history of mental illness.

Gallbladder heat mostly develops from exopathogenic disease and is therefore sub-acute, shorter course, and easier to treat. Clinical manifestations are related to heat disrupting the Gallbladder such as alternating chills and fever, yellow sclera and skin, a red tongue with yellow coating, and wiry rapid pulse.

The key points to distinguish these two patterns are as follows:
1) History of illness: mental illness vs. exopathogenic disease
2) Course of illness: chronic, long course vs. sub-acute, short course
3) Clinical symptoms: Alternating chills and fever, jaundice

Pattern	Gallbladder Stagnation with Phlegm Disturbance	Gallbladder Heat
Etiology and pathogenesis	Emotional stress stagnates qi, producing phlegm and heat, disrupts Gallbladder	Exopathogenic factors invasion or due to emotional stress, leads to qi stagnation that transforms into heat
Symptoms — Common	Irritability, short temper, tinnitus or ear pain, dry mouth, bitter taste in the mouth, hypochondriac distention or pain, red face, nausea or vomiting, constipation, scanty dark yellow urine, insomnia or dream-disturbed sleep, red tongue with yellow coating, rapid pulse	
Symptoms — Main	Fright, timidity, susceptibility, panic, and easily started	Alternating chills and fever, jaundice
Symptoms — Different	History of mental illness, yellow greasy coating, slippery pulse	History of exopathogenic disease, alternating chills and fever, yellow sclera and skin, wiry pulse
Mental condition	More severe	Mild
Characteristics	Chronic, longer course, recurrent	Sub-acute, shorter course
Treatment strategy	Regulate qi, transform phlegm, clear heat from the Gallbladder	Clear heat from the Gallbladder, harmonize *shào yáng*
Herbal formulas	Wen Dan Tang	Xiao Chai Hu Tang

Table 9.7 Comparison of Gallbladder Stagnation with Phlegm Disturbance and Gallbladder Heat

Comparison: Gallbladder Stagnation with Phlegm Disturbance vs. Heart Fire Blazing

Gallbladder stagnation with phlegm disturbance (膽鬱痰擾 *dǎn yū tán rǎo*) and Heart fire blazing (心火上炎 *xīn huǒ shàng yán*) are both excess heat conditions that present with a bitter taste in the mouth, irritability, restlessness, insomnia, dream-disturbed sleep, a red tongue, and a rapid pulse. However, they have different clinical manifestations due to a difference in pathological location.

Since the Gallbladder stores bile, its major symptoms are a bitter taste in the mouth and jaundice. The Gallbladder is the organ of justice (中正之官 *zhōng zhèng zhī guān*). It favors peace, calm, and quiet. Pathogenic heat harassing inside will disrupt the Gallbladder, leading to timidity and susceptibility to fright and being easily startled. Other symptoms related to the Gallbladder and its channel include alternating chills and fever, red eyes, hypochondriac pain, dizziness, and tinnitus.

The Heart houses the *shén* and its major symptoms involve excess heat disrupting the *shén*, which leads to irritability, vexation, insomnia, manic behavior, or delirium. Other symptoms related to excess heat in the Heart include mouth ulcers, tongue sores, canker sores, and urinary tract infections.

The key points to distinguish these two patterns are as follows:
1) Chief complaints: bitter taste in the mouth vs. *shén* disturbance
2) *Shén* disturbance: timidity, fright, easily startled vs. irritable, vexation, manic behavior
3) Alternating chills and fever vs. fever only
4) Tongue and pulse

Pattern	Gallbladder Stagnation with Phlegm Disturbance	Heart Fire Blazing
Etiology	Emotional stress, improper diet, exopathogenic heat invasion	
Pathogenesis	Excess heat accumulation inside steams upward	
	Failure to store bile	Failure to store *shén*
Characteristics	Acute or sub-acute, excess, heat	
Symptoms — Common	Bitter taste in mouth, irritable, restlessness, insomnia, dream-disturbed sleep, red tongue with yellow coating, and a rapid pulse	
Symptoms — Main	Bitter taste in the mouth, jaundice	Insomnia, agitation, anxiety, manic behavior, delirium
Symptoms — Different	Severe bitter taste in the mouth	Mild bitter taste in the mouth
	Alternating chills and fever	Fever or heat
Symptoms — Other	Dizziness, hypochondriac pain, tinnitus	Canker sores, tongue sores, UTI
Emotions	Frequent sighing	Short temper
Treatment strategy	Clear heat from the Gallbladder	Purge fire from the Heart
Herbal formulas	Wen Dan Tang	Xie Xin Tang

Table 9.8 Comparison of Gallbladder Stagnation with Phlegm Disturbance and Heart Fire Blazing

Comparison: Gallbladder Stagnation with Phlegm Disturbance vs. Phlegm-Fire Harassing the Heart

Gallbladder stagnation with phlegm disturbance (膽鬱痰擾 *dǎn yū tán rǎo*) and phlegm-fire harassing the Heart (痰火擾心 *tán huǒ rǎo xīn*) both have symptoms of *shén* disturbances, such as irritability, restlessness, palpitations, and insomnia, as well as symptoms of heat-phlegm, such as red face, thirst, bitter taste in the mouth, a red tongue with yellow greasy coating, and a slippery and rapid pulse.

However, the clinical manifestation of phlegm fire harassing the Heart is more severe. In this case, the Heart is the organ disrupted by heat-phlegm. Besides a red face, harsh breathing, constipation, and yellow urine, there is also manic behavior such as agitation, uncontrollable laughing or crying, and shouting. In comparison, Gallbladder stagnation with phlegm disturbance is more mild and has less heat signs. This pattern presents mainly with fright, timidity, susceptibility, panic, and being easily started. Additionally, this pattern involves qi failing to disperse, causing oppression in the chest, distention in the hypochondrium, and nausea.

The key points to distinguish these two patterns are as follows:
1) Severity of mental condition
2) Etiology

Pattern	Gallbladder Stagnation with Phlegm Disturbance	Phlegm-Fire Harassing the Heart
Etiology and pathogenesis	Emotional stress stagnates qi, producing phlegm and heat, disrupts Gallbladder	Emotional stress or exopathogenic heat invasion combined with phlegm harasses the Heart, disturbs *shén*
Symptoms – Common	Irritability, restlessness, insomnia, red face, thirst, bitter taste in the mouth, palpitations, red tongue with yellow greasy coating, slippery and rapid pulse	
Symptoms – Different	Fright, timidity, susceptibility, panic, and easily startled.	Manic agitation, incoherent and slurred speech, mental confusion, rash behavior, uncontrollable laughing or crying, shouting
Symptoms – Other	Distention in the chest or hypochondrium, nausea or vomiting, dizziness, tinnitus	Constipation, scanty and dark urine, fever
Mental condition	Mild	Severe
Treatment strategy	Regulate qi, transform phlegm, clear heat from the Gallbladder	Regulate qi, transform phlegm, clear heat from the Heart
Herbal formulas	Wen Dan Tang	Huang Lian Wen Dan Tang

Table 9.9 Comparison of Gallbladder Stagnation with Phlegm Disturbance and Phlegm-Fire Harassing the Heart

Summary of Gallbladder Disease Patterns

Key points: bitter taste in the mouth, timidity, startles easily, lack of courage and initiative, paranoia, indecisiveness, lack of good judgment, jaundice

	Patterns	Clinical Manifestations – Common	Clinical Manifestations – Different
Deficiency	Gallbladder Qi Deficiency	Dizziness, nervousness, timidity, startles easily, paranoia, lack of courage and initiative, indecisiveness, insomnia, dream-disturbed sleep, shortness of breath, pale tongue, thin wiry or weak pulse	
Excess	Gallbladder Heat	Irritability, tinnitus or ear pain, insomnia or dream-disturbed sleep, hypochondriac distention pain, bitter taste in the mouth, thirst, red face, nausea and vomiting, constipation, scanty dark yellow urine, red tongue with yellow coating, wiry and rapid pulse	Alternating chills and fever, yellow sclera and skin
Excess	Gallbladder Stagnation with Phlegm Disturbance		Chest distress, palpitations, thick, yellow, greasy tongue coating, slippery wiry pulse, history of mental illness

Table 9.10 Summary of Gallbladder disease patterns

Chapter 10
Urinary Bladder Disease Patterns

Physiological characteristics and functions of the Urinary Bladder

The Urinary Bladder is a cystic hollow organ that lies in the lower abdomen under the Kidney and in front of the Large Intestine. It is connected to the Kidney by the ureters from above and below to the urethra, which opens externally by means of the urinary orifice (溺竅 *nì qiào*). The Urinary Bladder channel begins at the inner corner of the eye, rising up through the eyebrow over the skull and runs along the back of the body from head to heal, with two parallel branches flowing along each side of the spine. It is the longest channel in the body and contains the most points. An internal branch connects with the Kidney and forms an external-internal relationship.

The main functions of the Urinary Bladder are storage and excretion of urine. It is the facility of aggregation for fluids and therefore is also called the Minister of Water Resource Control (州都之官 *zhōu dū zhī guān*) and 'viscera of body fluids' (津液之臟 *jīn yè zhī zàng*).

1 | Storing urine

After reabsorption and transformation, the fluid wastes are sent by the Small Intestine to the Urinary Bladder, which further transforms the waste into urine. The Urinary Bladder acts as a container that temporarily holds the fluid waste until it is full.

2 | Excreting urine

Fluid wastes are discharged from the body through the Urinary Bladder's qi transformation function (膀胱氣化 *páng guāng qì huà*) when a sufficient quantity has been accumulated. This function of the Urinary Bladder is performed with the assistance of the Kidney qi.

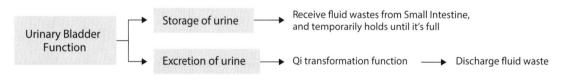

Chart 10.1 Summary of Urinary Bladder functions

Common etiological factors in Urinary Bladder patterns

The excess pattern of the Urinary Bladder is mostly caused by exopathogen invasion, improper diet and treatment, or other diseases. The deficiency pattern of the Urinary Bladder is usually due to chronic illness or weak constitution. The following are common etiological factors for Urinary Bladder disease patterns:
(1) Exopathogenic heat or damp-heat invasion
(2) Improper diet
(3) Chronic illness with improper treatment
(4) Weak constitution, aging

Pathological changes and major clinical manifestations of the Urinary Bladder

Pathological changes of the Urinary Bladder are mostly due to the organ failing to store urine such as frequency of urination, incontinence of urine and enuresis; as well as being unable to excrete urine such as anuria, urgency of urination and dysuria.

1 | Difficult urination

Definition: Dysuria (癃 *lóng*): a mild condition that suggests difficult urination. The urine passes only as drops and in small quantities overall. It is usually a chronic condition.

Anuria (閉 *bì*): a severe condition in which there is an absence of discharged urine, even though there is an urge to urinate. It is usually an acute condition. Although there are some differences between dysuria and anuria, they both refer to difficulty in eliminating urine, and thus the two words together, *lóng bì* (癃閉), are simply translated as urinary blockage.

Etiology and pathomechanism: Exopathogen invasion, improper diet, chronic illness, and aging can lead to Urinary Bladder qi transformation dysfunction, resulting in its inability to excrete urine, or difficult urination.

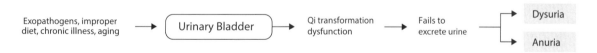

Chart 10.2 Etiology and pathomechanism of difficult urination

2 | Frequent urination or urinary incontinence

Definition: Frequent urination is the need to urinate more often than usual, while urinary incontinence involves any involuntary leakage of urine. Also related is enuresis, which is spontaneous urination while sleeping but having good bladder control while awake. This is usually seen in children.

Etiology and pathomechanism: Storing urine is a major function of the Urinary Bladder. Exopathogen invasion, improper diet, such as overconsumption of alcohol and spicy or greasy foods, or a lack of food intake, chronic illness, weak constitution, and aging can all lead to the Urinary Bladder failing to control fluids, resulting in urinary incontinence, frequent urination, or enuresis.

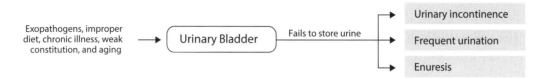

Chart 10.3 Etiology and pathomechanism of frequent urination or urinary incontinence

4 | Other signs and symptoms related to Urinary Bladder

Lower abdominal pain and distention also may relate to Urinary Bladder dysfunction.

Physiological Function	Pathological Change	Clinical Manifestation
Storage of urine	Failure to store and hold	Frequent urination, urinary incontinence, enuresis
Excretion of urine	Failure to excrete urine	Dysuria and anuria

Table 10.1 Physiological functions, pathological changes, and clinical manifestations of the Urinary Bladder

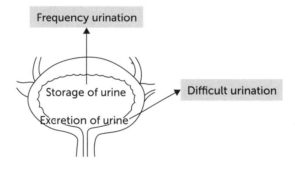

Chart 10.4 Bladder function and pathological symptoms

Common patterns in Urinary Bladder disease

There are only two common patterns of Urinary Bladder disease: excess type, which is Urinary Bladder Damp-Heat, and deficiency type, which is Urinary Bladder Deficiency Cold.

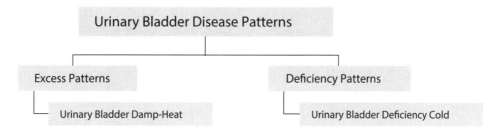

Chart 10.5 Common Urinary Bladder disease patterns

	Etiology	Patterns
Deficiency	Chronic illness, constitution, aging, physical or sexual overstrain	Urinary Bladder Deficiency Cold
Excess	Exopathogens invasion, improper diet	Urinary Bladder Damp-Heat

Table 10.2 Classification of common Urinary Bladder patterns

1 Urinary Bladder Deficiency Cold Pattern | 膀胱虛寒 |

Definition: A group of signs and symptoms due to Kidney yang deficiency failing to warm, leading to a disorder of the Urinary Bladder's storage and excretion functions.

Clinical manifestations: Frequent clear and copious urination, bedwetting, urinary incontinence, difficult urination, intolerance of cold, cold limbs, lassitude, listlessness, a pale tongue with white moist coating, and a deep and weak pulse.

Key points: Frequent clear and copious urination, urinary incontinence, plus yang deficiency signs and symptoms.

Etiology and pathogenesis: This pattern usually arises from Kidney yang deficiency, which is most commonly due to aging but can also be caused by a weak constitution, long-term physical and sexual overstrain, and chronic illness.

The Kidney yang is unable to give the Urinary Bladder enough qi to control fluids and therefore the fluids 'leak out,' such as in urinary incontinence and enuresis. Yang deficiency leads to the Urinary Bladder's failure to store urine, resulting in frequent urination. However, if yang deficiency impairs the Urinary Bladder's qi transformation function, the organ becomes unable to excrete urine, resulting in dysuria and anuria. Additionally, yang deficiency fails to warm and promote, manifesting with intolerance of cold, cold limbs, lassitude, listlessness, a pale tongue, and a deep weak pulse.

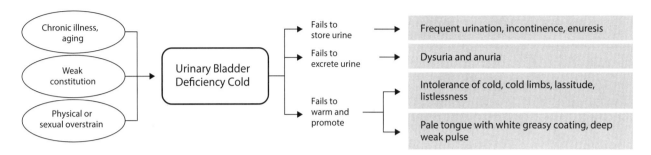

Chart 10.6 Etiology and pathogenesis of Urinary Bladder Deficiency Cold

TCM Disease	Western Disease	Herbal Formulas		Acupuncture	
Enuresis (遺尿)	Primary nocturnal enuresis, ADHD, psychological stress	Ji Sheng Shen Qi Wan, Suo Quan Wan	Sang Piao Xiao San	BL-22, BL-23, BL-28, GV-4, CV-4, ST-36	GV-20, CV-20, SP-6
Dysuria/anuria (癃閉)	Uroschesis, UTI, prostatitis, prostate enlargement, kidney stone, cystitis, renal failure		Ji Sheng Shen Qi Wan		Moxa
Urinary incontinence (小便失禁)	Menopause, pregnancy, MS, chronic UTI, hysterectomy, prostatitis, enlarged prostate, interstitial cystitis, overactive bladder, pelvic floor disorder		Tu Si Zi Wan		GV-20

Table 10.3 Diseases and treatments related to Urinary Bladder Deficiency Cold

Comparison: Urinary Bladder Deficiency Cold vs. Kidney Yang Deficiency

Urinary Bladder deficiency cold (膀胱虛寒 *páng guāng xū hán*) and Kidney yang deficiency (腎陽虛 *shèn yáng xū*) both have symptoms of frequent, clear, and copious urination, bedwetting, urinary incontinence, or difficult urination. The same treatment strategy and herbal formulas can also be applied to both patterns.

Kidney yang deficiency failing to warm causes qi failing to transform, leading to the dysfunction of the Urinary Bladder's ability to store and excrete, which results in the pattern of Urinary Bladder deficiency cold. Thus Urinary Bladder deficiency cold can be considered one of the results of Kidney yang deficiency. Kidney yang deficiency is therefore a prerequisite for Urinary Bladder deficiency cold.

Furthermore, Kidney yang deficiency encompasses not only abnormal urination, but also lower back pain, early morning diarrhea, loose stools, sexual dysfunction, menstrual disorders, and infertility. Urinary Bladder deficiency cold focuses only on abnormal urination.

The key point to distinguish these two patterns is the presence of Kidney related signs and symptoms.

Pattern	Urinary Bladder Deficiency Cold	Kidney Yang Deficiency
Etiology	Weak constitution, aging, chronic illness, physical or sexual overstrain, malnutrition, improper treatment	
Pathogenesis	Yang deficiency fails to warm and transform qi, disrupts storage and excretion	
Symptoms — Common	Frequent clear and copious urination or bedwetting, or incontinence, or difficult urination, intolerance of cold, cold limbs, lassitude, and listlessness. A pale tongue with white moist coating and a deep and weak pulse	
Symptoms — Different		Soreness and weakness in the lower back and groin, early morning diarrhea, loose stools, sexual dysfunction, menstrual disorders, infertility
Symptoms — Urination		Frequent nocturnal urination
Treatment strategy	Warm the yang, tonify the Kidney, assist qi to transform water, promote urination, shut off urinary frequency, stop leakage	
Herbal formulas	Ji Sheng Shen Qi Wan, Suo Quan Wan	

Table 10.4 Comparison of Urinary Bladder Deficiency Cold and Kidney Yang Deficiency

Comparison: Urinary Bladder Deficiency Cold vs. Small Intestine Deficiency Cold

Urinary Bladder deficiency cold (膀胱虛寒 *páng guāng xū hán*) and Small Intestine deficiency cold (小腸虛寒 *xiǎo cháng xū hán*) both result from yang deficiency causing frequent, clear, and copious urination, intolerance of cold, cold limbs, lassitude, listlessness, a pale tongue with a white moist coating, and a deep and weak pulse. However, the locations of these two patterns are different, and therefore they differ in clinical manifestation, treatment strategy, and herbal formula selection.

Urinary Bladder deficiency cold is due to Kidney yang deficiency failing to warm the Urinary Bladder, impairing qi transformation, and disrupting storage and excretion, which results in abnormal urination, including frequent, clear, and copious urination, difficult urination, bedwetting, and urinary incontinency.

Small Intestine deficiency cold results from yang qi deficiency that leads to the lack of motive force in the Small Intestine. It fails to reabsorb fluids, and to separate the clear from the turbid, which causes excess fluids to pour down to the Large Intestine and Urinary Bladder, resulting in loose stools and abnormal urination. This pattern can also develop from Spleen and Stomach yang deficiency, in which case it would present with gastrointestinal symptoms.

The key points to distinguish these two patterns are as follows:
1) Urination:
    - Urinary Bladder deficiency cold: frequent, clear, and copious urination, difficult urination, bedwetting, and urinary incontinency
    - Small Intestine deficiency cold: only frequent, clear, and copious urination
2) Presence of loose stools

Pattern	Urinary Bladder Deficiency Cold	Small Intestine Deficiency Cold
Etiology	Weak constitution, aging, chronic illness, malnutrition, improper treatment	
	Sexual overstrain	Exopathogenic cold invasion, history of Spleen and Stomach deficiency
Pathogenesis	Yang deficiency fails to warm the Urinary Bladder, impairs qi transforming, disrupts storage and excretion	Yang deficiency in Small Intestine, lacks motive force for absorption, fails to separate clear from turbid, excess fluid pours down
Symptoms — Common	Frequent clear and copious urination, intolerance of cold, cold limbs, lassitude, listlessness, pale tongue with a white moist coating, deep weak pulse	
Symptoms — Different	Difficult urination, bedwetting, urinary incontinence	Loose stools, borborygmus
Organs	Urinary Bladder, Kidney	Small Intestine, Spleen, Stomach, Kidney
Treatment strategy	Warms the yang, tonifies the Kidneys, assists the qi in transforming water, shuts off urinary frequency, and stops leakage	Warms and tonifies the middle burner
Herbal formulas	Ji Sheng Shen Qi Wan, Suo Quan Wan	Wu Zhu Yu Tang, Fu Zi Li Zhong Wan

Table 10.5 Comparison of Urinary Bladder Deficiency Cold and Small Intestine Deficiency Cold

2 Urinary Bladder Damp-Heat Pattern | 膀胱濕熱証 |

Definition: A group of signs and symptoms caused by damp-heat accumulation in the Urinary Bladder, leading to a disorder of its urine storage and discharge function.

Clinical manifestations: Frequent urination, urgent urination with burning pain, dark-colored, bloody, or cloudy urine, stones in the urine, dribbling urination, or discontinuation of urination in mid-stream, possibly accompanied by fever and chills, low back pain, red tongue with yellow coating, and a slippery rapid pulse.

Key points: Frequent, urgent, burning and painful urination, plus damp-heat signs and symptoms.

Etiology and pathogenesis: This pattern can be due to exopathogenic damp-heat invading and penetrating the Urinary Bladder, or to improper diet such as overconsumption of alcohol and hot, spicy, greasy foods that generate damp-heat. This damp-heat pours down to the Urinary Bladder, and impairs the organ's qi transformation function.

Damp-heat accumulation in the Urinary Bladder impairs the function of the organ, resulting in the failure of qi transformation. As a result, heat and fluid wastes pour down, irritate the urethra, and cause urgent, painful, and frequent urination. If damp-heat congeals and consumes fluids, fluid wastes condense and form stones. When stones form and obstruct the Urinary Bladder or Kidney channels and vessels, they can cause low back pain. When heat injures blood vessels, it leads to hematuria or blood in the urine.

Damp-heat accumulation can also steam outward, resulting in an increased body temperature, a red tongue with yellow greasy coating, and a slippery rapid pulse. If damp-heat invades from the exterior, it may be accompanied by chills and fever along with a superficial pulse

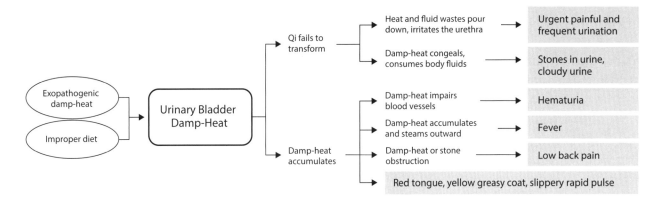

Chart 10.7 Etiology and pathogenesis Urinary Bladder Damp-Heat

TCM Disease	Western Disease	Herbal Formulas		Acupuncture	
Painful urinary dribbling (淋証)	UTI, gonorrhea, chlamydia, cystitis, prostatitis, urethritis, vulvovaginitis	Ba Zheng San, Wu Ling San	Xiao Ji Yin Zi, Zhu Ling Tang	SP-6, SP-9, BL-22, BL-66, ST-28, CV-3	BL-28, LR-2, KI-3, LI-4
Urinary blockage (癃閉)	Uroschesis, UTI, prostatitis, prostate enlargement, kidney stone, cystitis		Qian Lie Kang, Jie Jie Wan		BL-28, SP-9
Cloudy Urine (尿濁)	UTI, gonorrhea, cystitis, prostatitis, kidney stone, kidney failure, diabetic schistosomiasis		Bi Xie Fen Qing Yin		CV-6, BL-23, GV-20

Table 10.6 Diseases and treatments related to Urinary Bladder Damp-Heat

Comparison: Urinary Bladder Damp-Heat vs. Small Intestine Excess Fire

Urinary Bladder damp-heat (膀胱濕熱 *páng guāng shī rè*) and Small Intestine excess fire (小腸實火 *xiǎo cháng shí huǒ*) both present with frequent, urgent, burning, and painful urination, and both can develop from improper diet, such as overconsumption of alcohol or spicy, greasy foods. However, their location and pathogeneses are different, and therefore they have some differences in clinical manifestations.

Besides improper diet, Urinary Bladder damp-heat can also be due to poor hygiene in the genital area, allowing exopathogenic factors to directly invade. Damp-heat invasion impairs the Urinary Bladder, resulting in a failure to transform qi and excrete urine, which can lead to difficult urination. If damp-heat scorches and consumes fluids, fluid wastes, dampness, and impurities can condense and form stones, resulting in 'stone *lín*' (石淋 *shí lín*) or 'cloudy *lín*' (膏淋 *gáo lín*). And, since the Urinary Bladder is internally-externally paired with the Kidney, there may be Kidney symptoms, such as lower back pain.

Small Intestine excess fire is usually caused by emotional stress and long-term anxiety. The pathogensis for this pattern is excessive heat invasion that impairs the Small Intestine's ability to separate the clear from the turbid, causing heat to combine with excess fluid, which then pours down to the Large Intestine and Urinary Bladder. This results in loose stools and abnormal urination. Since the Small Intestine is internally-externally paired with the Heart, there may be symptoms related to Heart fire, such as mouth ulcers, tongue sores, insomnia, and irritability.

The key points to distinguish these two patterns are as follows:
1) Urination:
    - Urinary Bladder damp-heat: UTI and urinary blockage (*lóng bì*) symptoms such as various forms of painful urinary dribbling (heat, bloody, stone, turbid)
    - Small Intestine excess fire: only UTI, heat or bloody urinary dribbling
2) Kidney symptoms vs. Heart and gastrointestinal symptoms

Pattern		Urinary Bladder Damp-Heat	Small Intestine Excess Fire
Etiology		Improper diet, overconsumption of alcohol and spicy greasy foods	
		Exopathogenic factor invasion due to poor hygiene in the genital area	Emotional strain, anxiety, excessive stress
Pathogenesis		Damp-heat invasion impairs Urinary Bladder, fails to transform qi	Small Intestine fails to separate clean from turbid, which pours down to Large Intestine and Urinary Bladder
Symptoms	Common	Frequent, urgent, burning, painful urination, dark urine, blood in the urine, thirst, may have chills and fever, tongue is red with yellow coating, pulse is slippery and rapid	
	Different	Stone in the urine, cloudy urine, difficult urination, or even urinary blockage (*lóng bì*)	
	Other	Low back pain	Irritability, insomnia, canker sores, tongue sores, loose stools
Painful urinary dribbling		Hot painful urinary dribbling, bloody painful urinary dribbling, stone painful urinary dribbling, turbid painful urinary dribbling	Hot painful urinary dribbling, bloody painful urinary dribbling
Treatment strategy		Clear heat, promote urination, unblock painful urinary dysfunction	
Herbal formulas		Ba Zheng San	Dao Chi San

Table 10.7 Comparison of Urinary Bladder Damp-Heat and Small Intestine Excess Fire

Summary of Urinary Bladder Disease Patterns

Key points: abnormal urination, such as frequent, burning, or difficult urination		
Patterns		**Clinical manifestations**
Deficiency	Urinary Bladder Deficiency Cold	Frequent clear and copious urination, bedwetting, urinary incontinence, intolerance of cold, cold limbs, lassitude, listlessness, pale tongue with white moist coating, deep and weak pulse
Excess	Urinary Bladder Damp-Heat	Frequent urination, urgent urination with burning pain, dark-colored, bloody, or cloudy urine, stones in the urine, dribbling urination or discontinuation of urination mid-stream, possibly accompanied by fever and low back pain, red tongue with yellow coating, slippery and rapid pulse

Table 10.8 Summary of Urinary Bladder disease patterns

Part 3

COMPOUND PATTERNS

The *zàng fǔ* organs are related to one another not only in physiological functions but also over the entire course of disease development. When a pathological change occurs in one organ, disease can arise in other associated organs. If a disease pattern involves more than one *zàng fǔ* organ, it is called a compound or complex *zàng fǔ* pattern. In this chapter, the most common compound *zàng fǔ* patterns will be discussed.

CONTENTS

CHAPTER 11: HEART AND LUNG, 210

CHAPTER 12: HEART AND SPLEEN, 212

CHAPTER 13: HEART AND LIVER, 215

CHAPTER 14: HEART AND KIDNEY, 218

CHAPTER 15: HEART AND SMALL INTESTINE, 224

CHAPTER 16: SPLEEN AND LUNG, 227

CHAPTER 17: SPLEEN AND KIDNEY, 230

CHAPTER 18: SPLEEN AND STOMACH, 233

CHAPTER 19: LUNG AND KIDNEY, 236

CHAPTER 20: LIVER AND KIDNEY, 240

CHAPTER 21: LIVER AND SPLEEN/STOMACH, 244

CHAPTER 22: LIVER AND LUNG, 249

CHAPTER 23: LIVER AND GALLBLADDER, 252

Methods to identify compound *zàng fǔ* patterns

In compound *zàng fǔ* patterns there is a priority in the patterns involved, typically with one pattern being primarily responsible for the chief complaints of the patient. The pattern priority may change during the disease development process as indicated by changes in the signs and symptoms. Thus treatments should be adjusted accordingly to target the primary organ.

When identifying compound *zàng fǔ* patterns, the following guidelines should be followed:
- Identify which *zàng fǔ* organs have undergone pathological changes, which organ is the primary organ, which is the secondary, or which are of equal importance.
- Determine the order of the organs involved, whether the pathological changes in the separate *zàng fǔ* organs occurred at the same time, or if one came earlier than the others.
- Find any causative factors such as exopathogens or internal deficiencies; determine how they are transmitting and the relationship between the organs undergoing pathological changes such as internal-external pairs or cycles of generating, controlling, insulting or overacting.

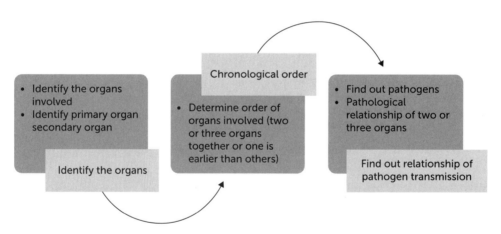

Chart Intro-1   Guideline to identify compound *zàng fǔ* organ patterns

There are three major steps for compound *zàng fǔ* pattern identification:
1. Use key signs and symptoms to identify the organs involved and then, along with the patient's chief complaints, determine the primary organ and secondary organ.
2. Analyze clinical signs and symptoms to understand the nature of the disease, its pathological changes, and its causative factors such as heat, cold, excess, deficiency, wind, phlegm, or blood stasis.
3. Conclude diagnosis based on the pathological relationship of two or three organs.

Introduction

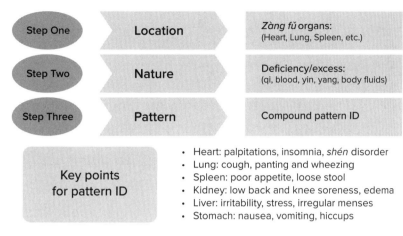

Chart Intro-2 Steps for compound pattern identification

Common compound *zàng fǔ* patterns

Because compound *zàng fǔ* patterns involve two or more organs, there are various pattern combinations. Some of them are commonly seen in the clinic while others are rare. The following fifteen patterns are the most common.

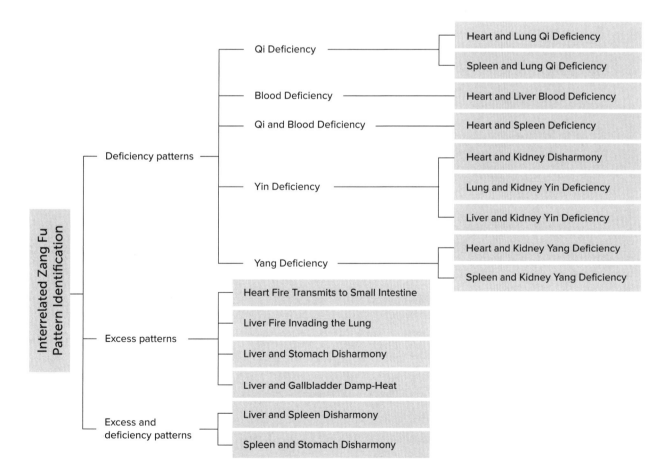

Chart Intro-3 Common compound *zàng fǔ* patterns

Chapter 11
Heart and Lung

Pathophysiological relationship between the Heart and Lung

The Heart governs blood and the Lung controls qi, so the relationship between the Heart and Lung essentially relates to the qi and blood, which means the Lung qi assists the Heart in promoting blood circulation while the Heart blood carries the Lung qi in order to distribute it throughout the entire body.

The Lung governs qi and controls respiration. The gathering qi (宗氣 zōng qì) is a combination of the clear qi (清氣 qīng qì) inhaled from the natural environment and absorbed from food qi (谷氣 gǔ qì). It provides the power to maintain qi and blood circulation.

Pathologically, the Lung and Heart also affect each other. If Lung qi is deficient, the gathering qi will also be insufficient, which then provides less power to propel qi and blood circulation. This can lead to qi and blood stagnation, manifesting with cough, shortness of breath, tightness in the chest, palpitations, and purple lips. On the other hand, if Heart qi is deficient, then Lung qi will fail to descend and disperse, manifesting with palpitations, tightness in the chest, panting, difficulty breathing, and pale lips.

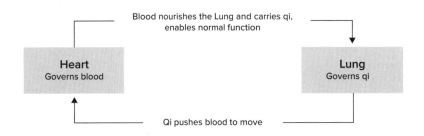

Chart 11.1 Physiological relationship of the Heart and Lung

1 Heart and Lung Qi Deficiency Pattern | 心肺氣虛証 |

Definition: A group of signs and symptoms characterized by qi deficiency of the Heart and Lung, presenting palpitations, cough, panting, and shortness of breath as the cardinal symptoms.

Clinical manifestations: Palpitations, coughing or panting, shortness of breath, and fatigue, all of which are aggravated by exertion. There may also be chest oppression, copious thin sputum, pale complexion, dizziness, spontaneous sweating, a weak and low voice, a pale tongue with a white coating, and a deep and weak pulse.

Key points: Palpitations, coughing and panting, difficulty breathing, plus qi deficiency signs and symptoms.

Etiology and Pathogenesis: Chronic illness with coughing or wheezing consumes Lung qi, which then affects the Heart qi. Additionally, aging, long-term excessive pensiveness and worrying, and a weak constitution can all impair the generation of qi and blood leading to Lung and Heart qi deficiency.

When the Heart qi is deficient it cannot provide enough power to propel qi and blood. This deficiency also fails to support the Heart *shén*, presenting physical and emotional symptoms of palpitations, and dizziness.

When Lung qi is deficient there is not enough qi to supply the Lung to perform its functions, leading to shortness of breath. The Lung is then unable to disperse qi downward, which accumulates in the chest, leading to rebellious qi, chest oppression, coughing, panting, and difficulty breathing.

Lung qi deficiency also causes fatigue, weakness, low voice, and the loss of control in securing the body's surface, which presents with spontaneous sweating. Since physical or mental exertion further consumes qi, the symptoms will worsen with exertion. The facial complexion will be pale and the pulse will be weak and deep.

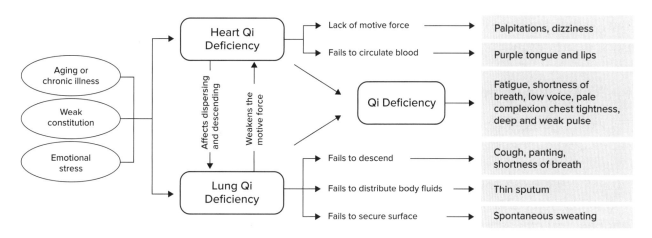

Chart 11.2 Etiology and pathogenesis of Heart and Lung Qi Deficiency

TCM Disease	Western Disease	Herbal Formulas		Acupuncture	
Cough (咳嗽)	COPD, CHF, cor pulmonale, chronic bronchitis, emphysema, chronic asthma	Bao Yuan Tang, Sheng Mai San, Bu Fei Tang	Bu Fei Tang	LU-7, LU-9, CV-6, CV-12, CV-17, BL-13, BL-15, GV-12, ST-36, HT-5, PC-5	LU-1, LU-5, LU-11, CV-22
Fatigue (虚劳)	COPD, asthma, CHF, emphysema, Lyme disease, hypothyroidism		Bu Fei Tang plus Bao Yuan Tang		GV-20, CV-4
Sweating (汗証)	Hyperthyroidism, vegetative never function disturbance, anxiety, HIV/AIDS		Yu Ping Feng San plus Gui Zhi Gan Cao Tang		KI-7, LU-4, GV-20, GV-14
Syncope (暈厥)	Hypotension, hypoglycemia, arrhythmia, bradycardia, anxiety, emotional shock, dehydration		Du Shen Tang, Si Wei Hui Yang Yin		GV-26

Table 11.1 Diseases and treatments related to Heart and Lung Qi Deficiency

Chapter 12
Heart and Spleen

Pathophysiological relationship between the Heart and Spleen

The relationship between the Heart and Spleen manifests in two ways: the production of blood and the maintenance of normal blood circulation.

1 | Production of blood

The Heart governs blood while the Spleen governs transportation and transformation. The Spleen can be considered the source of qi and blood because it transforms or distills food qi from ingested food and sends it upward to the Lungs, where it combines with gathering qi that is then pushed to the Heart and transformed into blood. The Heart's yang qi then provides the propulsion to distribute this blood to the rest of the body. When the Spleen function is normal, there is adequate transportation and transformation of food qi and thus proper production of blood, which means the Heart is well nourished and can maintain normal function.

Pathologically, this relationship between the Heart and Spleen means that a deficiency in one can lead to a deficiency in the other. For instance, overthinking and worrying weakens the Spleen, which loses its ability to properly transform and transport food qi for the production of blood in the Heart. This can eventually lead to blood deficiency in both the Heart and Spleen.

Chapter 12: Heart and Spleen

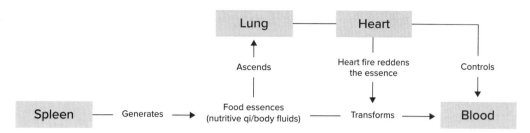

Chart 12.1 Heart and Spleen produce blood

2 | Maintain blood circulation

Blood circulation requires the regulated actions of a number of internal organs as well as the coordination of the Heart and Spleen. The 'Heart governs blood,' propelling blood circulation, while the 'Spleen controls blood,' keeping blood inside the vessels.

Pathologically, a disturbance of the Heart not only affects blood circulation, leading to blood stagnation or deficiency, but can also affect the transportation and transformation functions of the Spleen. Conversely, if Spleen functions are impaired, it will fail to keep blood within the vessels, resulting in bleeding and easy bruising. Profuse or long-term bleeding will eventually lead to Heart blood deficiency. Such a condition is known as Heart and Spleen deficiency pattern.

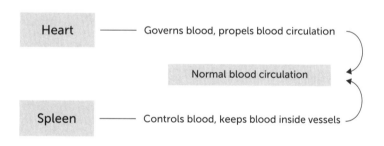

Chart 12.2 Heart and Spleen relationship to blood circulation

1 | Heart and Spleen Deficiency Pattern | 心脾兩虛証 |

Definition: A group of signs and symptoms characterized by a combination of Heart blood deficiency and Spleen qi deficiency. The Heart *shén* loses nourishment while the Spleen loses its proper function of transportation and transformation as well as controlling blood.

Clinical manifestations: Palpitations, poor memory, poor concentration, insomnia, dream-disturbed sleep, poor appetite, abdominal bloating and loose stools, fatigue, dizziness, subcutaneous bleeding, light and scanty menstrual bleeding, spotting or prolonged menstrual bleeding, a pale tender tongue, and a thin weak pulse.

Key points: Co-existence of palpitations, insomnia, poor appetite, and bleeding or bruising.

Etiology and pathogenesis: Improper diet, overthinking and worrying, chronic illness and bleeding can all impair the Spleen's function, leading to Spleen qi deficiency, which impairs its ability to cause food qi to ascend for the generation of blood, resulting in Heart blood deficiency.

The Heart houses the *shén*, which needs to be nourished by a sufficient supply of blood. Thus Heart blood deficiency results in an unsettled *shén* that manifests with symptoms such as palpitations, insomnia, and dream-disturbed sleep. Furthermore, when this deficiency results in blood failing to ascend to the brain, it can lead to dizziness, poor memory, and poor concentration.

Meanwhile, the Spleen's impaired functions of transportation and transformation gives rise to poor appetite, loose stools, abdominal bloating, and distention. The deficient Spleen qi fails to keep blood in the vessels, leading to bleeding problems such as easy bruising, subcutaneous bleeding, abnormal menstrual bleeding, and spotting. Moreover, this general lack of nourishment due to both qi and blood deficiency means that there will be fatigue and lassitude, a pale complexion and tongue, and a weak and thin pulse.

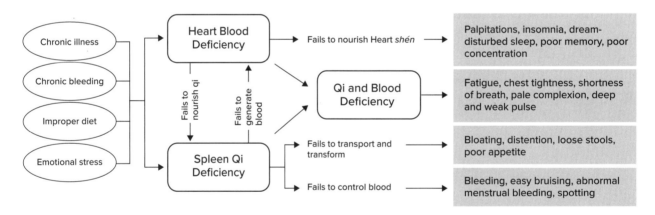

Chart 12.3 Etiology and pathogenesis of Heart and Spleen Deficiency

TCM Disease	Western Disease	Herbal Formulas		Acupuncture	
Fatigue (虛勞)	COPD, asthma, CHF, emphysema, Lyme disease, hypothyroidism	Si Wu Tang	Gui Pi Tang, Shi Quan Da Bu Tang	ST-36, GV-4, CV-4, CV-6, BL-24	HT-7, PC-6, CV-4, CV-12, CV-14, BL-15, BL-20, ST-36, SP-6
Palpitations (驚悸怔忡)	Arrhythmia, anemia, coronary artery disease, cor pulmonale, panic attack, menopause syndrome	Si Wu Tang plus Tian Wang Bu Xin Dan		HT-6, HT-7, HT-8, CV-14, BL-15	
Insomnia (不寐)	Menopause syndrome, depression, anxiety, neurosis	Yang Xin Tang		HT-5, HT-6, HT-7, Anmian, BL-15	
Forgetfulness (健忘)	Dementia, Alzheimer's, sleep apnea, depression, hypothyroidism, ADD/ADHD	Yi Qi An Shen Tang		BL-20, BL-23, KI-7 Sishengcong	
Bleeding (出血)	Thrombocytopenic purpura, chronic ITP, allergic purpura, aplastic anemia	Huang Tu Tang		BL-43, CV-6	
Dizziness and vertigo (眩暈)	Anemia, hypotension, hypoglycemia, BPPV	Ren Shen Yang Rong Tang		GV-20, GB-20, GB-34	
Metrorrhagia (崩漏)	PCOS, hypothyroidism, perimenopause, vaginal atrophy	Huang Tu Tang		Zigongxue, SP-1, SP-3, SP-10	

Table 12.1 Diseases and treatments related to Heart and Spleen Deficiency

Chapter 13

Heart and Liver

Pathophysiological relationship between the Heart and Liver

The relationship between the Heart and Liver manifests in two ways: blood circulation and mental or emotional activities.

1 | Maintain blood circulation

The Heart and Liver support and cooperate with each other to maintain normal blood circulation. The 'Heart governs blood,' propellng blood through the vessels, while the 'Liver stores blood,' regulating its volume. When there is sufficient Heart blood and exuberant qi, blood will move through the vessels normally and there will be enough blood stored in the Liver. When there is sufficient blood stored in the Liver, it can regulate the volume of blood in order to meet the physiological needs of the body and help the Heart in propelling the movement of blood.

Pathologically, this relationship between the Heart and Liver means that a deficiency in one can lead to a deficieny in the other. If Heart blood is deficient, not enough blood is sent to the Liver for storage and nourishment. This disrupts the Liver's ability to regulate blood, resulting in dizziness, blurred vision, numbness, twitching, or spasms. Conversely, if Liver blood is deficient, less volume of blood circulates in the body and eventually causes Heart blood deficiency, leading to blood deficiency in both the Heart and Liver.

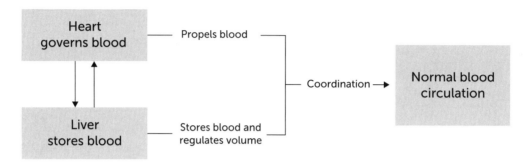

Chart 13.1 Heart and Liver regulate blood circulation

2 | Mental/emotional activities

The Heart houses the *shén* and is responsible for all mental and emotional activities. The Liver is involved as well by ensuring the smooth flow of qi to regulate the mental and emotional activities, keeping the *shén* settled and stored in the Heart. Conversely, when the Heart *shén* is normal, it helps the Liver to ensure a smooth flow of qi. Thus the Heart and Liver support and cooperate with each other to maintain normal mental and emotional activities.

Only when the Heart and Liver are in harmony can the mental and emotional activities be normal. When the Heart *shén* is disturbed, the Liver is unable to maintain a smooth flow of qi, resulting in Liver qi stagnation. Likewise, if emotional stress causes Liver qi stagnation, it may cause the Heart to become disturbed and unsettled, presenting with irritability, anxiety, anger, depression, palpitations, or insomnia.

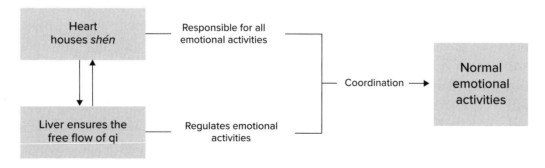

Chart 13.2 Heart and Liver relationship to emotional activities

1 Heart and Liver Blood Deficiency Pattern | 心肝血虛証 |

Definition: A group of signs and symptoms characterized by blood deficiency in both the Heart and Liver, presenting with symptoms resulting from the Heart and Liver losing nourishment.

Clinical manifestations: Palpitations, poor memory, poor concentration, insomnia, dream-disturbed sleep, dry eyes, blurry vision, dry and withered nails, numbness, twitching, or spasms of the extremities, irritability, dizziness, tinnitus, pale facial complexion, light and scanty menstruation or amenorrhea, a pale tongue with a white coating, and a thin and weak pulse.

Key points: Palpitations, poor memory, numbness, irritability, plus blood deficiency signs and symptoms.

Etiology and pathogenesis: Chronic illness, improper diet, bleeding, or long-term excessive pensiveness and mental overstrain consumes blood, leading to blood deficiency in both the Heart and Liver. Insufficient blood to nourish the Heart *shén* leads to palpitations, poor memory, poor concentration, insomnia, and dream-disturbed sleep. Meanwhile, insufficient blood to nourish the Liver results in dry withered nails, muscle cramps or spasms, and numbness of the extremities, since the nails are the 'surplus of the tendons,' which are nourished by Liver blood. This deficiency in Liver blood may also cause irritability due to Liver qi stagnation.

Additionally, a deficiency in blood can fail to nourish the brain and orifices, causing blurry vision, dizziness, and tinnitus. It can also fail to fill the Penetrating and Conception vessels, causing light and scanty menstruation or amenorrhea. This blood deficiency is further evidenced by a pale complexion, a pale tongue, and weak thin pulse.

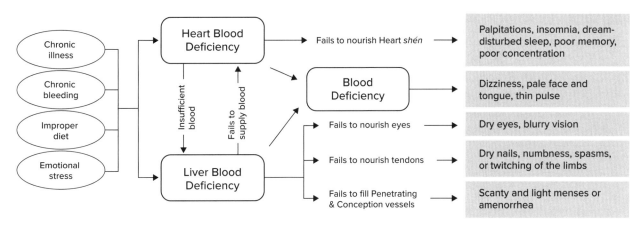

Chart 13.3 Etiology and pathogenesis of Heart and Liver Blood Deficiency

TCM Disease	Western Disease	Herbal Formulas		Acupuncture
Insomnia (不寐)	Menopause syndrome, depression, anxiety, neurosis	Suan Zao Ren Tang	Gui Pi Tang	Anmian, HT-5, HT-6 Yintang
Palpitations (驚悸)	Arrhythmia, anemia, coronary artery disease, cor pulmonale, panic attack, menopause syndrome	Tian Wang Bu Xin Dan		PC-6, CV-17
Fatigue (虛勞)	COPD, asthma, CHF, emphysema, Lyme disease, hypothyroidism	Gui Pi Tang, Ba Zhen Tang		GV-20, CV-6
Dizziness and vertigo (眩暈)	Anemia, hypotension, hypoglycemia, BPPV	Dang Gui Bu Xue Tang, Bai Wei Tang		GV-20, GB-20, GB-34
Spasms (痙病)	Convulsion, Parkinson's disease, Wilson's disease, Huntington's disease, Tourette's syndrome	Bu Gan Tang, Da Ding Feng Zhu		GB-20, GB-34, GB-31
Menstrual disorder (月經病)	Menorrhagia, polymenorrhea, metrorrhagia, amenorrhea, oligomenorrhea	Ba Zhen Tang		CV-6, LR-3

Acupuncture column additional points: HT-7, PC-6, CV-4, CV-14, BL-17, BL-18, BL-20, BL-23, LR-8, SP-6, ST-36

Table 13.1 Diseases and treatments related to Heart and Liver Blood Deficiency

Chapter 14
Heart and Kidney

Pathophysiological relationship between the Heart and Kidney

The Heart is located in the upper part of the body, pertains to yang, and is associated with fire, while the Kidney is located in the lower part of the body, pertains to yin, and is associated with water. This mutually supportive and restraining relationship between these two opposites manifests in three aspects: the harmony between yin and yang, the mutual generation of essence (精 jīng) and blood, and the regulation of mental and emotional activities.

1 | Harmony of yin and yang

Under normal conditions, the harmony between the Heart and Kidney means that there is a relative balance between the upper and lower, yin and yang, and fire and water. In each case, the opposing forces aid and control each other to ensure the normal physiological function of the

Heart and Kidney. This balance is shown in the interaction between the yin and yang of the Heart and Kidney.

Physiologically, Heart yang descends to the Kidney where it supports the Kidney yang to warm the Kidney water, preventing it from being too cold or freezing over. Meanwhile, the Kidney yin ascends to the Heart where it assists the Heart yin to anchor the Heart yang, preventing hyperactivity that could lead to a flaring of fire. This relationship of mutual communication and control is known as the 'interaction of the Heart and Kidney' (心肾相交 *xīn shèn xiāng jiāo*) or the 'mutual assistance of fire and water' (水火交融 *shuǐ huǒ jiāo róng*).

Pathologically, when either the Heart or the Kidney's own yin and yang become imbalanced, the harmony between the Heart and Kidney will be disrupted. When Heart yang is deficient, Heart fire cannot descend to warm the Kidney. The Kidney yang then fails to evaporate fluids, causing an overflow of water that can attack the Heart, giving rise to palpitations and edema. A deficient Kidney yang can also fail to evaporate Kidney yin, which cannot ascend to nourish the Heart yin for anchoring the Heart yang. In both cases, the Heart yin loses nourishment and becomes unable to restrain Heart yang. This leads to a hyperactivity of the Heart that can present with irritability, insomnia, and seminal emissions.

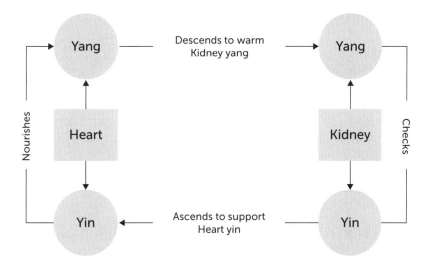

Chart 14.1 Harmony between the Heart and Kidney

2 | Generate essence and blood

The Heart governs blood and the Kidney stores essence. Essence and blood promote and nourish each other; essence can generate blood and blood can transform into essence. Pathologically, if Kidney essence is deficient, Heart blood will become deficient. Conversely, Heart blood deficiency can lead to Kidney essence deficiency.

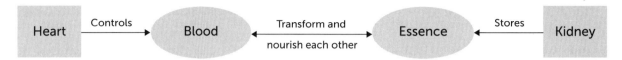

Chart 14.2 Essence and blood mutually transform and nourish

3 | Regulate emotional activities

The Heart houses the spirit or *shén*, responsible for mental and emotional activities, while the Kidney stores wisdom or *zhì*, which encompasses knowledge and self-awareness. A healthy mental and emotional state requires sufficient wisdom to avoid inappropriate thoughts and feelings such as anxiety and irrational fears. Kidney essence provides the material to nourish the *shén*, thus *shén* is the manifestation of essence. Kidney essence also engenders the marrow and blood that fills the brain and is thus the material basis of mental and emotional activities.

Pathologically, deficiency of blood or Kidney essence may cause abnormal mental and emotional functions. When Heart blood is deficient, it consumes Kidney essence, leading to the loss of nourishment for the *shén*. When Kidney essence is impaired, it also fails to fill the marrow and blood of the brain, causing abnormal mental and emotional functions such as poor memory, dizziness, insomnia and dream-disturbed sleep.

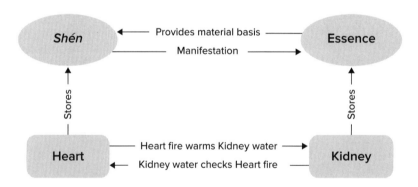

Chart 14.3 Heart and Kidney regulating mental and emotional activities

1 Heart and Kidney Yang Deficiency Pattern | 心腎陽虛 |

Definition: A group of signs and symptoms characterized by an insufficiency of Heart and Kidney yang, manifesting with blood stagnation due to a lack of Heart yang's motive force and dampness accumulation due to the Kidney yang's weakened function of warming and transforming fluids.

Clinical manifestations: Palpitations, edema on the face and lower extremities, scanty or difficult urination, intolerance of cold, cold limbs, physical and mental fatigue, sleepiness, dark and dim facial complexion and purplish lips, a pale and purple tongue, a white slippery tongue coating, and a deep, faint, and thin pulse.

Chapter 14: Heart and Kidney

Key points: Palpitations, edema, urinary disorder, plus yang deficiency signs and symptoms.

Etiology and pathogenesis: Chronic illness, aging, or overstrain can damage the yang of both the Heart and Kidney. A long-term yang deficiency can eventually affect the Heart's yang qi, resulting in both Heart and Kidney yang deficiency.

There are two mechanisms that can cause palpitations: the Heart's lack of motive force due to yang deficiency, and water attacking the Heart due to water retention caused by Heart and Kidney yang deficiency. Heart yang deficiency means a lack of warming and motive force, leading to blood stagnation, which gives rise to dark purplish lips, tongue, and complexion. Yang deficiency also causes a lack of power to supply blood to the rest of the body, resulting in lassitude and mental fatigue.

Kidney yang deficiency results in failure to transform qi and to control the opening and closing of the two lower yin orifices, leading to water metabolism disorders such as water retention, edema, and scanty or difficult urination. Yang deficiency also fails to warm the body, causing intolerance of cold and cold limbs, and is further evidenced by a pale tongue with a deep and weak pulse.

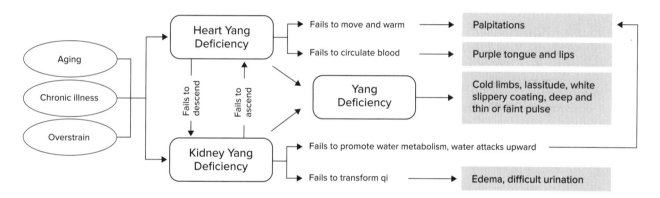

Chart 14.4 Etiology and pathogenesis of Heart and Kidney Yang Deficiency

TCM Disease	Western Disease	Herbal Formulas		Acupuncture	
Edema (水腫)	Chronic nephritis, COPD, CHF, chronic kidney failure, malnutrition	Shen Fu Tang, Gui Zhi Jia Ren Shen Fu Zi Tang	Bao Yuan Tang plus Zhen Wu Tang	HT-5, PC-6, BL-15, BL-23, CV-4, CV-6, CV-17, GV-4, GV-14, KI-3, KI-7	SP-9, BL-20, BL-23, CV-4, CV-9, KI-7, ST-36
Palpitations (驚悸)	Arrhythmia, anemia, coronary artery disease, cor pulmonale, panic attack, menopause syndrome		Ling Gui Zhu Gan Tang, Si Ni Tang, or Gui Zhi Gan Cao Long Gu Mu Li Tang		HT-6, HT-7, HT-8, CV-14, BL-19
Chest pain (胸痺)	MI, angina, cor-pulmonale, myocarditis, pericarditis, CAD, pulmonary embolism		Zhi Shi Xie Bai Gui Zhi Tang		HT-5, HT-7, BL-44, CV-4, GV-20

Table 14.1 Diseases and treatments related to Heart and Kidney Yang Deficiency

2 Heart and Kidney Disharmony Pattern | 心腎不交 |

Definition: A group of signs and symptoms characterized by a lack of coordination between Heart fire and Kidney water, manifesting as yin deficiency with yang excess of the Heart and Kidney.

Clinical manifestations: Palpitations, insomnia, vexation, dream-disturbed sleep, dizziness, tinnitus, dry mouth, malar flush, five-center heat, night sweats, soreness and weakness of the lower back and knees, seminal emissions, a red tongue with little or no coating, and a thin, rapid pulse.

Key points: Insomnia, palpitations, soreness and weakness of the lower back and knees, plus yin deficiency signs and symptoms.

Etiology and pathogenesis: Long-term qi stagnation caused by excessive worry, thinking, or depression generates pathogenic heat or fire, which then damages the Heart and Kidney yin. Sexual hyperactivity, aging, or chronic illness may also consume Kidney yin, leading to a relative excess of yang that rises up and disturbs the Heart *shén*, thereby undermining the coordination between Heart fire and Kidney water.

Kidney yin deficiency creates a relative excess of Heart yang. If Kidney water cannot restrain Heart fire, the fire will disturb the *shén*, giving rise to vexation, palpitations, dizziness, insomnia, and dream-disturbed sleep. Meanwhile, Kidney yin deficiency fails to nourish the brain and bones, causing poor memory with soreness and weakness of the lower back and knees. When the insufficient yin cannot anchor yang, the floating yang reddens the cheeks. This deficiency heat also causes night sweats and five-center heat. If deficiency fire disturbs the chamber of sperm (精室 *jīng shì*), seminal emissions can result. The tongue and pulse will show signs of yin deficiency such as a red tongue with scanty coating and a thin, rapid pulse.

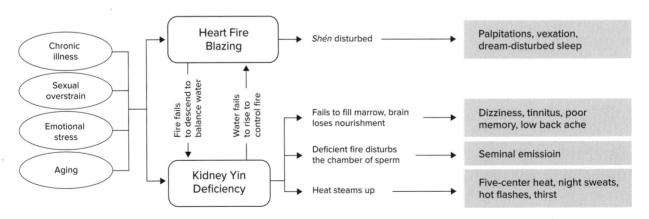

Chart 14.5 Etiology and pathogenesis of Heart and Kidney Disharmony

TCM Disease	Western Disease	Herbal Formulas		Acupuncture	
Insomnia (不寐)	Menopause syndrome, depression, anxiety, neurosis	Tian Wang Bu Xin Dan, Jiao Tai Wan, Liu Wei Di Huang Wan	Jiao Tai Wan, Huang Lian E Jiao Tang	HT-5, HT-6, HT-7, BL-15, CV-4, CV-15, GV-24, KI-3, KI-6, KI-10, SP-6	Anmian, Yintang
Palpitations (驚悸)	Arrhythmia, anemia, coronary artery disease, cor pulmonale, panic attack, menopause syndrome		Tian Wang Bu Xi Dan		PC-6, CV-17
Seminal emissions (遺精)	Spermatorrhea		Zhi Bai Di Huang Wan		KI-12, CV-6
Forgetfulness (健忘)	Dementia, Alzheimer's, hypothyroidism, ADD/ADHD, sleep apnea, depression		Liu Wei Di Huang Wan		Sishencong

Table 14.2 Diseases and treatments related to Heart and Kidney Disharmony

Comparison: Heart and Kidney Disharmony vs. Heart Fire Blazing

Heart and Kidney disharmony (心腎不交 *xīn shèn bù jiāo*) and Heart fire blazing (心火上炎 *xīn huǒ shàng yán*) both present with insomnia and palpitations, because both patterns involve pathogenic heat disrupting the *shén*. However, they require different treatment strategies because one arises from deficiency and the other from excess.

The root of Heart and Kidney disharmony is Kidney yin deficiency, which fails to control and keep Heart fire in check. In this pattern, the primary organ is the Kidney and the major complaints will involve Kidney yin deficiency. This is more commonly seen in elderly patients or those suffering from chronic illness.

Heart fire blazing, on the other hand, is a condition of excess that develops from emotional stress or overconsumption of alcohol and spicy greasy foods. In this pattern, the primary organ is the Heart, and therefore symptoms can include canker sores, mouth ulcers, irritability, anxiety, or even manic behavior. This is relatively short course and seen in younger patients.

The key points to distinguish these two patterns are as follows:
1) Presence of Kidney yin deficiency related symptoms
2) Presence of excess heat related symptoms
3) Status of the *shén*
4) Tongue and pulse

Pattern	Heart and Kidney Disharmony	Heart Fire Blazing
Etiology	Aging, sexual overstrain, chronic illness	Emotional stress, improper diet
Pathogenesis	Kidney yin cannot restrain Heart fire, which rises up and disturbs the *shén*	Pathogenic heat flares up and disturbs the *shén*, which becomes unsettled
Characteristics	Deficiency, chronic, longer course, relatively mild, more common in older patients	Excess, acute or sub-acute, short course, mild to severe, more common in younger patients
Symptoms – Common	Insomnia, palpitations, red tongue, rapid pulse	
Symptoms – Different	Tinnitus, dry mouth, malar flush, five-center heat, night sweats, soreness and weakness in the lower back and knees	Canker sores, irritability, vexation, thirst with desire for cold drinks, manic behavior, delirium
Tongue	Red cracked tongue with little or no coating	Red tongue with yellow coating
Pulse	Rapid and thin	Rapid and forceful
Treatment strategy	Enrich Kidney yin, harmonize Kidney and Heart, calm the *shén*	Drain heat from the Heart, calm the *shén*
Herbal formulas	Tian Wang Bu Xin Dan	Xie Xin Tang, Dao Chi San, Zhu Sha An Shen Wan

Table 14.3 Comparison of Heart and Kidney Disharmony and Heart Fire Blazing

Chapter 15
Heart and Small Intestine

Pathophysiological relationship between the Heart and Small Intestine

The Heart is a *zàng* organ while the Small Intestine is a *fǔ* organ. They are connected to each other via internal channel pathways and share an exterior-interior relationship.

When Heart fire is excessive, it can 'pour downward' through the internal channel pathway to the Small Intestine, leading to a burning sensation during urination, scanty and dark colored urine, or urinary tract infection. Conversely, excessive heat in the Small Intestine may also rise upward through the internal channel pathway to the Heart, giving rise to Heart fire and mental restlessness, irritability, and canker sores.

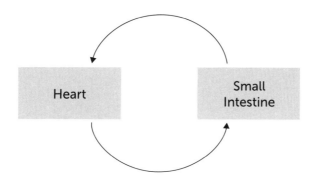

Chart 15.1 Physiological relationship between Heart and Small Intestine

1 Heart Fire Transmits to the Small Intestine Pattern | 心火下移小腸証 |

Definition: A group of signs and symptoms characterized by excessive Heart fire that transmits heat to the Small Intestine through the internal channel pathway, resulting in burning and painful urination. It is also known as 'Heart fire pouring downward.'

Clinical manifestations: Insomnia, irritability, anxiety, restlessness, canker sores, dry mouth, thirst and a preference for cold drinks, scanty dark urine with burning pain, a deep red tongue, and a forceful rapid pulse.

Key points: Canker sores, restlessness, anxiety, or burning pain during urination, plus heat signs and symptoms.

Etiology and pathogenesis: This pattern mostly occurs with excessive or long-term emotional stress that stagnates qi and generates heat; or improper diet, such as overconsumption of spicy, acrid, or greasy foods, and alcohol.

When pathogenic heat flares up, disturbing the *shén*, it can cause irritability or insomnia. If pathogenic heat flares up along the Heart channel, which opens to the tongue, it can decompose the tissues and flesh of the tongue and mouth, causing a red tongue, sore throat, canker sores, or mouth sores. When pathogenic heat impairs body fluids it can cause thirst and a desire to drink cold water. This impairment of body fluids also leads to yellow and scanty urination.

The Small Intestine governs fluids (主液 *zhǔ yè*) and is responsible for separating the clear from the turbid. Thus if excess heat transmits from the Heart to the Small Intestine, clear fluids fail to be separated and reabsorbed, resulting in excessive fluids combined with heat pouring down to the Bladder, disrupting the Bladder's qi transforming function. This causes frequent urination with burning, urgency, and pain. If heat injures the blood vessels, there may also be hematuria.

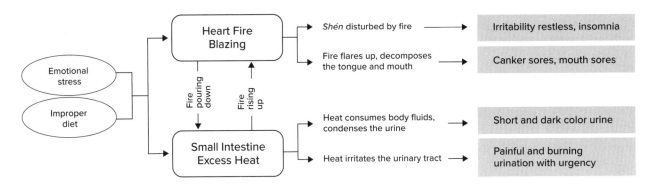

Chart 15.2 Etiology and pathogenesis of Heart Fire Transmits to the Small Intestine

TCM Disease	Western Disease	Herbal Formulas		Acupuncture	
Hot painful urinary dribbling (熱淋)	Cystitis, bladder infection, kidney infection, pyelonephritis, urethritis, interstitial cystitis	Dao Chi San	Ba Zheng San, Zhu Ling Tang	SI-2, SI-5, HT-5, HT-8, ST-39	CV-3, CV-4, BL-23, BL-28, KI-3
Hematuria (血淋)	UTI, pyelonephritis, prostatitis, glomerulonephritis, vasculitis, kidney or bladder stone or cancer		Xiao Ji Yin Zi		BL-22, BL-23, BL-27, PC-7, PC-8
Mouth sores (口瘡)	Cold sores, herpes simplex, stomatitis, Behcet's disease, Crohn's disease, celiac disease		Dao Chi San		SI-1, PC-8

Table 15.1 Diseases and treatments related to Heart Fire Transmits to the Small Intestine

Comparison: Heart Fire Transmits to the Small Intestine vs. Small Intestine Excess Fire

Heart fire transmitting to the Small Intestine (心火下移小腸 xīn huǒ xià yí xiǎo chǎng) and Small Intestine excess fire (小腸實火 xiǎo chǎng shí huǒ) are similar in etiology, pathogenesis, and nature. Thus they are almost identical in clinical manifestation, exhibiting urgency, frequency, burning and painful urination, thirst with a desire for cold water, a red tongue with a yellow coating, and a rapid pulse.

However, the primary organ under pathological change in Small Intestine excess fire is the Small Intestine, while the secondary organ is the Heart. In Heart fire transmitting to the Small Intestine it is the other way around. Thus the symptoms of Small Intestine excess fire are more focused on urinary tract infections, while the symptoms of Heart fire transmitting to the Small Intestine are more focused on irritability, restlessness, insomnia, canker sores, and tongue ulcers.

The key point in distinguishing these two patterns are the primary symptoms: urinary tract infection vs. *shén* disturbance

Pattern		Small Intestine Excess Fire	Heart Fire Transmitting to Small Intestine
Etiology	Common	Improper diet, emotional stress	
	Different	Exopathogenic factors invasion	Emotional stress is the primary factor
Pathogenesis		Excess heat disturbs the *shén*, disrupts the Small Intestine, which fails to separate clear from turbid	
Characteristics		Acute, excess, and heat	
Symptoms	Common	Frequent, burning, urgent, and painful urination, yellow and scanty urine, irritability, thirst, preference for cold drinks, canker sores, tongue ulcers, red tongue, rapid pulse	
	Primary	Urinary tract infection	*Shén* disturbance, canker sores, mouth sores
Treatment strategy		Clear heat, drain fire, promote urination	
Herbal formulas		Dao Chi San, Ba Zheng San	

Table 15.2 Comparison of Small Intestine Excess Fire and Heart Fire Transmitting to Small Intestine

Chapter 16
Spleen and Lung

Pathophysiological relationship between the Spleen and Lung

The relationship between the Spleen and Lung mainly centers on two aspects: the production of gathering qi or *zōng qì* and the regulation of water metabolism.

1 | Produce gathering qi

Gathering qi (宗氣 *zōng qì*) is the major source of post-natal qi in the body. *Zōng* means original, basic, or fundamental. It has been translated as essential qi, ancestral qi, chest qi, or pectoral qi. Additionally, it is also known as big qi (大氣 *dà qì*) or moving qi (動氣 *dòng qì*). It is responsible for promoting the Lung's respiration by moving through the respiratory tract, guiding qi and blood to stimulate the heartbeat, regulating the heart's rate and rhythm.

Gathering qi derives from the interaction of food qi (谷氣 *gǔ qi*) with clear air (清氣 *qīng qi*). The Spleen transforms food into essence qi (精氣 *jīng qi*) and then transports it to the Lung, where it is combined with clear air that is inhaled by the Lung. Thus the classic Chinese texts say: "The Spleen is the source of qi formation" and "The Lung is the pivot of governing the qi."

Physiologically, the Lung and Spleen mutually support and coordinate with each other, and they likewise have a pathological relationship. If the Spleen qi is impaired, it fails to transform and transport qi to the Lung, resulting in Lung qi deficiency, which leads to qi deficiency of both the Lung and Spleen. This condition is called 'earth not producing metal'. If Lung qi is deficient long enough, it will fail to distribute essence and body fluids to the whole body such that a deficiency of Spleen qi ensues, leading to further Spleen and Lung qi deficiency.

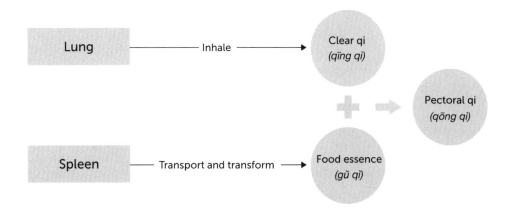

Chart 16.1 Lung and Spleen produce pectoral qi

2 | Regulate water metabolism

Water metabolism involves various *zàng fǔ* organs with the Spleen and the Lung being the two most important. The Spleen transports and transforms water while the Lung is the upper source of water and regulates the water passages. Thus coordination of the Lung and Spleen plays an important role in maintaining the balance of water metabolism.

When Spleen qi is deficient, transportation and transformation will be impaired. This means that ingested fluids will not be transformed into body fluids, but will instead remain inside the body, becoming pathological fluid retention, such as dampness or phlegm. Phlegm obstructing the Lung qi will affect its function of dispersing and descending, which will cause cough with phlegm. Thus the ancients said: "The Spleen is the source of phlegm formation, while the Lung is the container of phlegm." Conversely, when there is Lung qi deficiency, water waste from metabolism cannot descend for excretion but instead accumulates internally, generating dampness and impairing the Spleen's function.

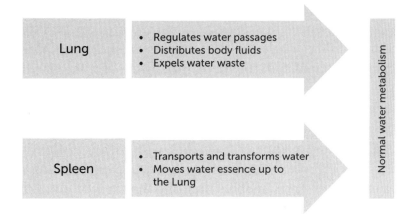

Chart 16.2 Lung and Spleen regulate water metabolism

1 Spleen and Lung Qi Deficiency Pattern | 脾肺氣虛証 |

Definition: A group of signs and symptoms characterized by qi deficiency both in the Lung and Spleen. It manifests with a dysfunction of the Spleen's transportation and transformation as well as the failure of the Lung's dispersing and descending functions.

Clinical manifestations: Chronic cough or panting with profuse sputum, a feeble voice, aversion to speaking, shortness of breath, general fatigue, poor appetite, abdominal bloating and distention, loose stools, pale complexion and tongue, and a deficient pulse. Edema is seen in severe cases.

Key points: Poor appetite, loose stools, cough, panting, shortness of breath, plus qi deficiency signs and symptoms.

Etiology and pathogenesis: Aging or chronic cough consumes Lung qi, which can no longer properly disperse and move qi downward, and thereby encumbers the function of the Spleen qi. Conversely, if an improper diet impairs the Spleen, it cannot properly produce qi and thereby affects the Lung qi. When both Spleen and Lung qi are deficient, water and fluid metabolism is abnormal, leading to the accumulation of dampness and phlegm in the body.

Both Lung and Spleen deficiency can produce phlegm, which is responsible for coughing with expectoration of sputum. Lung qi deficiency causes a loss of power to disperse and descend, giving rise to a feeble voice, shortness of breath, cough, or panting, while Spleen deficiency causes poor appetite. When either the Spleen or Lung is severely deficient, water metabolism will be affected, resulting in water retention and edema. Qi deficiency is further confirmed by a pale complexion and a deficient pulse.

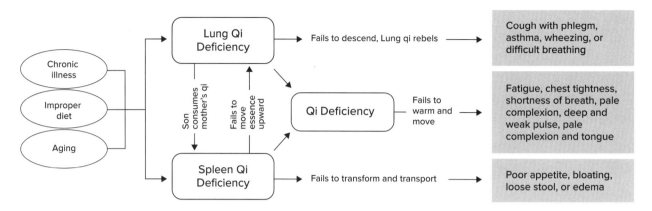

Chart 16.3 Etiology and pathogenesis of Spleen and Lung Qi Deficiency

TCM Disease	Western Disease	Herbal Formulas		Acupuncture
Cold, flu (感冒)	Common cold, flu, upper respiratory tract infection, early stage of infectious disease, such as meningitis, whooping cough	Liu Jun Zi Tang, Qi Wei Bai Zhu San	Shen Su Yin	LU-5, LU-7, LU-9, GB-20, BL-12
Cough (咳嗽)	Chronic bronchitis, emphysema, COPD, CHF, allergy asthma, sarcoidosis, cystic fibrosis, lung cancer		Bai Zhu Tang	CV-22, GV-14, SP-9, LU-1
Asthma (喘証)	Bronchial asthma, COPD, emphysema, pneumonia, CHF, silicosis, anxiety attack, allergic asthma		Su Zi Jiang Qi Tang	Dingchuan, CV-17, CV-22, KI-1, LU-1
Fatigue (虚勞)	COPD, asthma, emphysema, hypothyroidism		Bu Zhong Yi Qi Tang	SP-2, SP-3, SP-5

Acupuncture column also includes: ST-36, SP-3, BL-20, BL-13, LU-9, GV-12, BL-21

Table 16.1 Diseases and treatments related to Spleen and Lung Qi Deficiency

Chapter 17
Spleen and Kidney

Pathophysiological relationship between the Spleen and Kidney

The Kidney is the congenital root or source of pre-natal essence while the Spleen is the acquired root or source of post-natal essence. The Spleen and Kidney mutually nourish each other and coordinate in the regulation of water metabolism.

1 | Generate and store essence

The Spleen plays a vital role in the digestion and absorption of food. The warming and promoting function of the Kidney yang supports the Spleen in distilling food qi and moving it upward to the

Lung for distribution to the entire body, including the Kidney. Thus, the congenital promotes the acquired and the acquired nourishes the congenital.

However, when Kidney yang is deficient, it fails to warm the Spleen yang, leading to Spleen yang deficiency. Conversely, long-term deficiency of Spleen yang will eventually impair the Kidney yang, leading to yang deficiency of both the Spleen and Kidney.

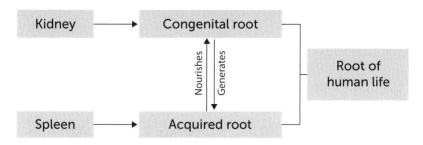

Chart 17.1 Kidney and Spleen as root of human life

2 | Regulate water metabolism

The Spleen's transportation and transformation function for distributing body fluids to the entire body relies on the warming function of the Kidney. The Kidney governs water and controls the opening and closing of the lower two yin orifices (urethra and anus), which also requires the cooperation of the Spleen.

Pathologically, if the Spleen qi is insufficient it fails to transform and transport water, leading to the accumulation of dampness; if Kidney qi is deficient and unable to transform qi, it also results in water retention, causing water metabolism disorders, and presents clinically with scanty urine, edema, abdominal bloating and distention, and loose stools.

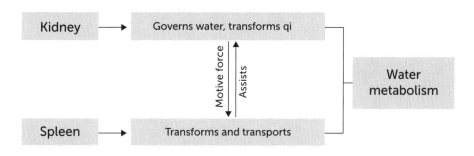

Chart 17.2 Kidney and Spleen for water metabolism

1 | Spleen and Kidney Yang Deficiency Pattern | 脾腎陽虛証 |

Definition: A group of signs and symptoms characterized by yang deficiency in both the Kidney and Spleen with a loss of warming and transforming functions, resulting in loose stools or edema as the cardinal signs and symptoms.

Clinical manifestations: Pale complexion, cold limbs and body, shortness of breath, lassitude, soreness and weakness of the lower back and knees, lower abdominal cold pain, chronic loose stools, or early morning diarrhea, poor appetite, watery stools with undigested food, edema, and difficult urination, a pale and tender tongue with a white slippery coating, and a deep, weak, and slow pulse.

Key points: Edema, loose stools, poor appetite, abdominal or lower abdominal pain that is relieved by warmth, plus yang deficiency signs and symptoms.

Etiology and pathogenesis: Chronic illness, aging, and improper diet consumes qi and impairs Kidney yang. Chronic diarrhea and loose stools or living and working in humid and damp environments can damage Kidney and Spleen yang.

If the Spleen yang declines and the Spleen fails to produce food essence to nourish the Kidney, the Kidney yang will also decline. If the Kidney yang is deficient, the *mìng mén* fire will fail to support and warm the earth, which will further impact the Spleen yang. In fact, either Spleen yang deficiency or Kidney yang deficiency can develop into the yang deficiency patterns of both the Spleen and the Kidney if they last long enough.

Spleen yang deficiency impairs the transportation and transformation function of the Spleen, leading to a deficiency of qi and blood. This manifests with a pale face, shortness of breath, lassitude, aversion to talking, and a weak pulse. This deficiency of yang also impairs the warming and motive functions of the Kidney, causing cold limbs and a general cold sensation in the body.

Spleen and Kidney yang deficiency leads to a relative excess of yin internally, resulting in qi and cold stagnation and abdominal cold pain. Without proper Spleen and Kidney yang, food cannot be digested and absorbed, resulting in poor appetite, diarrhea, and loose stools. Dampness and fluids accumulate because they are not adequately transformed and transported. Additionally, the impairment of the Kidney's qi transformation function will lead to difficult urination and edema.

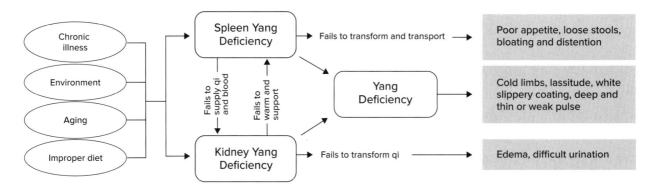

Chart 17.3 Etiology and pathogenesis of Spleen and Kidney Yang Deficiency

TCM Disease	Western Disease	Herbal Formulas		Acupuncture	
Fatigue (虛勞)	Adrenal fatigue, hypothyroidism, Lyme disease, EBV, renal failure, fibromyalgia, malnutrition	Fu Zi Li Zhong Wan, You Gui Wan	You Gui Wan	SP-3, SP-6, SP-9, CV-4, CV-6, CV-9, CV-12, GV-4, ST-28, ST-36, BL-20, BL-21, BL-22, BL-23, BL-25, BL-52, KI-3, KI-7	GV-20, Moxa
Diarrhea (泄瀉)	Colitis, IBS, Crohn's disease, IBD, celiac disease		Si Shen Wan		CV-3, ST-25, LR-13
Edema (水腫)	Chronic nephritis, CHF, chronic renal failure, malnutrition, COPD		Zhen Wu Tang		CV-10, GV-23, LI-6
Ascites (膨脹)	Cirrhosis, heart failure, constrictive pericarditis, nephrotic syndrome, Kwashiorkor		Shen Qi Wan		LI-6
Atrophy (痿証)	Sequelae of encephalitis or polio, MS, MG, tumors in CNS, myelitis, progressive muscular drystrophy, progressive myodystrophy		Gui Pi Tang plus You Gui Wan		Huatuojiaji, SP-9, ST-31, ST-32, ST-40, ST-42, GB-34, LI-2, LI-3, LI-4, LI-10, LI-11, LI-14, TB-5
Hematochezia (便血)	IBD such as diverticulosis, Crohn's disease, Behcet's disease, colitis, or hemorrhoids, rectum cancer		Huang Tu Tang		BL-24, BL-36, BL-57, BL-58, KI-7

Table 17.1 Diseases and treatments related to Spleen and Kidney Yang Deficiency

Chapter 18
Spleen and Stomach

Pathophysiological relationship between the Spleen and Stomach

Both the Spleen and Stomach are located in the middle burner and are interconnected by a membrane in the abdomen, forming an interior and exterior relationship. They coordinate and cooperate to maintain the normal digestive function. The relationship between the Spleen and Stomach manifests in three aspects: coordination of ingestion, transportation, and transformation; complementary ascending and descending movements; and the regulation of dryness and dampness.

1 | Coordinate ingestion, transportation, and transformation

The Spleen governs transportation and transformation, and the Stomach governs reception and decomposition. The Stomach prepares the food for the Spleen to transport and transform, while the Spleen sends body fluids to the Stomach to support its proper function. Dysfunction of Stomach in reception will lead to an aversion to food, gastric discomfort, or sensations of hunger. Dysfunction of the Spleen's transporting and transforming functions may result in abdominal distention, bloating, and loose stools.

2 | Complementary ascending and descending movements

The Spleen governs ascending and the Stomach governs descending. The Spleen moves the food and water essence upward to the Heart and Lung. The Stomach moves the digested water and food downward to the Small Intestine. Ascending and descending requires mutual cooperation of the Spleen and Stomach. If the Spleen qi descends rather than ascends, there may be diarrhea, loose stools, and rectal prolapse. If the Stomach qi ascends rather than descends, there may be nausea, vomiting, hiccups, or belching.

3 | Regulate dryness and dampness

The Spleen is a yin organ. It needs yang warmth to enable transportation and transformation. It favors dryness and disfavors dampness. The Stomach is a yang organ. It needs to be nourished by body fluids in order to receive and decompose. It favors moisture and disfavors dryness. Being yin and yang in nature respectively, each needs the other, and conditions the other. The Stomach yang protects the Spleen from an invasion of dampness, while the Spleen yin protects the Stomach from being impaired by dryness.

Pathologically, if transportation and transformation of the Spleen and Stomach become dysfunctional, symptoms may arise such as aversion to food or lost appetite, bloating and distention, and diarrhea or loose stools. If the ascending and descending functions are compromised, the resulting symptoms may include vomiting, nausea, hiccups, or loose stools. If the regulation of dryness and dampness becomes disordered, this can cause bloating, gas, poor appetite, loose stools, or constipation.

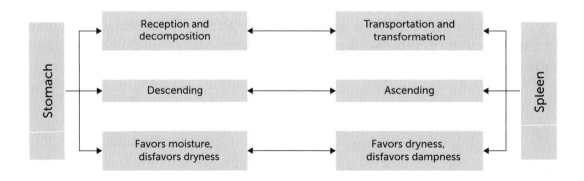

Chart 18.1 Physiological relationship between the Stomach and Spleen

1 Spleen and Stomach Disharmony Pattern | 脾胃不和証 |

Definition: A group of signs ands symptoms that presents when the Spleen and Stomach have lost their cooperating and coordinating relationship, characterized by poor appetite, belching, nausea, and irregular bowel movements.

Clinical manifestations: Aversion to food, poor appetite, nausea, vomiting, belching, hiccups, epigastric pain, abdominal bloating and distention, diarrhea, loose stools or constipation, a thick greasy tongue coating, and a slippery pulse.

Key points: Aversion to food, poor appetite, nausea, belching, irregular bowel movements, plus general gastrointestinal signs and symptoms.

Etiology and pathogenesis: Irregular or improper diet such as overeating greasy or raw and cold foods; long-term excessive pensiveness, worry, or overthinking; physical overstrain; improper or overuse of treatment strategies such as purgatives or emetics. All of these conditions can lead to Spleen and Stomach disharmony.

Dampness accumulation impairs the Spleen, blocking proper generation of qi, blood, and body fluids, while dryness and lack of nourishment impairs the Stomach, preventing proper decomposition of food and movement of waste downward. Thus Spleen and Stomach disharmony can result in irregular bowel movements, constipation, or diarrhea.

The Spleen and Stomach work together as a pivot in the center of the body with the Spleen ascending and the Stomach descending to keep qi moving smoothly. A disorder of either organ will disrupt this movement of qi, resulting in rebellious Stomach qi or sinking Spleen qi. This can present with nausea, vomiting, hiccups, abdominal bloating, loose stools, and even uterine or rectal prolapse. Additionally, when the Spleen's transportation and transformation is impaired, there can be epigastric pain and poor appetite.

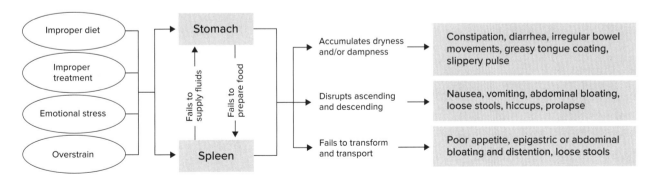

Chart 18.2 Etiology and pathogenesis of Spleen and Stomach Disharmony

TCM Disease	Western Disease	Herbal Formulas		Acupuncture	
Epigastric pain (胃脘痛)	Atrophic gastritis, gastroneurosis, GERD, peptic ulcer, gastric carcinoma	Shen Ling Bai Zhu San, Ban Xia Xie Xin Tang	Bao He Wan	CV-6, CV-12, ST-36, SP-3, SP-6, BL-20, BL-21	PC-6, KI-3, ST-44
Vomiting (嘔吐)	Food poisoning, gastroenteritis, stomach flu, gastritis, motion sickness, pregnant		Xuan Fu Dai Zhe Tang		PC-6, ST-25, CV-17
Diarrhea (泄瀉)	Food poisoning, gastroenteritis, SIBO, stomach flu, celiac disease, IBS, IBD		Zhi Shi Dao Zhi Wan		CV-3, CV-4, ST-25, LR-13

Table 18.1 Diseases and treatments related to Spleen and Stomach Disharmony

Chapter 19
Lung and Kidney

Pathophysiological relationship between the Lung and Kidney

The Lung and Kidney relationship involves water metabolism and respiration. Lung yin and Kidney yin mutually nourish each other.

1 | Maintain water metabolism

The Lung is the 'upper source of water' (肺為水之上源 *fèi wéi shuǐ zhī shàng yuán*); it disperses and descends, regulates the water passages, and distributes body fluids to the entire body, including the Kidney. The Kidney is the 'lower source of water' (腎為水之下源 *shèn wéi shuǐ zhī xià yuán*) and a water organ; it governs water metabolism, transforms qi, moves the pure body fluids upward, and the turbid downward. This evaporating and transforming function of the Kidney also assists the Lung's dispersing and descending function. Thus, the Lung and Kidney work together to maintain balanced water metabolism.

Pathologically, dysfunction of the Lung or Kidney not only affects water metabolism, but also each organ's separate functions. When the Kidney fails to transform qi, the retention of water can develop into an overflow into the Lung, a condition known as 'cold-water shooting into the Lung' (寒水射肺 *hán shuǐ shè fèi*). It presents with edema, severe cough, and asthmatic breathing (see p. 53 for more details).

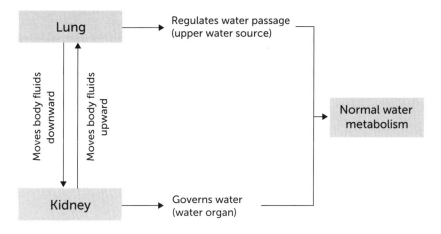

Chart 19.1 Lung and Kidney coordinate water metabolism

2 | Maintain normal respiration

The Lung governs qi and is responsible for respiration while the Kidney receives and anchors qi and is the root of qi. Only when Kidney qi is vigorous can air or 'clear qi' (清氣 *qīng qì*) be inhaled and sent downward by the descending function of the Lung to be received by the Kidney, maintaining even and deep respiration. Thus the Lung and Kidney work together in close communication to achieve proper respiratory function.

Pathologically, when the Kidney qi is insufficient and fails to receive or 'grasp qi,' this results in qi that cannot descend, leading to breathing difficulty on inhalation. Prolonged deficiency of Lung qi also causes a failure to move qi downward, which affects Kidney qi. Signs and symptoms include coughing, shortness of breath, panting, rapid or shallow breathing, and difficult breathing.

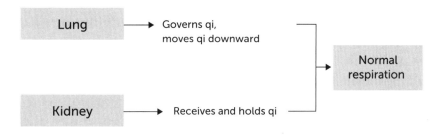

Chart 19.2 Lung and Kidney coordinate with respiration

3 | Lung and Kidney yin mutually nourish and replenish each other

The Lung pertains to metal, metal generates water, and water nourishes metal. When Lung yin is sufficient, it descends to fill the Kidney yin. When Kidney yin is sufficient, and as the root of yin for the entire body, it upwardly nourishes Lung yin. Thus Lung and Kidney yin mutually nourish and replenish each other, enabling these two organs to maintain balance and coordination.

Pathologically, if Lung yin is insufficient, there is not enough body fluids descending to nourish the Kidney, which can lead to Kidney yin deficiency. If Kidney yin is insufficient, it cannot evaporate enough body fluids upward to replenish the Lung yin, eventually leading to Lung yin deficiency.

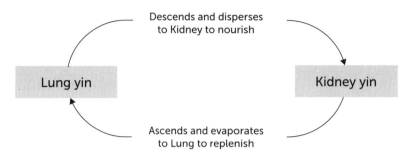

Chart 19.3 Lung and Kidney yin mutually nourishes

1 Lung and Kidney Yin Deficiency Pattern | 肺腎陰虛 |

Definition: A group of signs and symptoms characterized by the Lung losing its dispersing and descending function, leading to the Kidney losing yin nourishment. This insufficiency of Lung and Kidney yin generates internal pathogenic heat.

Clinical manifestations: Dry cough with little or no sputum, sputum that may contain blood, hoarse voice, soreness and weakness of the lower back and knees, malar flush, night sweats, low-grade fever in the afternoon or evening, fatigue, nocturnal emissions, five-center heat, insomnia, scanty urination, and constipation. The tongue is red with scanty or no coating and the pulse is thin and rapid.

Key points: Cough with scanty sputum, soreness and weakness of the lower back and knees, plus yin deficiency signs and symptoms.

Etiology and pathogenesis: Chronic illness with coughing or the later stage of febrile diseases may exhaust Lung yin, causing it to lose its ability to disperse and move body fluids downward to nourish the Kidney. Furthermore, chronic illness, aging, improper diet, and sexual overstrain may impair or exhaust the Kidney yin, which then affects the Lung yin and results in yin deficiency of both the Lung and Kidney.

The Lung's inability to disperse and descend when it is not nourished by sufficient yin leads to qi and body fluids accumulating in the Lung, causing cough with sputum. Yin deficiency generates heat, which damages blood vessels and consumes body fluids, resulting in scanty sputum that contains blood. The vocal cords also lose nourishment from Lung yin deficiency and may be further affected by deficiency heat, resulting in a hoarse voice.

Kidney yin deficiency will fail to nourish and strengthen the bones and marrow, giving rise to soreness and weakness of the lower back and knees. When a deficiency of yin is unable to contain the yang, the floating yang makes the cheeks red. This deficiency heat might also cause night sweats and five-center heat. If deficiency fire disturbs the chamber of sperm (精室 *jīng shì*), it can result in nocturnal emissions. The tongue and pulse will indicate signs of yin deficiency.

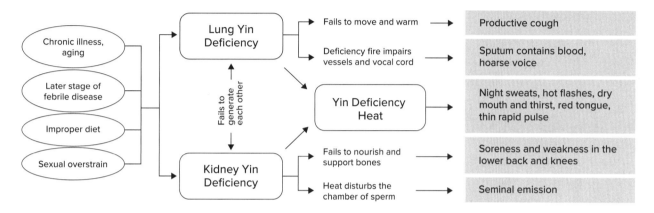

Chart 19.4 Etiology and pathogenesis of Lung and Kidney Yin Deficiency

TCM Disease	Western Disease	Herbal Formulas		Acupuncture
Cough (咳嗽)	Chronic bronchitis, emphysema, COPD, CHF, allergy asthma, lung TB, GERD, allergic rhinitis, lung cancer	Yue Hua Wan	Bai He Gu Jin Tang	CV-22, BL-13, GV-14, SP-9, LU-7
Asthma (喘証)	Bronchial asthma, URTI, LRTI such as bronchitis, pneumonia, allergic asthma	Qi Wei Du Qi Wan		Dingchuan, CV-17, CV-22, KI-1, GV-14, LU-1
Dysphonia (失音)	URTI caused by common cold or flu, such as pharyngitis, laryngitis	Bai He Gu Jin Tang	KI-3, KI-6, KI-13, LU-1, LU-7, LU-9, CV-4, SP-6, BL-43	LU-6, LU-10, LI-4, LI-10, ST-6, HT-6, HT-7
Fatigue (虛勞)	COPD, asthma, CHF, emphysema, Lyme disease, hypothyroidism	Da Bu Yuan Jian		BL-43, ST-36
Diabetes (消渴)	Diabetes, hyperthyroidism	Er Dong Tang		Yishuxue

Table 19.1 Diseases and treatments related to Lung and Kidney Yin Deficiency

Chapter 20
Liver and Kidney

Pathophysiological relationship between the Liver and Kidney

Ancient Chinese sources say "the Liver and Kidney are of the same source" (乙癸同源 *yī guǐ tóng yuán*). This statement manifests in three aspects: essence and blood share the same source, the coordination of conducting and storage, and mutual control of yin and yang.

1 | Store essence and blood

The Liver stores blood and the Kidney stores essence. Blood and essence are both generated from food qi and can transform into each other. Kidney essence can be transformed into Liver blood, while Liver blood can be transformed into Kidney essence.

2 | Coordinate coursing and storage

The Liver has an outward action of coursing and discharging while the Kidney has an inward action of sealing and storing. The Liver ensures the smooth flow of qi, which enables proper Kidney function to store essence, while the Kidney's sealing function prevents Liver qi from overly discharging. Thus the opposing functions of the Liver and Kidney mutually support and control each other. They also regulate the menstrual cycle in females and ejaculation in males.

3 | Mutually control yin and yang

The relationship between yin and yang of the Kidney and Liver is that of mutual generation and control. When Liver yin is abundant, it nourishes Kidney yin, and when Kidney yin is abundant, it nourishes Liver yin. Since yin anchors yang, sufficient Liver and Kidney yin not only nourishes each other, but prevents both the rising of excess Liver yang and the hyperactivity of Kidney fire. This enables the yin and yang of the Liver and Kidney to remain in balance.

Pathologically, insufficient Kidney essence can lead to Liver blood and yin deficiency while Liver blood and yin deficiency can consume Kidney essence, causing dizziness, vertigo, tinnitus, poor hearing, and soreness and weakness of the lower back and knees.

If Liver blood and yin as well as Kidney essence are insufficient, or Liver and Kidney yin is deficient with fire, there may be a disruption in the balance between the Liver's coursing and discharging of qi and the Kidney's storage of essence, resulting in irregular menstrual cycles, dysmenorrhea, or amenorrhea in women, and nocturnal emissions, premature ejaculation, or difficult ejaculation in men.

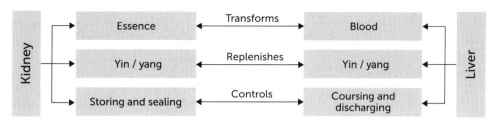

Chart 20.1 Kidney essence and Liver blood transform into each other

1 Liver and Kidney Yin Deficiency Pattern | 肺腎陰虛 |

Definition: A group of signs and symptoms characterized by the inability to control yang due to yin deficiency of the Liver and Kidney, which manifests with deficiency heat that disturbs the Liver and Kidney.

Clinical manifestations: Dizziness or vertigo, blurry vision, tinnitus, poor memory, dry mouth and throat, hypochondriac pain, soreness and weakness of the lower back and knees, five-center heat, night sweats, low-grade fever in the afternoon or evening, spermatorrhea in males, and scanty and short menstruation in females. The tongue will have a red or cracked body along with a scanty coating and the pulse will be thin and wiry.

Key points: Soreness and weakness of the lower back and knees, hypochondriac pain, tinnitus, dizziness, seminal emissions, plus yin deficiency heat signs and symptoms.

Etiology and pathogenesis: Chronic illness, aging, or long-term improper diet causes an insufficiency of yin and body fluids, emotional stress causes qi stagnation with yang excess that consumes yin, sexual hyperactivity impairs the Kidney essence, and long-term febrile diseases damages the Liver and Kidney yin.

When deficient Liver yin fails to nourish its orifice and channel there can be blurry vision and hypochondriac pain. When Liver yang is not anchored due to Liver yin deficiency, it flares up and rises to the head, causing dizziness and vertigo. And, when the Penetrating and Conception vessels are not filled due to Liver yin deficiency, there is scanty and short menstruation in women.

When deficient Kidney yin fails to nourish its orifices, bones, and marrow there is tinnitus, poor memory, and soreness and weakness of the lower back and knees. When Kidney yang is not anchored due to Kidney yin deficiency, it floats up to the face, causing malar flush. The deficiency heat also causes night sweats and five-center heat. If deficiency fire disturbs the chamber of sperm there is spontaneous emission. The tongue and pulse will be consistent with yin deficiency.

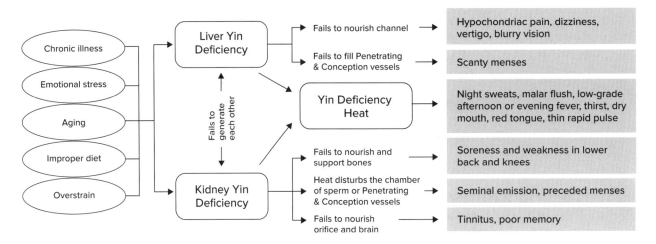

Chart 20.2 Etiology and pathogenesis of Liver and Kidney Yin Deficiency

TCM Disease	Western Disease	Herbal Formulas		Acupuncture
Hypochondriac pain (脇痛)	Chronic hepatitis, costochondritis, cholecystitis, intercostal neuralgia, shingles	Yi Guan Jian	Yi Guan Jian	TB-5, GB-34, GB-40, LR-3, BL-19
Lumbago (腰痛)	Sciatica, herniated disc, spinal stenosis, arthritis, degeneration	Zuo Gui Wan		Yaoyanxue, BL-40
Fatigue (虛勞)	Adrenal fatigue, Lyme disease, hypothyroidism, CFS, EBV, anemia, malnutrition, fibromyalgia	Da Bu Yin Wan		ST-36, CV-6, GV-20
Bleeding (血証)	Hematochezia, hemorrhoids, ITP, menorrhagia and metrostaxis, thrombocytopenic purpura	Zi Shui Qing Gan Yin		SP-10, LR-2, KI-2
Dizziness, vertigo (眩暈)	Hypertension, hypotension, BPPV, vestibular migraine, anemia, anxiety	Qi Ju Di Huang Wan		GV-20, GB-20, GB-34
Preceded menses (月經先期)	Perimenopause syndrome, PCOS, stress	Liang Di Tang		SP-10, SP-8, LR-2, KI-2
Amenorrhea (閉經)	PCOS, menopause, anorexia or bulimia, stress, thyroid malfunction	Gui Shen Wan		SP-4, SP-8, CV-4, LI-4
Dysmenorrhea (痛經)	Endometriosis, uterus fibroids, PID, STI, adenomyosis, IUD	Tiao Gan Tang		LR-2, CV-3, CV-6, GB-34

Acupuncture column (second formula column): KI-3, KI-6, KI-13, LU-7, LU-1, LU-9, CV-4, SP-6, BL-43

Table 20.1 Diseases and treatments related to Liver and Kidney Yin Deficiency

Comparison: Liver and Kidney Yin Deficiency vs. Liver Yang Rising

Liver yang rising (肝陽上亢 *gān yáng shàng kàng*) and Liver and Kidney yin deficiency (肝腎陰虛 *gān shèn yīn xū*) can be difficult to differentiate. The Liver and Kidney are of the same source

(肝肾同源 *gān shèn tóng yuán*) and thus have a close physiological and pathological relationship. Since 'water nourishes wood' (水能涵木 *shuǐ néng hán mù*), Kidney nourishes Liver, and deficiency in one leads to deficiency in the other. When a condition starts with Liver yang rising due to hyperactive yang, it may eventually consume both Liver and Kidney yin. Conversely, a condition that starts with Liver and Kidney yin deficiency may eventually fail to anchor Liver yang. Thus to differentiate these two patterns, the primary pathology must be determined.

A sturdy constitution exhibiting a hyperactive condition with anger, irritability, short temper, insomnia, dizziness, red face, headache, tinnitus, and a wiry forceful pulse indicates that Liver yang rising is the primary pathology. Over time, this can develop into Liver and Kidney yin deficiency as the excess yang consumes yin.

A weak constitution, improper diet, sexual overstrain, chronic illness, and a failure to recuperate results in Liver and Kidney yin deficiency that can lead to a relative yang excess. Yin deficiency signs are primarily seen here, presenting as five-center heat, hot flashes, night sweats, soreness and weakness of the lower back and knees, dry throat, dry red tongue, and a wiry, thin, and rapid pulse. There may be emaciation or distention headaches, but irritability and short temper are not as obvious.

Key points to distinguish these two patterns are as follows:
1) Upper body vs. lower body:
    Liver yang rising symptoms are more upper body, such as dizziness and top-heaviness; Liver and Kidney yin deficiency symptoms are more lower body, such as soreness and weakness in the lower back and knees
2) Sub-acute vs. chronic
3) Liver and Kidney yin deficiency exhibits obvious deficiency heat

Pattern		Liver Yang Rising	Liver and Kidney Yin Deficiency
Pathogenesis		Liver and Kidney yin deficiency, water unable to nourish wood	
		Liver yang rising, qi and blood move upward	Yin and essence insufficiency, deficiency fire disturbs the interior
Characteristics		Root deficiency, branch excess, sub-acute, more severe, more common in younger patients	Deficiency, chronic, mild, more common in older patients
Symptoms	Common	Dizziness, vertigo, tinnitus, poor memory, dry mouth and throat, insomnia, dream-disturbed sleep, hypochondriac pain, soreness and weakness of the lower back and knees	
	Different	Red face and eyes, distention headache, eye pain, top-heavy sensation, irritability, anger	Malar flush, five center heat, nocturnal emissions, scanty menstruation
Herbal formulas		Tian Ma Gou Teng Yin	Zhen Gan Xi Feng Tang

Table 20.2 Comparison of Liver yang rising and Liver and Kidney yin deficiency

Chapter 21
Liver and Spleen/Stomach

Pathophysiological relationship between the Liver and Spleen/Stomach

The relationship between the Liver and Spleen manifests in two aspects: digestion and circulation of blood.

1 | Digestion

The Liver governs coursing and discharging (疏泄 *shū xiè*) and regulates the ascending and descending of the Spleen and Stomach qi. It also promotes the Gallbladder to secrete bile, which further helps the Spleen and Stomach in digestion. The Spleen governs transportation and transformation (運化 *yùn huà*), distilling food qi for generating qi and blood, which nourishes the Liver to properly course and discharge. Thus the Liver and Spleen work together to maintain normal digestion.

Pathologically, if Liver qi is stagnated and unable to course and discharge it will disrupt the ascending and descending function of the Spleen and Stomach, leading to poor transportation and transformation with symptoms such as poor appetite, abdominal bloating, distention, and loose stools. On the other hand, if the Spleen's transportation and transformation function is impaired, dampness will accumulate, which can generate heat. This damp-heat steams up and disrupts the Liver and Gallbladder, ultimately undermining their functions in promoting bile, causing qi stagnation that results in poor appetite and jaundice.

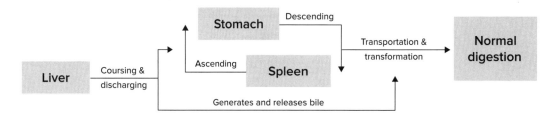

Chart 21.1 Liver, Spleen, and Stomach cooperate to maintain normal digestion

2 | Maintain normal blood circulation

Liver stores blood and regulates the volume of blood while the Spleen generates blood and controls blood by keeping it inside the vessels. Liver and Spleen work together to keep blood circulating regularly.

Pathologically, if Spleen qi deficiency fails to generate enough blood, or Spleen qi deficiency fails to control blood and causes bleeding, the Liver blood will become deficient and manifest with poor appetite, fatigue, dizziness, blurry vision, numbness, tingling, and scanty menstruation. If Liver qi stagnation fails to maintain the free coursing of qi, the Spleen cannot properly transform and transport food qi for generation of qi and blood, eventually leading to a Spleen qi deficiency.

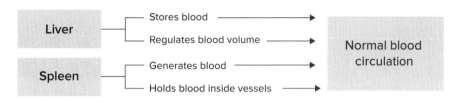

Chart 21.2 Liver and Spleen maintain normal blood circulation

1 Liver and Spleen Disharmony Pattern | 肝脾不和証 |

Definition: A group of signs and symptoms characterized by Liver qi stagnation that transversely attacks the Spleen, leading to Spleen qi is deficiency. It is also called 'Liver overacting on the Spleen' or 'wood overacting on earth.'

Clinical manifestations: Distention and pain in the abdominal and hypochondriac region, frequent sighing, depression, irritability, short temper, poor appetite, bloating, leukorrhea, loose stools with an incomplete sensation, watery stools, borborygmus, gas, and abdominal pain and diarrhea that is relieved after bowel movement. The tongue has a white coating and the pulse is wiry or weak.

Key points: Distention and pain in the abdominal and hypochondriac region, borborygmus, irregular bowel movements, and poor appetite, plus general gastrointestinal signs and symptoms.

Etiology and pathogenesis: The most common cause of this pattern is emotional stress that disrupts the Liver's coursing and discharging function. Other causes include long-term worrying, overthinking, improper diet, overstrain, or chronic illness, which can all deplete and damage the Spleen qi.

The Liver is responsible for the smooth flow of qi throughout the entire body. When Liver qi is stagnated, it may counterflow and attack the Spleen, disrupting its function of transportation and transformation. The Spleen is responsible for generating qi and blood. If it is impaired, it will fail to generate enough blood to nourish and store in the Liver, which then compromises the Liver's function, causing further Liver qi stagnation.

When Liver qi stagnation predominates, it disrupts the ascending and descending function of the Spleen and Stomach, slowing peristalsis, which leads to constipation with dry bitty stools. The qi stagnation can affect the Liver channel, resulting in hypochrondriac distention pain as well as chest oppression such that the patient needs to sigh frequently to release the sensation of pressure. It can also present with anger and irritability, emotions associated with the Liver.

When Spleen qi is deficient, there are transportation and transformation function disorders. These result in the accumulation of dampness in the interior, which blocks the movement of qi, causing bloating, poor appetite, and abdominal pain that is relieved by the passage of gas. When dampness is stagnated in the intestinal tract, it causes borborygmus and loose stools. The dampness accumulation also causes leukorrhea.

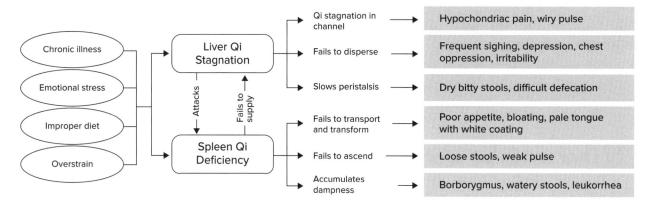

Chart 21.3 Etiology and pathogenesis of Liver and Spleen Disharmony

TCM Disease	Western Disease	Herbal Formulas		Acupuncture
Loose stools (泄瀉)	Chronic enteritis, Crohn's disease, chronic colitis, IBS, celiac disease, SIBO	Tong Xie Yao Fang	Xiao Yao San	CV-3, CV-4
Hypochondriac pain (脇痛)	Chronic hepatitis, costochondritis, chronic cholecystitis, intercostal neuralgia, hypochondriasis	Chai Hu Shu Gan Wan		TB-5, GB-40, BL-19
Ascites (膨脹)	Cirrhosis, heart failure, constrictive pericarditis, nephrotic syndrome, Kwashiorkor	Wei Ling Tang		LI-6
Abdominal pain (腹痛)	Diverticulitis, Crohn's disease, lead poisoning, celiac disease, IBS, PID, SIBO	Chai Hu Shu Gan Wan		SP-4, PC-6
Irregular menstrual cycle (月經不調)	Perimenopause syndrome, PCOS, eating disorder, malnutrition, stress, D&C, miscarriage	Xiao Yao San		LI-4, CV-4, Zigongxue
Leukorrhagia (帶下)	STD, vulvitis, candida infections, bacterial vaginosis	Long Dan Xie Gan Tang		GB-26, GB-27, GB-41, BL-30, BL-54, SP-9

Acupuncture points (spanning column): LR-3, LR-13, LR-14, GB-34, CV-6, CV-12, TB-6, PC-6, ST-25, ST-36, SP-4, SP-6, SP-15

Table 21.1 Diseases and treatments related to Liver and Spleen Disharmony

2 Liver and Stomach Disharmony Pattern │ 肝胃不和証 │

Definition: A group of signs and symptoms characterized by Liver qi stagnation that transversely attacks the Stomach, leading to rebellious Stomach qi. It is also called 'Liver overacting on the Stomach' or 'wood overacting on earth.'

Clinical manifestations: Distention and pain in the epigastric and hypochondriac region, belching, hiccups, nausea or vomiting, acid regurgitation, depression, irritability, frequent sighing, and an aversion to food. The tongue coating is thin white or thin yellow. The pulse is wiry or slightly rapid.

Key points: Distention and pain in the epigastric and hypochondriac region with nausea, hiccups, or belching, plus general gastrointestinal signs and symptoms.

Etiology and pathogenesis: Emotional stress, improper diet, and overstrain can all lead to a disharmony of the Liver and Stomach or essentially Liver qi stagnation with Stomach qi rebellion.

The Liver governs coursing and discharging and is responsible for keeping the qi of the whole body flowing smoothly. The Stomach governs the receiving and downward movement of food and drink. Under normal circumstances, the free-flowing Liver qi assists the Stomach qi to perform its descending function. However, when Liver qi stagnates, the proper directional flow of qi is disrupted and the Liver may transversely 'attack' the Stomach, causing Stomach qi to counterflow or 'rebel.' This can lead to nausea, vomiting, belching, hiccups, and aversion to food.

Furthemore, if fire is generated by this qi stagnation and rebellion it can cause acid regurgitation and epigastric discomfort. And, since the Liver channel courses through the hypochondrium, when Liver qi is stagnated, there is also distention and pain in the hypochondriac region. The tongue coating is yellow and the pulse is rapid.

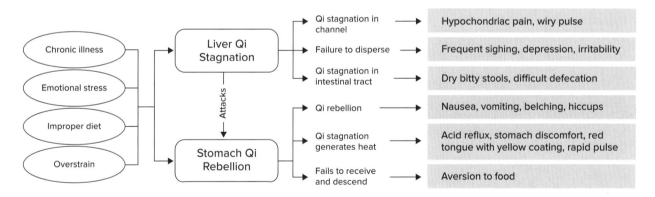

Chart 21.4 Etiology and pathogenesis of Liver and Stomach Disharmony

TCM Disease	Western Disease	Herbal Formulas		Acupuncture	
Epigastric pain (胃脘痛)	Atrophic gastritis, gastroneurosis, peptic ulcer, GERD, gastric carcinoma, pyloric obstruction	Chai Hu Shu Gan Wan	Si Ni San, Xiao Yao San	LR-14, GB-34, CV-12, CV-10, CV-13, ST-19, ST-21, ST-34, ST-36, BL-21	PC-6
Vomiting (嘔吐)	Food poisoning, gastroenteritis, stomach flu, panic attack, pregnancy		Si Qi Tang		PC-6
Hiccups (呃逆)	GERD, stroke, MS, Diabetes, kidney failure, steroids		Ju Pi Zhu Ru Yin		BL-17

Table 21.2 Diseases and treatments related to Liver and Stomach Disharmony

Comparison: Liver and Spleen Disharmony vs. Liver and Stomach Disharmony

Liver and Spleen disharmony (肝郁脾虚 *gān yū pí xū*) and Liver and Stomach disharmony (肝胃不和 *gān wèi bù hé*) are both caused by Liver qi stagnation. Thus depression, irritability, short temper, hypochondriac pain and distention, poor appetite, and a wiry pulse are commonly seen in both patterns. When Liver qi stagnates, it can horizontally attack the Spleen or Stomach, disrupting the Spleen's function of transportation and transformation, or the Stomach's function of descending and decomposition.

Although, the Spleen and Stomach are both located in the middle burner and are an internal-external pair, they are different in their qi dynamics. Spleen qi ascends while Stomach qi descends. Thus when the Spleen is attacked by rebellious Liver qi, Spleen qi cannot ascend, and there will be diarrhea or loose stools. When the Stomach is attacked, Stomach qi cannot descend, and there will be nausea, vomiting, belching, and acid reflux.

The key point to distinguish these two patterns is loose stools vs. nausea and vomiting.

Pattern		Liver and Spleen Disharmony	Liver and Stomach Disharmony
Pathogenesis		Liver qi stagnation causes failure of Spleen to transport and transform	Liver qi attack causes Stomach qi rebellion
Symptoms	Common	Depression, irritability, easy to anger, hypochondriac pain and distention, poor appetite, and wiry pulse	
Symptoms	Different	Abdominal pain, borborygmus, loose stools with tenesmus, abdominal pain before diarrhea that improves after bowel movement, alternating constipation and loose stools	Belching, nausea, vomiting, acid regurgitation, bloating, and discomfort in the stomach area
Treatment strategy		Spread Liver qi, strengthen Spleen, nourish blood	Spread Liver qi, harmonize blood, alleviate pain
Herbal formulas		Xiao Yao San, Si Ni San	Chai Hu Shu Gan Wan

Table 21.3 Comparison of Liver and Spleen Disharmony and Liver and Stomach Disharmony

Chapter 22
Liver and Lung

Pathophysiological relationship between the Liver and Lung

The relationship between the Liver and Lung manifests in the regulation of the ascending and descending activities of qi.

1 | Regulate qi ascending and descending

The Lung is located in the upper burner and it governs, disperses, and moves qi downward. The Liver is located in the lower burner and it courses, discharges, and moves qi upward. Ancient Chinese theory says: "The Liver qi ascends on the left, while the Lung qi descends on the right." The descent of Lung qi and ascent of Liver qi rely on each other. The Lung qi needs to descend for the Liver qi to ascend and vice versa.

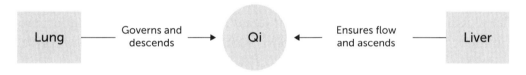

Chart 22.1 Lung and Liver coordinate qi movement

2 | Channel connection

The Liver channel passes through the diaphragm and enters the Lung from beneath, thus the Lung and the Liver physiologically coordinate with each other, but also influence each other in pathology. When Liver qi stagnates, it may generate heat, which rises upward along the Liver channel to consume the Lung yin. This leads to a deficiency of Lung yin and causes dry cough and hemoptysis. This is known as 'wood fire insulting metal' (木火刑金 *mù huǒ xíng jīn*) or 'Liver fire attacking the Lung.' Conversely, if the Lung fails to descend and distribute the qi, the Liver qi will be unable to ascend, resulting in Liver qi stagnation, thus in addition to cough there may be hypochondriac pain and depression.

1 Liver Fire Invading the Lung Pattern | 肝火犯肺証 |

Definition: A group of signs and symptoms characterized by Liver fire rising, causing rebellious Lung qi and manifesting with paroxysmal cough and hypochondriac pain.

Clinical manifestations: Burning pain in the hypochondria, irritability, easily angered, dizziness, distention headaches, red face and eyes, bitter taste in the mouth, paroxysmal cough, or even cough with blood, scanty, yellow, sticky sputum, a red tongue with thin yellow coating, and a wiry and rapid pulse.

Key points: Cough, or cough with blood, burning pain sensation in the chest or hypochondriac region, irritability and easily angered, accompanied by internal excess heat symptoms.

Etiology and pathogenesis: Exopathogenic attack combined with pre-existing emotional stress, especially anger, impairs the Liver and causes its qi to stagnate. Qi stagnation then transforms into fire or pathogenic heat. This accumulates in the Liver channel and flares up through the channel to affect the Lung.

The Liver ensures the free flow of qi. If the Liver qi stagnates over a long period of time it can generate heat, which turns into Liver fire. When Liver fire flares up, it causes headaches, red face and eyes, dizziness and thirst. Liver fire also can steam up bile from the Gallbladder resulting in a bitter taste in the mouth. The Liver channel courses through the hypochondriac region, so there is burning pain there as well.

If the Liver fire flares up through the channels and affects the Lung, it can consume the Lung yin and disrupt its descending and distributing function, leading to paroxysmal cough or difficult breathing and phlegm. If heat also injures the blood vessels, a cough with blood occurs. The red tongue body with a yellow coating, wiry and rapid pulse are all signs of Liver fire.

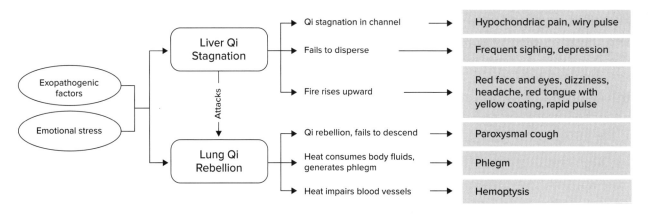

Chart 22.2   Etiology and pathogenesis of Liver Fire Invading the Lung

TCM Disease	Western Disease	Herbal Formulas		Acupuncture	
Cough (咳嗽)	Pneumonia, acute or chronic bronchitis, bronchiectasis, pertussis, COPD, emphysema, GERD	Qing Jin Hua Tan Tang, Dai Ge San	Dan Qing Yin	LR-2, LR-3, LR-14, CV-17, CV-22, PC-6, LU-7, LI-11	CV-22, BL-13, GV-14, ST-9, LU-1, LU-9
Hemoptysis (咳血)	Bronchitis, pneumonia, tuberculosis, bronchiectasis, pulmonary edema, lung cancer, cystic fibrosis		Xie Bai San		LU-6

Table 22.1 Diseases and treatments related to Liver Fire Invading the Lung

Comparison: Liver Fire Invading the Lung vs. Heat Congesting the Lung

Liver fire invading the Lung (肝火犯肺 *gān huǒ fàn fèi*) and heat congesting the Lung (熱邪壅肺 *rè xié yōng fèi*) are both caused by pathogenic heat impairing the Lung's dispersing and discending functions, resulting in cough, asthma, dyspnea, cough with blood, a red tongue, and a rapid pulse. However, they have diffferent clinical manifestations and treatment strategies because they differ in etiology, location of pathology, and course of illness.

Liver fire invading the Lung is usually caused by long-term or severe emotional stress that impairs the Liver and stagnates qi, which then transforms into fire or pathogenic heat. This heat accumulates and travels up the Liver channel to affect the Lung. The primary pathological organ is the Liver, the secondary is the Lung, and thus the symptoms related to Liver dysfunction are the major complaints, including burning pain in the hypochondrium, irritability, short temper, dizziness, distention headaches, red face and eyes, and a bitter taste in the mouth.

Heat congesting the Lung is caused by pathogenic heat invading the Lung directly or by unresolved pathogenic cold entering and transforming into heat, which means the patient may have a history of chills and fever. In this pattern, the Lung is the primary and only organ involved, and therefore only symptoms related to the Lung will be the main complaints, including cough, dyspnea, asthma, rapid breathing, and pain in the chest.

The key points to distinguish these two patterns are as follows:
1) Sub-acute or chronic, longer course vs. acute, short course
2) Emotional stress vs. exopathogenic factors
3) Condition of cough: Paroxysmal cough that is induced or aggravated by emotional stress vs. harsh, coarse, hacking, choking cough.
4) Presence of Liver related symptoms: burning pain in hypochondrium, irritability, anger, dizziness, distention

Pattern	Liver Fire Invading the Lung	Heat Congesting the Lung
Etiology	Emotional stress	Exopathogenic factors invasion
Pathogenesis	Liver qi transforms to fire, follows the Liver channel up to invade the Lung, results in Lung dysfunction	Excess heat congests the Lung, disrupts Lung's descending and dispersing function, results in Lung qi rebellion
Characteristics	Excess, heat, sub-acute or chronic, longer course, milder	Excess, heat, acute, short course, severe
Symptoms — Common	Cough, asthma and dyspnea, or cough with blood, red tongue with rapid pulse	
Symptoms — Cough	Paroxysmal cough, induced or aggravated by emotional stress	Harsh, coarse, hacking, choking, loud cough
Symptoms — Other	Burning pain in the hypochondria, irritability, short temper, dizziness, distention headaches, red face and eyes, bitter taste in the mouth	High fever with flaring nostrils, chest, or cough with pus and blood
Treatment strategy	Soothe Liver qi, clear heat from the Liver, stop cough	Clear heat from the Lung, regulate Lung qi, stop cough
Herbal formulas	Qing Jin Hua Tan Tang, Dai Ge San	Bai Hu Tang, Xie Bai San, Ma Xing Shi Gan Tang

Table 22.2 Comparison of Liver Fire Invading the Lung and Heat Congesting the Lung

Chapter 23
Liver and Gallbladder

Pathophysiological relationship between the Liver and Gallbladder

The relationship between the Liver and Gallbladder is very close from both the anatomical and physiological points of view. The Liver is located on the right side beneath the diaphragm and the Gallbladder is attached and located between the hepatic lobes. Through the channels, they share an internal-external relationship. The relationship between the Liver and Gallbladder manifests in the digestion of food and emotional activities.

1 | Food digestion and absorption

Bile is one of the body's most important fluids for digestion and is involved in the decomposition, transformation, and transportation process. It is generated by a surplus of Liver qi, which collects in the Gallbladder to form bile. The storage and secretion of bile is the responsibility of the Gallbladder, which must coordinate with the Liver's coursing and discharging function.

Pathologically, if the Liver fails to course and discharge, the Gallbladder's function of bile secretion will be impaired. If the Gallbladder is unable to secrete bile, the bile will accumulate and generate heat, which will disrupt the Liver. The Liver will fail to ensure the free flow of qi, causing damp-heat in the Liver and Gallbladder that can develop into Liver and Gallbladder fire.

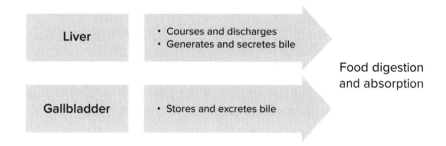

Chart 23.1 Liver and Gallbladder coordinate food digestion and absorption

2 | Maintain normal emotional activity

In addition, the Liver governs strategic thinking and is associated with emotional activity, while the Gallbladder governs decision making and judgment, and is associated with courage. Thus only when the Liver and Gallbladder coordinate and cooperate with each other can one make the right decisions.

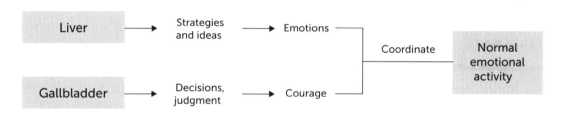

Chart 23.2 Physiological relationship between Liver and Gallbladder in emotional activity

1 Liver and Gallbladder Damp-Heat Pattern | 肝膽濕熱証 |

Definition: A group of signs and symptoms characterized by damp-heat stagnation in both the Liver and Gallbladder and their channels, which manifests as yang type jaundice.

Clinical manifestations: Alternating chills and fever, distention pain in the hypochondriac region, bitter taste in the mouth, nausea, thirst without a large fluid intake, poor appetite, alternating constipation and loose stools, yellow urine, jaundiced body and eyes, abdominal distention, fever, vaginal discharge or itching, and scrotal itching or swelling. The tongue coating is yellow and greasy and the pulse is wiry and rapid.

Key points: Hypochondriac distention, poor appetite, abdominal bloating, yellow skin and eyes, genital itching, plus damp-heat signs and symptoms.

254 Part 3: Compound Patterns

Etiology and pathogenesis: Improper diet, such as overeating sweet and greasy foods and overconsumption of alcohol, can lead to the accumulation of damp-heat. External damp-heat invasion can also cause Liver and Gallbladder stagnation and dysfunction.

Exopathogenic damp-heat invasion and accumulation of dampness transforms into heat, which rises and steams the Liver and Gallbladder. When damp-heat steams upward, the bile will secrete abnormally from the Gallbladder and flow upward and outward, bringing a yellow color to the eyes and skin. When bile ascends to the mouth, there is a bitter taste. Meanwhile, Liver qi failing to ensure smooth flow of qi in the Liver channel gives rise to distending pain in hypochondriac region.

When dampness accumulation leads to Spleen dysfunction it disrupts the ascending and descending of qi, causing poor appetite, nausea, vomiting, and abdominal distention. When dampness is more prevalent, the stools are loose; when heat is more prevalent, the stools are dry. If the heat consumes body fluids there is thirst, but if there is also dampness, then large fluid intake will cause nausea.

When damp-heat assails the Gallbladder, a *shào yáng* (half exterior and half interior) organ, there can be alternating chills and fever. When damp-heat pours downward, the urine is yellow, scanty, and turbid. And when damp-heat pours down through the Liver channel to the genitals, there can be painful swelling and burning of the testicles in men, or yellow and foul vaginal discharge in women.

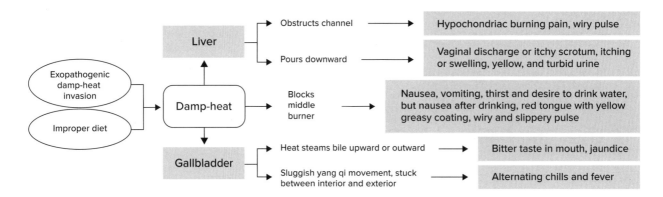

Chart 23.3 Etiology and pathogenesis of Liver and Gallbladder Damp-Heat

TCM Disease	Western Disease	Herbal Formulas		Acupuncture	
Hypochondriac pain (脇痛)	Chronic hepatitis, intercostal neuralgia, costochondritis, cholecystitis, shingles	Yin Chen Hao Tang, Long Dan Xie Gan Tang	Long Dan Xie Gan Tang	GB-24, LR-3, LR-5, LR-14, CV-12, Dannangxue, GV-9, BL-19, BL-20, LI-11, TB-6, ST-19, SP-9	LR-13
Jaundice (黃疸)	Acute cholecystitis, baby jaundice, Gilbert's syndrome, obstruction or inflammation of the bile duct		Yin Chen Hao Tang		LI-4
Scrotum eczema (陰囊濕疹)	Scrotum eczema, psoriasis, or fungal or bacteria infections		Long Dan Xie Gan Tang		SP-10
Vaginal itching (陰癢)	Vaginitis, yeast infection, STD, bacterial vaginosis, menopause				
Leukorrhagia (帶下)	STD, vulvitis, candida infections, bacterial vaginosis				
Turbid painful urinary dribbling (濁淋)	Urinary tract infections, cystitis, gonorrhea, bladder infection		Chen Xiang San		
Urinary blockage (癃閉)	Kidney or bladder stones, BPH		Ba Zheng Sang		BL-22, BL-28, GV-4, CV-4

Table 23.1 Diseases and treatments related to Liver and Gallbladder Damp-Heat

Comparison: Liver and Gallbladder Damp-Heat vs. Gallbladder Heat

Gallbladder heat (膽熱 *dǎn rè*) and Liver and Gallbladder damp-heat (肝膽濕熱 *gān dǎn shī rè*) both involve pathogenic heat disrupting Gallbladder function, and thus both present with a bitter taste in the mouth and hypochondriac pain.

Gallbladder heat is caused by emotional stress or the invasion of exopathogenic factors and tends to be acute and short course. Liver and Gallbladder damp-heat is usually caused by over-consumption of alcohol and greasy, raw, or cold foods. Thus it tends to be more chronic and long course.

Since fire tends to rise upward, while dampness sinks downward, symptoms related to heat congesting in the Gallbladder mostly appear in the upper body, such as red face, irritability, dizziness, tinnitus, and headaches. Symptoms related to Liver and Gallbladder damp-heat mostly appear in the lower body, such as loose stools, vaginal discharge or itching, and scrotal itching or swelling.

Key points to distinguish these two patterns are as follows:
1) Acute, short course vs. chronic, long course
2) Heat vs. damp-heat
3) Tongue and pulse

Pattern	Liver and Gallbladder Damp-Heat	Gallbladder Heat
Etiology and pathogenesis	Overconsumption of alcohol, greasy, raw, or cold foods, exopathogenic dampness invasion that transforms into damp-heat	Emotional stress or exopathogenic factors invasion that transforms into heat
Characteristics	Chronic, long course, excess	Acute, short course, excess
Organs	Liver and Gallbladder	Gallbladder
Symptoms — Common	Bitter taste in the mouth, hypochondriac pain and distention, alternating chills and fever, thirst, anorexia, nausea, vomiting, yellow urine, jaundice	
Symptoms — Different	Thirst without desire to drink lots of water	Dry mouth, thirst with desire to drink lots of water
Symptoms — Other	Constipation or loose stools, abdominal distention, vaginal discharge or itching, scrotal itching or swelling	Irritability, short temper, tinnitus, ear pain, headache, insomnia or dream-disturbed sleep, red face, constipation
Tongue	Red tongue, yellow greasy coating	Red tongue, yellow coating
Pulse	Wiry, rapid, slippery	Wiry, rapid
Treatment strategy	Drain excess fire from the Liver and Gallbladder, clear and drain damp-heat from the lower burner	Regulate qi, transform phlegm, clear the Gallbladder
Herbal formulas	Long Dan Xie Gan Tang	Huang Lian Wen Dan Tang

Table 23.2 Comparison of Gallbladder Heat and Liver and Gallbladder Damp-Heat

Part 4

QUESTIONS & ANSWERS
FOR DEEPER INSIGHT

CONTENTS

THE QUESTIONS IN SUMMARY, 258

CHAPTER 24: THE QUESTIONS AND ANSWERS, 260

The Questions in Summary

1. What is wind-cold-dampness invading the body's surface (風寒濕襲表 *fēng hán shī xí biǎo*)? ⋯ 258

2. What is the difference between wind-cold-dampness invading the body's surface (風寒濕襲表 *fēng hán shī xí biǎo*) and wind-cold-dampness painful obstruction disorder (風寒濕痹証 *fēng hán shī bì zhèng*)? ⋯ 259

3. What is dampness (濕 *shī*), water (水 *shuǐ*), thin mucus (飲 *yǐn*), and phlegm (痰 *tán*)? ⋯ 260

4. What is water qi encroaching on the Heart pattern (水氣凌心 *shuǐ qì líng xīn*)? ⋯ 266

5. How to distinguish water qi encroaching on the Heart (水氣凌心 *shuǐ qì líng xīn*) from Heart yang deficiency (心陽虛 *xīn yáng xū*)? ⋯ 269

6. How to distinguish Water Qi Encroaching on the Heart (水氣凌心 *shuǐ qì líng xīn*) from Cold-Water Shooting into the Lung (寒水射肺 *hán shuǐ shè fèi*)? ⋯ 271

7. What is Kidney Water Invading the Spleen (腎水泛脾 *shèn shuǐ fàn pí*)? ⋯ 273

8. What is the relationship of the following five patterns: Kidney Yang Deficiency (腎陽虛 *shèn yáng xū*), Kidney Yang Deficiency with Water Effusion (腎虛水泛 *shèn xū shuǐ fàn*), Water Qi Encroaching on the Heart (水氣凌心 *shuǐ qì líng xīn*), Cold-Water Shooting into the Lung (寒水射肺 *hán shuǐ shè fèi*), and Kidney Water Invading the Spleen (腎水泛脾 *shèn shuǐ fàn pí*)? ⋯ 274

9. Does the pattern Lung Yang Deficiency exist? If so, what is its clinical manifestation, etiology, and pathogenesis? ⋯ 275

10. Does the pattern Lung Blood Deficiency exist? If so, what is its clinical manifestation, etiology, and pathogenesis? ⋯ 277

11. Dryness Invading the Lung, Lung Yin Deficiency, and Liver Fire Invading the Lung all share the major symptoms of dry cough, cough with scanty sputum, or cough with blood, but how are these three patterns different from each other? ⋯ 280

12. What is the pathogenesis of Liver Qi Stagnation and Liver Qi Rebellion? How are they different? ⋯ 282

13. What is the clinical manifestation, etiology, and pathogenesis of Liver Fire? ⋯ 283

14. What is the difference between Liver heat and Liver fire? ⋯ 285

15. What are the pathological changes of the Liver? ⋯ 286

16. What is the clinical manifestation of internal wind? ⋯ 287

17. Does the pattern Liver Qi Deficiency exist? ⋯ 288

18. What is the clinical manifestation, etiology, and pathogenesis of Liver Qi Deficiency? ⋯ 291

19. Does the pattern Liver Yang Deficiency exist? ⋯ 292

20. What is the clinical manifestation, etiology, and pathogenesis of Liver Yang Deficiency? ⋯ 294

21. Why is Liver Qi Deficiency blamed on the Spleen? And how to distinguish Liver Qi Deficiency from Spleen Qi Deficiency? ⋯ 297

22. What are the similarities and differences between the patterns Liver Qi Stagnation, Liver Fire Blazing, and Liver Yang Rising? ⋯ 299

23. What are the similarities and differences between the patterns Liver and Gallbladder Damp-Heat and Damp-Heat Encumbering the Spleen? ⋯ 300

24. Why is Liver Yang Deficiency commonly blamed on the Kidney? How is Liver Yang Deficiency distinguished from Kidney Yang Deficiency? ⋯ 301

25. What are the different types of fever and their associated pathogenesis and *zàng fǔ* patterns? ⋯ 304

26. What is Stomach Qi Deficiency? ⋯ 308

27. What is Middle Qi Insufficiency (中氣不足 *zhōng qì bù zú*)? How does Stomach Qi Deficiency compare with Spleen Qi Deficiency? ⋯ 309

28. Since the Spleen favors dryness and disfavors dampness, does the pattern of Spleen Yin Deficiency exist? ⋯ 311

29. What is Stomach Excess with Spleen Deficiency? How to distinguish this pattern from Stomach Fire? ⋯ 313

30. Is the pattern Stomach Excess with Spleen Deficiency the same as Constrained Spleen? If not, how are they different? ⋯ 315

31. How does Damp-Heat in the Spleen and Stomach compare with Damp-Heat in the middle burner? ⋯ 317

32. What is Kidney essence and Kidney qi? What are Kidney yin, Kidney yang, true yin, true yang, primary yin, primary yang, *mìng mén* fire, and *mìng mén* water? How are they all related to each other? ⋯ 318

33. What is the concept of *mìng mén*? Where is it located and what is its form and function? ⋯ 319

34. What is the difference between Kidney Yang Deficiency (腎陽虛) and *mìng mén* Fire Decline (命門火衰)? ⋯ 321

36. Do Kidney excess patterns exist and why? ⋯ 323

37. In which conditions do we see the pattern Kidney Qi Failing to Secure (腎氣不固)? ⋯ 325

38. Kidney yin deficiency can cause both amenorrhea and menorrhagia. What is the pathogenesis of these conditions? ⋯ 325

39. What is the history and development of *zàng fǔ* pattern identification? ⋯ 327

40. What are the pattern identification methods and their relationships? ⋯ 331

Chapter 24
The Questions and Answers

1. What is wind-cold-dampness invading the body's surface (風寒濕襲表 *fēng hán shī xí biǎo*)?

Definition: A group of signs and symptoms caused by wind-cold combined with dampness invading the body's surface that disrupts the nutritive (營 *yíng*) and protective (衛 *wèi*) qi system, obstructs channels and collaterals, and clinically manifests with body aches, joint pain, chills, and fever.

Clinical manifestation: Cough with thin clear sputum, aversion to cold, fever, neck stiffness, tension headache, generalized body aches with a heavy sensation that is worse in the upper body, joint stiffness and pain, tiredness, nasal congestion and discharge with thin snivel, a thin white or slightly thick white tongue coating, and a superficial, tight, and slippery pulse.

Key points: Cough with thin clear sputum, tension headache, body aches with a heavy sensation, joint pain, plus exterior wind-cold signs and symptoms.

Etiology and pathogenesis: Jogging or walking in the rain, playing in the water, or taking a shower or bath without drying off, all can cause exopathogenic wind-cold and dampness to invade the body's surface.

Exopathogenic wind-cold invasion disrupts and impairs the nutritive and protective qi system, which manifests as chills and fever. When exopathogenic cold obstructs the channels and collaterals, it compromises the circulation of qi and blood. The resulting stagnation leads to body aches, headaches, neck stiffness, and a tight pulse. Although dampness is sticky, heavy, and has a tendency to sink downward, the upward and outward force of wind pushes dampness to the upper part of the body. The pathological changes of dampness in the upper body manifests as tension headache that feels like a tight band wrapped around the head, body aches accompanied by a sensation of heaviness, stiff and painful joints, a slightly thick tongue coating, and a slippery pulse.

The Lung, a 'delicate organ' in the upper body, governs qi, controls the skin and hair, and opens to the nose. When exopathogens invade the body, the Lung is usually the first organ to be affected. Exopathogens

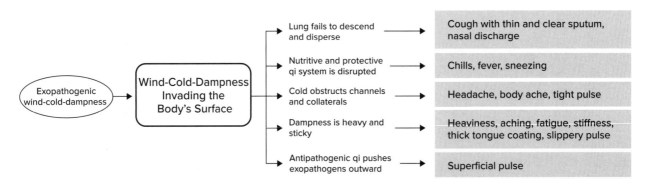

Chart 24.1.1 Etiology and pathogenesis of Wind-Cold-Dampness Invading the Body's Surface

compromise the Lung's dispersing and descending function, causing cough, nasal congestion, and nasal discharge. When the antipathogenic qi rises up against the exopathogens, it pushes the qi outward, causing a floating pulse. Since the pathogens exist on the superficial level and have not entered the deeper level of the *zàng fǔ* organs, the tongue's appearance will remain normal: a pink tongue body with a thin or slightly thick white coating.

TCM Disease	Western Disease	Herbal Formulas		Acupuncture	
Headache (頭痛)	Influences, meningitis or meningoencephalitis, coronavirus	Qiang Huo Sheng Shi Tang, Ren Shen Bai Du San	Ge Gen Tang	LU-7, LI-4, BL-12, BL-13, GB-20, GV-14, GV-16, TB-17, SP-9	Taiyang, GB-7, GB-8, BL-2
Cold, flu (感冒)	Bronchitis, URTI caused by common cold or flu, sinusitis, rhinitis, pharyngitis, laryngitis		Ma Huang Tang		LI-20, SI-7
Asthma (喘証)	Bronchial asthma, URTI, LRTI, bronchitis, pneumonia, lung abscess		San Ao Tang		LU-1, LU-3, LU-5, LU-9, BL-42, BL-44, CV-17, CV-22
Painful obstruction disorder (痹証)	Acute rheumatoid arthritis, acute gouty arthritis, acute bursitis, acute osteoarthritis		Gui Zhi Shao Yao Zhi Mu Tang		GB-34, SI-3, BL-62

Table 24.1.1 Diseases and treatments related to Wind-Cold-Dampness Invading the Body's Surface

2. What is the difference between wind-cold-dampness invading the body's surface (風寒濕襲表 *fēng hán shī xí biǎo*) and wind-cold-dampness painful obstruction disorder (風寒濕痹証 *fēng hán shī bì zhèng*)?

Pathogenic wind-cold and dampness invasion is the main etiological factor for both of these patterns, and therefore, they share signs and symptoms such as pain and stiffness of the limbs and joints that are relieved by warmth and aggravated by cold. However, there are differences in pathogenesis, clinical manifestations, and the location of the pathological change.

Wind-cold-dampness invading the body's surface is an exterior pattern, where the pathological change happens on the body's surface (肌表 *jī biǎo*), as in the Lung, skin, and interstitial spaces (腠理 *còu lǐ*). Thus coughing with chills, fever, and a superficial pulse are the major clinical symptoms. Although dampness is sticky, heavy, and has a tendency to sink downward, the upward and outward force of wind pushes dampness to the upper part of the body. The pathological changes of dampness occur in the upper body, where cold and dampness lodge in the muscle layers and manifest as neck stiffness; tension headache that feels like a tight band wrapped around the head; body aches accompanied by a sensation of heaviness; and joint pain, stiffness, or numbness.

In contrast, painful obstruction disorder due to wind-cold-dampness is an interior pattern, and thus there are chills but no fever. This pattern is caused by pathogenic wind-cold and dampness directly invading the channels and collaterals, blocking qi and blood, and causing the tendons and sinews to spasm. This results in pain and stiffness in the limbs and joints, and the sensation of pain moving from joint to joint. The pathological changes in this pattern tend to be located in the lower part of the body.

The key points to distinguish these two patterns are as follows:
1) Course of illness: acute and short course vs. chronic and long course
2) Presence of exterior signs and symptoms such as chills and fever
3) Location of pathological changes: upper body vs. lower body; body's surface vs. deeper in the joints
4) Tongue and pulse

Pattern		Wind-Cold-Dampness Invading the Body's Surface	Wind-Cold-Dampness Painful Obstruction Syndrome
Etiology		Wind, cold, and dampness	
Pathogenesis		Exopathogens disrupt nutritive and defensive qi system, impairing Lung function obstructing channels and collaterals	Exopathogens directly invade and obstruct the channels and collaterals, resulting in joint and limb pain
Characteristic		Acute, short course	Chronic, long course
Disease nature		Exterior, excess	Interior, excess
Pathological location		Body's surface: Lung, channels and collaterals, upper body	Channels and collaterals, lower body
Symptoms	Common	Pain, stiffness, and heaviness in the limbs and joints. Symptoms worse with cold and better with warmth.	
	Main	Chills and fever, cough, tension headache	Joint pain with sensation of pain moving from joint to joint
	Others	Nasal congestion, body aches with sensation of heaviness, neck stiffness with difficulty turning and moving	Numbness of limbs
Tongue and pulse		Normal tongue, possibly with a slightly thicker white tongue coating, a superficial and tight pulse	A thick white tongue coating, a slow or slippery pulse
Treatment strategy		Release the exterior, dispel wind and dampness	Invigorate the blood, unblock the collaterals, dispel cold and dampness
Herbal formulas		Qiang Huo Sheng Shi Tang, Jiu Wei Qiang Huo Tang, Ren Shen Bai Du San	Xiao Huo Luo Dan, Juan Bi Tang

Table 24.2.1 Comparison of Wind-Cold-Dampness Invading the Body's Surface and Wind-Cold-Dampness Painful Obstruction Syndrome

3. What is dampness (濕 shī), water (水 shuǐ), thin mucus (飲 yǐn), and phlegm (痰 tán)?

Dampness, water, thin mucus, and phlegm are all pathological products of water metabolism disorder, and form when the body fails to transform water and grain essences. Lung, Spleen, Kidney, and Triple Burner are the most important organs related to water metabolism; dysfunction in any of these zàng fǔ organs will result in the formation of dampness, water, thin mucus, and phlegm. These pathological fluids all belong to the category of yin-type pathogens. Although they are secondary to existing dysfunctions caused by primary pathogenic factors, once they form, they act as new pathogenic factors in the body, further obstructing

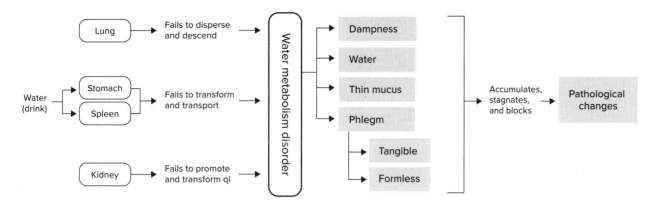

Chart 24.3.1 Pathogenesis of the products of water metabolism disorder

qi and blood circulation, blocking channels and collaterals, affecting the qi of *zàng fǔ* organs, and thereby causing dysfunction that leads to various kinds of complex pathological changes.

Dampness, water, thin mucus, and phlegm may have different names, but they all come from the same source, are very closely related, and can coexist and transform into each other. When dampness accumulates, it forms water; when water accumulates and stagnates, it forms thin mucus; when thin mucus congeals and scorches, it forms phlegm. They are different in shape, quality, location, pathogenic characteristics, clinical manifestations, and treatment methods.

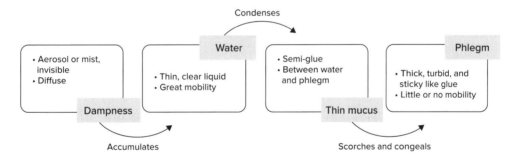

Chart 24.3.2 Pathogenesis of the products of water metabolism disorder

Dampness is invisible, an 'aerosol' or mist; it is diffuse in tissues and organs, and generally there is no obvious shape. Dampness spreads throughout the body in a diffuse state that easily traps the Spleen and is prone to staying in the lower burner. It blocks movement of qi, causing various kinds of signs and symptoms, and leads to long lingering courses of illness. When it affects the body's surface, it causes body soreness and aching; when it attacks the head, it causes a heavy wrapped-around headache; when it invades the skin, it causes exudate and erosion; when it accumulates in the middle burner, it leads to epigastric tightness and distention, bloating, nausea, and vomiting; and when it flows downward, it causes turbid urine, leukorrhea, loose stools, and diarrhea.

Dampness can invade from the exterior such as when living or working in humid environments and exposed to rain or water; or it can be generated internally by the failure of the Spleen's transportation and transformation function. Dampness is a heavy and turbid yin-type pathogen that is usually combined with heat or cold based on the constitution and course of illness.

Common patterns caused by dampness include damp-heat or cold-dampness encumbering the Spleen, Liver and Gallbladder damp-heat, wind-dampness invading the Lung, Large Intestine damp-heat or cold-dampness, and Urinary Bladder damp-heat. Clinical manifestations of dampness include chronic inflammation, food allergies or food sensitivities, certain kinds of autoimmune diseases, some water or lipid metabolism issues, and symptoms caused by the imbalance of microbial flora.

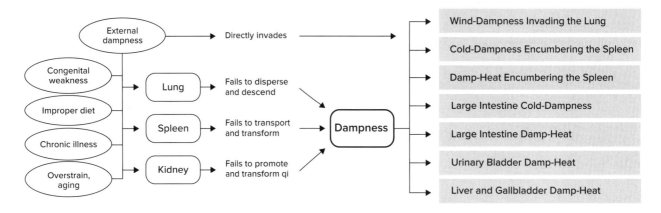

Chart 24.3.3 Etiology and pathogenesis of *zàng fǔ* patterns related to dampness

Water is clear, thin, heavy, and has great mobility. Water overflows on the body's surface and is characterized by edema. It is prone to going to the lower part of the body, but when combined with wind it can cause edema on the head and face, or even the entire body. When it accumulates in the abdominal cavity, it causes ascites. Based on its etiology, pathogenesis, and location, edema can be classified into yang edema and yin edema.

Yang edema is usually caused by external pathogenic invasions, is an excess condition, has a nature of heat, and its pathological location is mostly in the Lung and Spleen. Yang edema usually starts from the head and face, then spreads to the entire body, and is accompanied by an exterior pattern or heat signs and symptoms

Pattern	Yang Edema	Yin Edema
Etiology	Exopathogenic wind, water, dampness, damp-heat, heat toxicity	Chronic illness, physical overstrain, delayed or improper treatment of yang edema
Organs	Lung and Spleen	Spleen and Kidney
Nature	Heat, excess	Cold, deficiency
Course	Acute	Chronic
Edema characteristics	Starts from eyes, face, upper body	Starts from ankles, usually below the waist
Accompanying symptoms	Exterior symptoms, heavy limbs, abdominal distention	Intolerance of cold, fatigue, lower backache, poor appetite
Tongue	White greasy coating	Pale and tender tongue with slippery coating
Pulse	Superficial or deep, and forceful	Deep, slow, and forceless

Table 24.3.1 Comparison of yang edema and yin edema

such as chills, fever, red tongue, yellow tongue coating, and a superficial and rapid pulse. In contrast, yin edema is mostly related to Spleen and Kidney yang deficiency, is a deficiency condition, is cold in nature, and its pathological location is mostly in the Spleen and Kidney. Yin edema usually appears below the waist, and is accompanied by cold or deficiency signs and symptoms such as intolerance of cold, pale complexion, fatigue, a pale tongue, and a deep deficient pulse.

Common patterns caused by water include cold-water shooting into the Lung, Kidney yang deficiency with water effusion, Kidney water upwardly invading the Spleen, and water qi encroaching on the Heart. Water and thin mucus are all exudate produced by pathological changes of body organs; fluids leaking from blood vessels remain inside tissues and organs. It can be caused by kidney disease, cirrhosis, malnutrition, poor heart function, and allergic reactions.

Thin mucus is between water and phlegm; it is thicker and more turbid than water, but thinner and cleaner than phlegm; and it has less mobility than water, but more mobility than phlegm. It mostly accumulates in the gaps, cavities, or loose parts of the body such as the gastrointestinal tract, chest, diaphragm, and

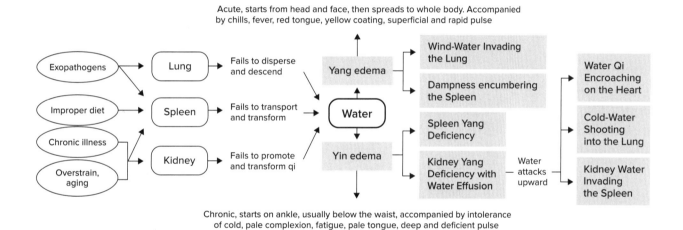

Chart 24.3.4 Etiology and pathogenesis of *zàng fǔ* patterns related to water

joints. The etiology and pathogenesis of thin mucus is the pre-existing condition of Heart and Lung yang deficiency, also known as chest yang deficiency (胸陽不振 *xiōng yáng bú zhèn*), or Spleen and Kidney yang deficiency. Along with external cold-dampness invasion or improper diet that results in *zàng fǔ* organ dysfunction and water metabolism disorder, such circumstances can lead to the accumulation of pathological fluids in certain parts of the body.

When thin mucus accumulates in the gastrointestinal tract, it is phlegm-thin mucus (痰飲 *tán yǐn*). Symptoms include abdominal bloating and distention, borborygmus, and vomiting with clear sticky fluids. *Zàng fǔ* patterns include Spleen and Stomach yang deficiency with phlegm-thin mucus accumulation, Large Intestine deficiency cold, Large Intestine cold-dampness, or Small Intestine deficiency cold.

When thin mucus accumulates in the chest and ribcage, it is suspended thin mucus (懸飲 *xuán yǐn*). Symptoms include chest pain and distention induced or aggravated by cough, sneezing, or deep breathing. *Zàng fǔ* patterns include exopathogens invading the Lung and chest, or thin mucus accumulation in the chest and ribcage (hypochondria).

When thin mucus overflows on the body's surface, it is spillage thin mucus (溢飲 *yì yǐn*). Symptoms include edema of the limbs, heaviness of the body, no sweating, and scanty urination. *Zàng fǔ* patterns include Kidney yang deficiency with water effusion, and Kidney yang deficiency with water upwardly invading the Spleen.

When thin mucus accumulates in the chest and diaphragm, it is propping thin mucus (支飲 *zhī yǐn*). Symptoms include chest oppression, cough with profuse, clear, thin sputum, shortness of breath or dyspnea and an inability to lie flat, and edema that is worse in the legs. *Zàng fǔ* patterns include thin mucus obstructing the Heart, water-dampness upwardly invading the Heart, and cold-water shooting into the Lung.

Thin mucus is exudate caused by various kinds of disease such as inflammation, kidney disease, cardiovascular disease, and allergic reactions.

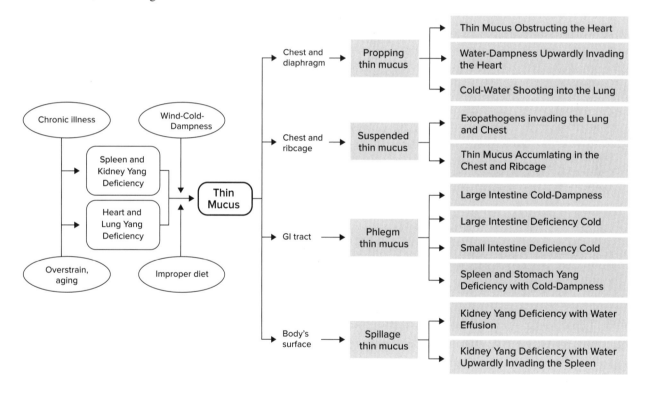

Chart 24.3.5 Etiology and pathogenesis of *zàng fǔ* patterns related to thin mucus

Phlegm's texture is thick, turbid, and sticky; it is like glue with low or no mobility. The common etiology for phlegm includes the invasion of exopathogens, improper diet, emotional stress, and overstrain that affects the qi transforming function of the Spleen, Lung, and Kidney. This dysfunction results in the accumulation of pathological fluids that cohere and condense into phlegm. It is mostly found in the Lung, however it can follow the ascending and descending of qi and travel throughout the entire body from the skin, muscles, tendons, bones, channels and collaterals to most of the internal organs. It obstructs channels and collaterals, stagnates qi and blood circulation, and causes dysfunction of *zàng fǔ* organs, leading to various kinds of disease.

In addition, phlegm can be subdivided into 'tangible phlegm' and 'formless phlegm.' Tangible phlegm refers to visible, audible, accessible, and palpable phlegm. It is thick and more condensed with low or no mobility, and can manifest as sputum, wheezing sound, scrofula, lumps, and nodules. Formless phlegm refers to phlegm that is stagnated in the *zàng fǔ* organs, channels and collaterals, and other tissues; it is invisible, inaudible, and not palpable. Instead, it is manifested in symptoms or syndromes specific to phlegm such as plum-pit syndrome, dizziness, vomiting, nausea, and manic behaviors. It can also appear in the tongue and pulse such as a thick and greasy or moldy tongue coating, and a rolling or wiry pulse.

Since phlegm is one of the products of water metabolism disorder, it is a yin-type pathogen. Phlegm can be formed by the stagnation and congealing of pathological fluids, but most phlegm is generated by heat scorching and condensing the pathological fluids. Thus phlegm is considered to be more of a yang pathogen. Phlegm may combine with other pathogens such as heat, cold, dampness, wind, and dryness. Common patterns caused by phlegm include phlegm obstructing the Lung, phlegm misting the Heart, phlegm-fire harassing the Heart, phlegm obstructing the Heart vessels, and Gallbladder stagnation with phlegm disturbance. Phlegm in traditional Chinese medicine includes a wide range of etiologies and pathogeneses such as various kinds of inflammation or sequelae of inflammation; allergic reactions; tissue exudates; immune or autoimmune diseases; water, fat, or carbohydrate metabolism disorders; cysts; and certain types of mental illness.

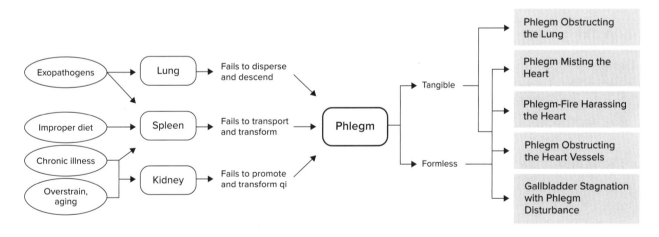

Chart 24.3.6 Etiology and pathogenesis of *zàng fǔ* patterns related to phlegm

Although damp, water, thin mucus, and phlegm have different names, they come from the same source, are very closely related, and can coexist and transform into each other. Thus it is difficult to separate them in many situations. Thus clinically, they are often referred to as water-dampness (水濕 *shuǐ shī*), water-thin mucus (水飲 *shuǐ yǐn*), phlegm-dampness (痰濕 *tán shī*), or phlegm-thin mucus (痰飲 *tán yǐn*). For example, there is a pattern called water-dampness invading upward (水濕上犯 *shuǐ shī shàng fàn*), a sub-pattern of water qi encroaching on the Heart (水氣凌心 *shuǐ qì líng xīn*), and ascites involves a pattern called water-thin mucus accumulation in the abdomen.

	Dampness, water, thin mucus, and phlegm come from the same source; they are the products of water metabolism disorder. They can combine, coexist, and transform into each other. They share similar tongue and pulse: thick, greasy, moldy, or slippery tongue coating, and a wiry or slippery pulse.
Dampness	• Shape: aerosol or mist, invisible, no shape • Location: diffuse into tissues and organs, mostly in the Spleen • Main symptoms: general heaviness, aching, diarrhea, loose stools, discharges
Water	• Shape: thin and clear liquid, heavy, high mobility • Location: body's surface, lower extremities • Main symptoms: edema
Thin mucus	• Shape: semi-liquid, between water and phlegm • Location: accumulates in the gaps, cavities, joints, and gastrointestinal tract • Main symptoms: propping thin mucus, suspended thin mucus, spillage thin mucus, phlegm-thin mucus
Phlegm	• Shape: turbid, sticky like glue, low mobility • Location: mostly in the Lung, but can be in entire body such as skin, bones, organs, channels and collaterals • Main symptoms: wide range including sputum, cysts, vertigo, hemiplegia, mental issues

Table 24.3.2 Summary of dampness, water, thin mucus, and phlegm

4. What is water qi encroaching on the Heart pattern (水氣凌心 *shuǐ qì líng xīn*)?

Definition: A group of signs and symptoms caused by water-thin mucus (水飲 *shuǐ yǐn*) accumulation, obstructing the Heart yang and manifesting as palpitations, panting, fatigue, weakness, cold limbs, edema, and difficult urination. This is a complex *zàng fǔ* pattern with two subtypes: thin mucus obstructing the Heart (飲阻于心 *yǐn zǔ yú xīn*) and water-dampness invading upward (水濕上犯 *shuǐ shī shàng fàn*).

Clinical manifestation: Palpitations, dizziness, nausea, vomiting, poor appetite, cold limbs, panting, thirst without desire to drink, edema, fatigue, weakness, a white slippery tongue coating, and a wiry and slippery pulse.

(1) **Thin mucus obstructing the Heart:** Productive cough with profuse white foaming phlegm, oppression and tightness in the chest, inability to lie down flat, and facial edema.
(2) **Water-dampness invading upward:** Whole-body edema that is worse in the lower extremities, abdominal bloating and distention, scanty or difficult urination, a pale and flabby tongue, and a deep, slow, and deficient pulse.

Etiology and pathogenesis: Water-thin mucus accumulating inside and obstructing Heart yang is the basic pathogenesis for both subtypes of water qi encroaching on the Heart. However, there are some differences in etiology and pathogenesis that distinguish one subtype from the other.

For the subtype of thin mucus obstructing the Heart there are two major causes. The first involves chronic cough impairing the descending and dispersing function of the Lung, leading to thin mucus accumulation in the upper burner. The second involves overstrain and overconsumption of greasy oily foods that damage the transforming and transporting function of the Spleen, leading to the accumulation of phlegm-thin mucus in the middle burner that moves upward and obstructs the Heart. Thus both Lung and Spleen qi deficiency play a role in this pattern.

For the subtype of water-dampness invading upward, there are three major causes. The first is congenital weakness that leads to primary yang deficiency, the second is overconsumption of cold foods impairing Spleen yang, and the third is exopathogenic cold-dampness invasion that damages yang qi and injures the Spleen's transforming and transporting function. All of these conditions result in dampness and water accumulation that upwardly invades the Heart. Thus, Spleen and Kidney yang deficiency is the root of this pattern.

When thin mucus accumulates inside, it can surge upward, assaulting and disrupting the Heart, causing palpitations. Thin mucus accumulation obstructs qi circulation, leading to shortness of breath, panting, and oppression and tightness in the chest.

If thin mucus accumulation affects Stomach function, there is nausea or vomiting. This water metabolism dysfunction will obstruct body fluid distribution, which cannot properly nourish the tongue, causing a sensation of thirst. However, since there is dampness and thin mucus accumulation internally, there is no desire to drink.

When the Kidney yang is deficient, its qi transforming function is impaired, leading to edema and difficult urination. In general, when yang is deficient, it cannot perform its warming function, causing an aversion to cold and cold limbs. For this type of thin mucus accumulation with yang deficiency, the tongue has a white greasy coating, and the pulse is thin and slippery.

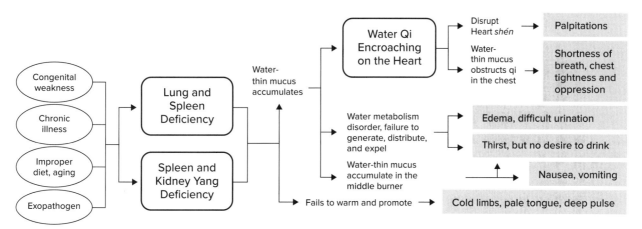

Chart 24.4.1 Etiology and pathogenesis of Water Qi Encroaching on the Heart

270   Zàng fǔ Pattern Identification

TCM Disease	Western Disease	Herbal Formulas		Acupuncture	
Palpitations (心悸)	CHF, panic attack, anxiety, hyperthyroidism, SVT, VT, arrhythmia	Ling Gui Zhu Gan Tang, Zhen Wu Tang	Gui Zhi Gan Cao Long Gu Mu Li Tang	HT-5, PC-6, BL-20, BL-23, BL-52, CV-6, CV-17, GV-14	BL-15, CV-14, CV-17, PC-6
Dizziness and vertigo (眩晕)	CHF, primary pulmonary hypertension, hypotension, arrhythmia		Ling Gui Zhu Gan Tang		GV-20
Cough and asthma (咳喘)	CHF, pulmonary edema, chronic bronchitis, asthma, emphysema, cor-pulmonary disease		Zhen Wu Tang		LU-5, LU-7, BL-13
Spillage of thin mucus (溢饮)	Kidney failure, uremia, CHF, glomerulonephritis, nephrotic syndrome		Ji Sheng Shen Qi Wan		ST-36

Table 24.4.1 Diseases and treatments related to Water Qi Encroaching on the Heart

The key points to distinguish the two subtypes of water qi encroaching on the Heart are as follows:
(1) Location of edema: facial edema vs. whole-body edema worse in the lower extremities
(2) Severity of gastrointestinal symptoms
(3) Productive cough with profuse white foaming phlegm and an inability to lie down flat vs. scanty or difficult urination

Pattern	Thin Mucus Obstructing the Heart	Water-Dampness Invading Upward
Etiology	Chronic cough, overstrain, improper diet	Exopathogenic cold-dampness attack, improper diet, congenital deficiency
Pathogenesis	Water-thin mucus accumulation inside, obstructs Heart yang	
	Spleen and Lung qi deficiency, fails to transform water-thin mucus, obstructs Heart yang	Spleen and Kidney yang deficiency, leads to water accumulation in the lower burner, water qi rebels upward, attacking the Heart
Symptoms	Palpitations, tightness and distress in the chest, fatigue, sweating, cold body and limbs, dizziness, nausea and/or vomiting, poor appetite, panting, thirsty but no desire to drink, edema, a white slippery tongue coating	
	Productive cough with profuse white foaming phlegm, oppression and tightness in the chest, inability to lie down flat, facial edema	Whole-body edema worse in the lower extremities, thirst but no desire to drink water, abdominal bloating and distention, scanty or difficult urination
Treatment strategy	Warm and transform water-thin mucus, promote and invigorate Heart yang	Warm and tonify Spleen and Kidney yang, move qi and promote urination
Herbal formulas	Ling Gui Zhu Gan Tang	Zhen Wu Tang

Table 24.4.2 Comparison of Thin Mucus Obstructing the Heart and Water-Dampness Invading Upward

5. How to distinguish water qi encroaching on the Heart (水氣凌心 shuǐ qì líng xīn) from Heart yang deficiency (心陽虛 xīn yáng xū)?

Water qi encroaching on the Heart is a group of signs and symptoms caused by Spleen and Lung qi deficiency failing to transform water-thin mucus, which obstructs Heart yang. It can also be due to Spleen and Kidney yang deficiency leading to water accumulation in the lower burner that rebels upward and invades the Heart. Both subtypes lead to palpitations, panting, fatigue, weakness, cold limbs, and whole body or local edema. The two subtypes of this complex zàng fǔ pattern are: thin mucus obstructing the Heart (飲阻於心 yǐn zǔ yú xīn) and water-dampness invading upward (水濕上犯 shuǐ shī shàng fàn).

Heart yang deficiency refers to a pattern where the insufficiency of Heart yang results in a lack of motive force for promoting blood and a decreased warming and nourishing function that leads to fright, continuous palpitations, chest distress with tightness or pain, shortness of breath, and cold limbs.

Spleen, Lung, and Kidney yang deficiency results in the accumulation of water-thin mucus, which can upwardly attack the Heart and Lung. This obstruction of the Heart yang is the pathogenesis of water qi encroaching on the Heart. Thus yang deficiency is the root, and water-thin mucus accumulation obstructing the Heart yang is the branch. It is pathologically located in the Heart, but related with the Lung, Spleen, and Kidney. In contrast, the pathogenesis for Heart yang deficiency is insufficient Heart yang that fails to nourish and warm the Heart shén, resulting in a lack of motive force to promote blood circulation and internal deficiency cold. However, long-term Heart yang deficiency can develop into Heart yang collapse or water qi encroaching on the Heart.

The key points to distinguish these two patterns are as follows:

(1) Clinical manifestations:

    Water qi encroaching on the Heart can be divided into three subgroups: (1) water-thin mucus attacking the Lung and Heart, obstructing the Heart yang, which then fails to promote blood circulation, leading to fright and/or continuous palpitations, cough, panting, shortness of breath, and chest distress and tightness; (2) water-thin mucus accumulation, resulting in edema and cough with profuse white foaming phlegm; and (3) failure of the Spleen's transportation and transformation function causing poor appetite, nausea or vomiting, fatigue, and low energy.

    Heart yang deficiency can be divided into two subgroups: (1) a series of symptoms due to Heart qi failing to promote blood circulation, leading to fright and/or continuous palpitations, chest distress and tightness that is worse with exertion, shortness of breath, spontaneous sweating, and pale facial complexion; and (2) cold due to yang deficiency such as cold limbs, or chest pain.

    The signs and symptoms of Heart yang deficiency, such as productive cough, edema, or poor appetite, are not related to multiple organ failure. In contrast, water qi encroaching on the Heart usually develops from the dysfunction of multiple organs such as Lung,

Spleen, and Kidney yang deficiency with water-thin mucus accumulation that obstructs Heart yang. Thus compared to the pattern Heart yang deficiency, water qi encroaching on the Heart is more severe, chronic, longer course, and has a poorer prognosis.

(2) Severity of symptoms:

Palpitations, chest distress and tightness, and cold body and limbs appear in both patterns. However, due to the difference in etiology and pathogenesis, there is a difference in the severity of the symptoms.

    a. Regarding palpitations, it is relatively milder in Heart yang deficiency compared to water qi encroaching on the Heart. Palpitations in Heart yang deficiency is caused by Heart failing to nourish and promote. According to *Standard for Diagnosis and Treatment* (證治準繩 *zhèng zhì zhǔn shéng*): "When there is yang deficiency, there is a feeling of emptiness in the chest area, which is similar to fright palpitations." In contrast, palpitations in water qi encroaching on the Heart is caused by water attacking fire (Heart yang), unsettling the Heart *shén*, so there is "fright palpitations and continuous palpitations, constant restlessness, and dysphoria."

    b. Chest distress and tightness in Heart yang deficiency is milder because it is caused by insufficiency of the gathering qi (宗氣 *zōng qì*) in the chest, failing to promote. In contrast, for water qi encroaching on the Heart, chest distress and tightness is caused by excess pathogens such as water-thin mucus attacking the Heart and Lung, leading to water-thin mucus accumulation in the upper burner. Thus there is chest distress with oppression or distention, panting, shortness of breath, and even an inability to lie down flat.

    c. Cold body and limbs are more severe in water qi encroaching on the Heart because Spleen and Kidney yang deficiency are the root of this pattern. The Spleen governs the limbs and muscles while the Kidney is the root of primary yang. Thus when the Spleen and Kidney yang are deficient, yang qi fails to distribute and warm, leading to extremely cold limbs (厥逆 *jué nì*).

(3) Characteristics of the illness:

    a. History of the illness

    b. Deficiency root with excess branch (本虛表實 *běn xū biǎo shí*) vs. deficiency

Pattern	Water Qi Encroaching on the Heart		Heart Yang Deficiency
	Thin Mucus Obstructing the Heart	Water-Dampness Invading Upward	
Etiology	Chronic cough, overstrain, improper diet	Exopathogenic cold-dampness attack, improper diet, congenital deficiency	Chronic illness, improper treatment, aging
Pathogenesis	Spleen and Lung qi deficiency fails to transform water-thin mucus and obstructs Heart yang	Spleen and Kidney yang deficiency leads to water accumulation in the lower burner, water qi rebels upward and attacks the Heart	Heart yang insufficiency, lack of motive force to promote blood, impairs the function of warming and nourishing
Organs	Spleen, Lung, Heart	Spleen, Kidney, Heart	Heart
Characteristics	Deficiency root, excess branch		Deficiency
	Complex, long-term illness, chronic cough, history of edema		Simple, mild, shorter history
Symptoms — Common	Palpitations, chest distress and tightness, fatigue, weakness, spontaneous sweating, cold body and limbs		
Symptoms — Others	Dizziness, nausea, vomiting, poor appetite, cold limbs, panting, thirst without desire to drink, edema		
	Productive cough with profuse white foaming phlegm, oppression and tightness in the chest, inability to lie down flat, facial edema	Whole-body edema worse in the lower extremities, thirst without desire to drink, abdominal bloating and distention, scanty or difficult urination	
Tongue	Pale flabby tongue with a white slippery coating		
Pulse	Deep, weak or wiry, slippery	Deep, slow, slippery	Deep, weak, or irregular
Treatment strategy	Warm and transform water-thin mucus, promote and invigorate Heart yang	Warm and tonify Spleen and Kidney yang, move qi and promote urination	Warm and tonify Heart yang
Herbal formulas	Ling Gui Zhu Gan Tang	Zhen Wu Tang	Shen Fu Tang, Bao Yuan Tang

Table 24.5.1 Comparison of Water Qi Encroaching on the Heart and Heart Yang Deficiency

6. How to distinguish Water Qi Encroaching on the Heart (水氣淩心 *shuǐ qì líng xīn*) from Cold-Water Shooting into the Lung (寒水射肺 *hán shuǐ shè fèi*)?

Both patterns can develop from thin mucus syndrome (飲証 *yǐn zhèng*), edema, or other diseases involving water metabolism disorder. Spleen and Kidney yang deficiency failing to promote water metabolism, resulting in water-thin mucus and/or phlegm accumulation upwardly attacking the Lung or Heart, is the pathology for these two patterns. Since their etiology and pathology are similar, their clinical manifestation is also similar. Symptoms include chest distress and tightness, panting, shortness of breath, difficulty lying down flat, facial or body edema, scanty or difficult urination, cold body and limbs, a pale tongue with slippery coating, and a deep and weak pulse.

Both patterns exhibit 'deficient root and excessive branch.' The root is Spleen and Kidney deficiency, while the branch is water-thin mucus accumulation upwardly attacking the Lung and/or Heart.

However, since water-thin mucus is attacking different organs in these two patterns, the major symptoms are different. Fright and continuous palpations are the chief complaints for water qi encroaching on the Heart, while productive cough with profuse white foaming phlegm, panting, and shortness of breath are the key symptoms for cold-water shooting into the Lung.

Cold-water shooting into the Lung is mostly induced by exopathogenic invasion such as exopathogenic cold attack when the patient has pre-existing water-thin mucus disorder. Thus it may be accompanied by chills and fever and the symptoms are more acute, severe, and can develop quickly. These two patterns may combine when the disease develops without control or proper treatment.

The key points to distinguish these two patterns:
(1) Major symptoms: Palpitations vs. coughing and wheezing
(2) Severity: water qi encroaching on the Heart results from chronic illness and develops gradually, while cold-water shooting into the Lung usually results from an acute exopathogenic invasion and develops quickly

Pattern		Water Qi Encroaching on the Heart	Cold-Water Shooting into the Lung
Etiology		Chronic cough or illness, overstrain, improper diet	Exopathogenic cold combined with water attack, improper diet, or chronic illness
Characteristic		Deficiency root, excess branch	
		Longer course	More acute and severe, develops quicker
Pathogenesis		Spleen and Kidney yang deficiency causes water-thin mucus accumulation and obstruction that attacks upward	
		Water-thin mucus obstructs Heart yang, which fails to promote and nourish the *Shén*	Water-thin mucus blocks the Lung qi, causing Lung qi rebellion
Symptoms	Common	Chest distress and tightness, shortness of breath, dyspnea, difficult to lie down float, facial or body edema, scanty or difficult urination, cold body and limbs, a pale tongue with a slippery coating, and a deep and weak pulse	
	Main	Fright and/or continuous palpitations, intermittent pulse	Productive cough with profuse white foaming phlegm, wheezing or asthma
	Others	Nausea, vomiting, poor appetite	Exterior symptoms such as chills, fever, and superficial pulse
Treatment strategy		Warm and transform water-thin mucus, promote and invigorate Heart yang	Warm the Lung, transform phlegm, stop cough
herbal formulas		Zhen Wu Tang, Ling Gui Zhu Gan Tang	Xiao Qing Long Tang

Table 24.6.1 Comparison of Water Qi Encroaching on the Heart and Cold-Water Shooting into the Lung

7. What is Kidney Water Invading the Spleen (肾水泛脾 *shèn shuǐ fàn pí*)?

Definition: A group of signs and symptoms marked by a long duration of Spleen and Kidney yang deficiency with severe edema in the lower extremities. This pattern is also called yin edema or 'main water pattern' (正水證 *zhèng shuǐ zhèng*).

Clinical manifestation: Repeated relapse of pitting edema that is worse below the waist; epigastric and abdominal distention and oppression; poor appetite; loose stools; fatigue; weak limbs; cold body and limbs; preference for warmth; aching cold sensation of the lower back and knees; scanty or difficult urination; a dull or pale complexion; a pale and flabby tongue with a white and slippery coating; and a deep, slow, and weak pulse.

Key points: Chronic repeated relapse of pitting edema that is worse below the waist, plus Spleen and Kidney yang deficiency signs and symptoms.

Etiology and pathogenesis: Long-term Spleen and Kidney yang deficiency causing water metabolism disorder; Kidney Yang deficiency with water effusion that leads to water upwardly attacking the Spleen; chronic illness with Spleen and Kidney yang deficiency; physical or sexual overstrain; and improper diet can all lead to yin edema. Yin edema can also develop from yang edema.

A long duration of Spleen and Kidney yang deficiency fails to warm and promote, leading to an intolerance of cold, a dull or pale complexion, cold body and limbs, aching cold sensation in the lower back and knees, fatigue, weak limbs, and repeated relapse of chronic pitting edema that is worse below the waist. The deficiency of Spleen yang involves a failure of its transportation and transformation function, which leads to epigastric and abdominal distention with oppression, poor appetite, and loose stools. The deficiency of Kidney yang involves failure of its qi transformation function, which leads to difficult or scanty urination.

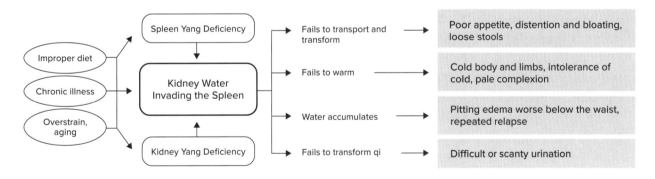

Chart 24.7.1 Etiology and pathogenesis of Kidney Water Invading the Spleen

TCM Disease	Western Disease	Herbal Formulas		Acupuncture	
Edema (水腫)	Chronic nephritis, CHF, chronic renal failure, malnutrition, COPD	Zhen Wu Tang	Shi Pi Yin	BL-20, BL-23, CV-9, CV-4, KI-7, ST-36, Moxa CV-4, CV-6	SP-3, SP-5, KI-3, KI-7
Diarrhea (泄瀉)	Crohn's disease, microscopic colitis, ulcerative colitis, celiac disease, parasite, irritable bower syndrome, hypothyroid, malnutrition		Si Shen Wan, Shen Ling Bai Zhu San		SP-3, CV-13, KI-3, KI-4, GV-4
Urinary blockage (癃閉)	Cystocele, UTI, benign prostatic hyperplasia, multiple sclerosis		Bu Zhong Yi Qi Tang, Shen Qi Wan		KI-5, GV-4, GV-20, CV-4
Spillage thin mucus (溢飲)	Kidney failure, uremia, CHF, glomerulonephritis, nephrotic syndrome		Ji Sheng Shen Qi Wan		SP-3, SP-9, KI-3

Table 24.7.1 Diseases and treatments related to Kidney Water Invading the Spleen

8. What is the relationship of the following five patterns: Kidney Yang Deficiency (腎陽虛 *shèn yáng xū*), Kidney Yang Deficiency with Water Effusion (腎虛水泛 *shèn xū shuǐ fàn*), Water Qi Encroaching on the Heart (水氣凌心 *shuǐ qì líng xīn*), Cold-Water Shooting into the Lung (寒水射肺 *hán shuǐ shè fèi*), and Kidney Water Invading the Spleen (腎水泛脾 *shèn shuǐ fàn pí*)?

When Kidney yang is deficient, it fails to warm and transform, leading to water-thin mucus accumulation, which is the primary pathogenesis for these five patterns. The resulting water metabolism disorder of water-thin mucus accumulation in the lower burner is the pattern called Kidney yang deficiency with water effusion. This manifests with general pitting edema that is worse in the lower extremities, cold body and limbs, scanty or difficult urination, a pale tongue with a slippery coating, and a deep thin pulse.

When the water-thin mucus accumulation in Kidney yang deficiency with water effusion attacks upward, it leads to various organ dysfunctions. For instance, when the water-thin mucus upwardly attacks the Heart, it leads to the pattern called water qi encroaching on the Heart, which manifests with palpitations and an inability to lie down flat. When the water-thin mucus upwardly attacks the Lung, the resulting pattern is called cold-water shooting into the Lung, which manifests with productive cough and profuse white foaming phlegm. When the water-thin mucus upwardly attacks the Spleen, it causes 'main water pattern' (正水證 *zhèng shuǐ zhèng*), or yin edema that manifests with repeated relapses of pitting edema that is worse below the waist, epigastric and abdominal distention and oppression, poor appetite, and loose stools. Thus Kidney yang deficiency is the root of all of these patterns, and Kidney yang deficiency with water effusion encompasses the other three patterns, which are its different clinical manifestations.

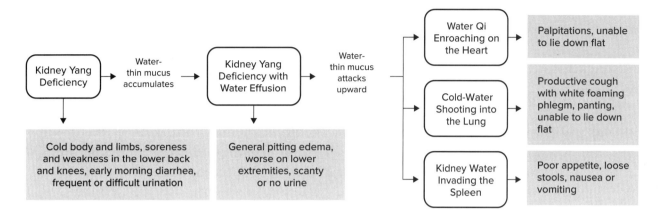

Chart 24.8.1 Water-thin mucus accumulation patterns related to Kidney Yang Deficiency

9. Does the pattern Lung Yang Deficiency exist? If so, what is its clinical manifestation, etiology, and pathogenesis?

All *zàng* organs have yin and yang, including the Lung. This concept was first mentioned in *Basic Questions* (素問 *sù wèn*), Chapter 14, which states: "Some diseases do not start from the exterior, but rather are caused by yang qi exhaustion of the five *zàng* organs, leading to water accumulation on the body's surface." It was also noted in *Basic Questions* (素問 *sù wèn*), Chapter 21, that "appropriate adjustments must be made based on the change of seasons and the variations of yin and yang of the five *zàng* organs." While the existence of yin and yang for the five *zàng* organs was acknowledged, there was only mention of Lung qi deficiency, Lung yin deficiency, and Lung cold, but no mention of Lung yang deficiency.

Lung yang governs warming and dispersing, while Lung yin controls cooling and descending. Lung yin and Lung yang are rooted in each other, interdependent, and mutually constraining, keeping each other balanced to ensure the proper Lung function of dispersing, descending, coordinating, and transforming qi. Compared to Lung yin, Lung yang has warming, promoting, dispersing, diffusing, and excitatory effects. Its existence is a precondition of Lung yin.

In the *Golden Cabinet* (金匱要略 *jīn guì yào lùe*), Chapter 7, Zhang Zhongjing stated that the herbal formula Licorice and Ginger Decoction (甘草乾薑湯 *gān cǎo gān jiāng tāng*) was used for "Lung atrophy" (肺痿 *fèi wěi*) caused by cold-thin mucus accumulating in the Lung that impairs Lung yang. He did not mention Lung yang deficiency, just Lung cold. However, starting in the Tang, Song, and Yuan dynasties, physicians and scholars began to clarify this concept and explore Lung yang and Lung yang deficiency. In the Ming and Qing dynasties, there were further discussions about the physiological functions and pathological changes of Lung yang, clinical symptoms of Lung yang deficiency, treatment strategies, and herbal prescriptions.

Definition: A group of signs and symptoms resulting from Lung yang deficiency failing to warm, promote, descend, and disperse.

Clinical manifestation: Chronic cough, profuse white clear sputum, panting, chest pain, shortness of breath, cold limbs, tendency to catch colds, intolerance of cold, a pale flabby tongue or a pale dusky tongue with teethmarks, a thin white or moist tongue coating, and a slow or slow and wiry pulse.

Key points: Lung qi deficiency symptoms, plus yang deficiency symptoms.

Etiology and pathogenesis: Invasion of exopathogenic factors, chronic illness, smoking, and improper diet can all cause Lung yang deficiency. There are five different pathogeneses involved in this pattern:
(1) Phlegm-thin mucus accumulation in the Lung blocks yang qi, leading to stagnation and obstruction of Lung yang, which fails to warm
(2) Pathogenic cold invades the Lung and impairs its yang
(3) Lung qi deficiency leads to Lung yang deficiency
(4) Lung yin deficiency leads to Lung yang deficiency
(5) Other organ dysfunctions resulting in Lung yang deficiency such as Heart and Spleen yang deficiency

Deficient Lung yang failing to descend and disperse can cause qi rebellion, which results in dyspnea, panting, cough, wheezing, and chest distress and pain. When deficient Lung yang fails to promote, there may be feeble breath, fatigue, aversion to talking, shortness of breath, low voice, tendency to catch colds, spontaneous sweating, and a weak pulse. And, when deficient Lung yang fails to warm, there may be cold limbs, profuse white thin sputum, a pale tongue, and a slow pulse.

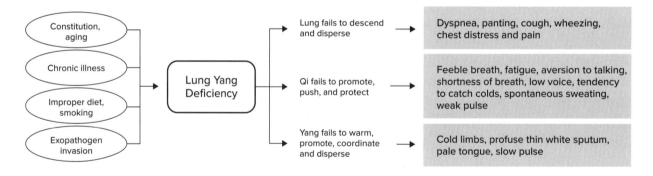

Chart 24.9.1 Etiology and pathogenesis of Lung Yang Deficiency

TCM Disease	Western Disease	Herbal Formulas		Acupuncture	
Asthma and wheezing (哮喘)	Bronchial asthma, COPD, emphysema, pneumonia, CHF, silicosis, anxiety attack, lung TB	Gan Cao Gan Jiang Tang	Bu Fei Tang	BL-13, BL-23, ST-36, GV-4, CV-4, LU-7, LU-9	Dingchuan, CV-17, CV-22, KI-1, GV-14, ST-9, LU-1
Lung atrophy (肺痿)	Pulmonary fibrosis, atelectasis, lung cirrhosis, bronchiectasis, silicosis, chronic bronchitis		Si Jun Zi Tang		LU-1, LU-2, CV-17

Table 24.9.1 Diseases and treatments related to Lung Yang Deficiency

10. Does the pattern Lung Blood Deficiency exist? If so, what is its clinical manifestation, etiology, and pathogenesis?

Lung blood deficiency is a long-forgotten and ignored pattern. Most traditional Chinese medicine scholars and practitioners think that this pattern does not exist and some believe that Lung blood deficiency is an intermediate transitional pattern between Lung qi deficiency and Lung yin deficiency. Emphasis is placed on the Lung's physiological function of controlling qi, regulating water passages, and distributing body fluids. Thus pathologically, the focus is on Lung qi, Lung yin, and body fluid deficiency, while Lung blood deficiency and Lung yang deficiency are rarely mentioned.

However, there are some scholars and practitioners who think that Lung blood deficiency pattern exists. Their reasoning is based on the following:

(1) 'The Lung joins the skin and hair' (肺合皮毛 *fèi hé pí máo*): the Lung controls and is associated with the body's surface. The clinical manifestation of blood deficiency is a pale or sallow complexion along with pale lips, eyelids, and nails—all symptoms on the body's surface. *Basic Questions* (素問 *sù wèn*), Chapter 10, states, "The Lung is associated with the skin and hair because it nourishes the skin and hair." Thus when the body's surface fails to be nourished by blood, it is closely related to the Lung; when the Lung's blood is deficient, the body's surface will not be nourished.

(2) 'The Lung is a blood organ' (肺為血臟 *fèi wéi xuě zàng*): the Lung not only controls qi, but also involves generating blood, as it is considered a blood organ. The *Spiritual Pivot* (靈樞 *líng shū*), Chapter 18, states:
> The middle burner is situated in the Stomach and under the upper burner. It receives food and water. After the process of evaporating and excreting dross, it retains the refined substances, extracting food and water essences to be sent upward to the Lung, where the essences will be transformed into blood to nourish the whole body.

This indicates that blood is first generated in the Lung and then distributed to the entire body to nourish all organs and tissues. *Basic Questions* (素問 *sù wèn*), Chapter 21, states:
> After food enters the Stomach and gets digested, its refined essences are distributed to the Liver to moisten the tendons, …the thick and condensed part of the essence is sent to the Heart to form nutritive qi and blood, which fills the vessels to the Lung. All vessels gather into the Lung, which then transports and distributes this essence to the entire body, including the skin and hair. Qi and blood combine and flow from small vessels confluent to big vessels; abundant qi and blood fill and circulate inside the big vessels, sending qi and blood to the other four *zàng* organs, the Heart, Liver, Spleen, and Kidney; and qi and blood maintain their balance.

Traditional Chinese Medicine Fundamental Theory (中醫基礎理論 *zhōng yī jī chǔ lǐ lùn*), a TCM university textbook, states:

All vessels gather into the Lung (肺朝百脈 *fèi cháo bǎi mài*) means that the blood of the entire body passes through the Lung, where air exchange is conducted by the breathing function of the Lung, enriching the blood with clear qi (清氣 *qīng qì*) that will then be transported to the entire body via the vessels.

Similarly, *Essence of Medicine Classic* (醫經精義 *yī jīng jīng yì*) states:
> The Heart is King, while the Lung is by its side, assisting the Heart… Blood from the Heart enters the Lung under Lung qi's assistance to blow out turbid qi (濁氣 *zhuó qì*) from the blood, redden the blood, and then return it to the Heart.

This means that the Lung participates in producing blood and is a blood organ. Thus there can be various causes of Lung blood deficiency.

(3) There are some classic TCM books that document treatment strategies, herbs, herbal formulas, or the pathogeneses of Lung blood deficiency:

In *Symptoms, Causes, Pulse, and Treatment* (症因脈治 *zhèng yīn mài zhì*, 1706), Qin Jingming said: "Cough due to blood deficiency requires replenishing blood, using Si Wu Tang (四物湯 *sì wù tāng*), Gui Shao Di Huang Tang (歸芍地黃湯 *guī sháo dì huáng tāng*), and Tian Di Jian (天地煎 *tiān dì jiān*), indicating that there were herbal formulas for cough caused by Lung blood deficiency.

In *Fine Formulas for Women* (婦人良方大全 *fù rén liáng fāng dà quán*, 1237), Chen Ziming explains a pathogenesis of a female patient: "Hard and dry stools caused by internal heat has led the patient to become gradually thinner, resulting in Spleen and Lung blood deficiency."

In the famous book *Comprehensive Outline of the Materia Medica* (本草綱目 *běn cǎo gāng mù*, 1590), Li Shizhen states: "Huang Qi tonifies Lung qi, while E Jiao nourishes Lung blood." The herbal formulas Six-Gentlemen of Metal and Water Decoction (金水六君子煎 *jīn shuǐ liù jūn zǐ jiān*), mentioned in *Collected Treatises of Jing-Yue* (景岳全書 *jǐng yuè quán shū*, 1624), and Lily Bulb Decoction to Preserve the Metal (百合固金湯 *bǎi hé gù jīn tāng*), mentioned in *Legacy Book of Shen-Zhai* (慎齋遺書 *shèn zhāi yí shū*, 16TH CENTURY), both have the function of nourishing the Lung yin and tonifying the Lung blood, and are used for Lung yin and Lung blood deficiency patterns.

(4) Some scholars use modern medicine to speculate the existence of Lung blood deficiency. Research affirms that the lungs have the function of storing blood. In fact, the lungs contain approximately 750-1,000 mL of blood, a volume that is higher than air exchange requires. This means that the lungs not only have the function of air exchange, but also blood storage. Thus under certain circumstances, there may be blood deficiency.

Clinical manifestations: Cough, dyspnea, shortness of breath, pale complexion, dizziness, blurry vision, a pale tongue, and a thin weak pulse. Lung blood deficiency is mostly combined with qi deficiency or yin deficiency, so based on the combination of the pathogenesis, the clinical manifestations are as follows:

(1) Lung blood deficiency caused by chronic or severe cough impairing the Lung collaterals: cough, hemoptysis, blood-stained sputum, or coughing up blood and pus.
(2) Lung blood deficiency combined with Lung qi deficiency: fatigue, shortness of breath, panting, worse with exertion, a weak voice, tendency to catch colds, a pale complexion, dizziness, blurry vision, palpitations, little or no sweating, pale lips, and a thin weak pulse.
(3) Lung blood deficiency combined with Lung yin deficiency: pale complexion, dizziness and blurry vision, palpitations, dry cough, shortness of breath, scanty and thick phlegm, cough with blood, dry mouth and throat, hoarseness, emaciation, low-grade fever in the afternoon or evening, night sweats, malar flush, pale lips, a red tongue, and a thin rapid pulse.

Etiology and pathogenesis: Insufficient production, excessive consumption, and bleeding are the three major causes of Lung blood deficiency. Congenital insufficiency, chronic illness with Spleen and Stomach dysfunction, and improper diet all diminish generation and transformation, which results in a lack of blood production. Disease, serious illness, injury to the vital qi, or long-term physical and mental overstrain excessively consume qi and blood. Lung blood deficiency can also develop from Lung yin deficiency or bleeding.

Hemoptysis is one of the causes of Lung blood deficiency and can also be worsened by Lung blood deficiency. The Lung is a blood organ that requires a sufficient amount of blood to properly perform its dispersing and descending function. When blood is insufficient, Lung qi can become rebellious, resulting in cough, panting, hemoptysis, or even coughing up both blood and pus.

Physically, qi and blood are closely related and interdependent; the relationship is described as 'qi is the commander of blood' (氣為血之帥 qì wéi xuě zhī shuài) and 'blood is the mother of qi' (血為氣之母 xuě wéi qì zhī mǔ). Qi generates blood and blood nourishes qi; pathologically, they affect each other. When blood is deficient, the lack of nourishment results in qi deficiency; and when qi is deficient, the failure to generate blood causes blood deficiency. Thus Lung blood deficiency commonly combines with Lung qi deficiency. When blood is deficient, there may be a pale complexion, pale lips, and a thin pulse. When qi is deficient, failing to push and promote, there may be a weak voice, feeble cough or panting, shortness of breath, fatigue, aversion to speaking, and a deficient pulse. Water metabolism can also be disrupted, leading to the accumulation of pathological fluids, generation of phlegm, and cough with thin white sputum. Additionally, when qi is deficient, it may fail to protect the exterior of the body, causing susceptibility to colds. Activity consumes qi, and thus symptoms are worse after exertion.

Blood and body fluids share the same source and transform into each other. Thus when blood is deficient, body fluids will also be deficient. Even though deficient qi fails to secure, the deficient body fluids in this pattern means that there may be little or no sweating.

Blood is part of yin, and thus blood deficiency can lead to yin deficiency, and they can occur together. Thus Lung blood deficiency is commonly combined with Lung yin deficiency. Blood deficiency fails to nourish the head and face resulting in dizziness, blurred vision, palpitations, and pale complexion and lips, while yin deficiency produces symptoms of internal heat such as low-grade fever in the afternoon or evening, malar flush, five center heat, night sweats, a red tongue, and a thin rapid pulse. Yin deficiency also leads to deficient body fluids, manifesting as dry mouth and throat.

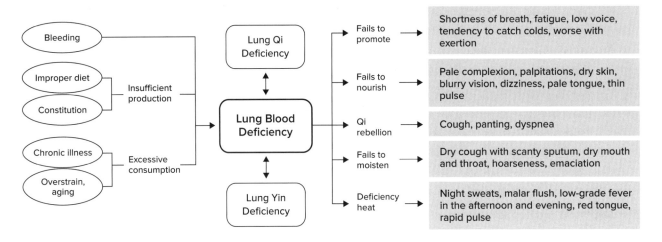

Chart 24.10.1 Etiology and pathogenesis of Lung Blood Deficiency

TCM Disease	Western Disease	Herbal Formulas		Acupuncture	
Cough (咳嗽)	Chronic bronchitis, emphysema, COPD, CHF, allergy asthma, lung TB, GERD, allergic rhinitis, lung cancer	Si Su Tant, Ren Shen Yin Zi, Jie Geng Tang	Gui Shao Di Huang Tang	ST-36, SP-6, LR-3, BL-11, BL-13, BL-17	CV-22, BL-13, GV-14, ST-9, LU-1, LU-7
Asthma and wheezing (哮喘)	Bronchial asthma, COPD, emphysema, pneumonia, CHF, silicosis, anxiety attack, lung TB		Sheng Mai San		Dingchuan, CV-17, CV-22, KI-1, GV-14, ST-9, LU-1
Consumptive disorder (肺痨)	Lung TB, lung cancer		Qing Hao Bie Jia San, Tian Di Jian		LU-5
Hemoptysis (咳血)	Bronchitis, bronchiectasis, CHF, TB, lung cancer or lung tumors, pneumonia, pulmonary embolism		Bai He Gu Jin Tang		LU-6
Atrophic lung disease (肺痿)	Stiff lung disease, atrophic emphysema, atelectasis, pulmonary fibrosis		Qing Zao Jiu Fei Tang		BL-42

Table 24.10.1 Diseases and treatments related to Lung Blood Deficiency

11. Dryness Invading the Lung, Lung Yin Deficiency, and Liver Fire Invading the Lung all share the major symptoms of dry cough, cough with scanty sputum, or cough with blood, but how are these three patterns different from each other?

Dryness invading the Lung is due to exopathogenic dryness attacking the Lung, causing it to lose both its moisture and its dispersing and descending function. This results in Lung qi rebellion and stagnation, which gives rise to coughing that is dry with scanty, sticky, or blood-stained sputum, and difficult expectoration. Meanwhile, there are other signs and symptoms caused by dryness such as dry skin; dry nose, lips, mouth, tongue, and throat; thirst; scanty urine; and dry stool. Chills and fever may also appear in the early stages. This pattern most often occurs in the fall and winter due to the use of heaters, or in dry climates. It is acute, short course, and an exterior pattern.

Lung yin deficiency is an endopathogenic disease that can result from febrile diseases, chronic illness, improper lifestyle, and improper treatments. Yin deficiency fails to nourish the Lung, leading to cough due to Lung qi rebellion. Yin deficient heat condenses the sputum, leading to cough producing scanty sticky phlegm. If heat injures the blood vessels, the cough may produce blood-stained sputum. The function of yin fluids is to nourish and moisten; therefore, when yin is deficient, there is dry mouth and throat, constipation, and dry stools. Meanwhile, there are also signs and symptoms of yin deficiency such as hot flashes, night sweats, five center heat, malar flush, a red tongue with little or no coating, and a thin rapid pulse. This pattern most often occurs in elderly patients; it is chronic, long course, and an interior deficiency pattern.

Liver fire invading the Lung, also called 'wood fire punishes metal' (木火刑金 *mù huǒ xíng jīn*), is due to emotional stress, especially anger, which impairs the Liver and causes qi stagnation that then transforms into fire or pathogenic heat. This accumulation in the Liver flares up through the channel and affects the Lung, consuming Lung yin, disrupting its descending and dispersing function, and leading to paroxysmal cough or difficult breathing. When the heat injures the blood vessels there may be coughing with blood. In this pattern, Liver qi stagnation transforming into heat is the primary pathogenesis, and therefore the major signs and symptoms may include burning pain in the hypochondrium, irritability, short temper, dizziness, distending headaches, red face and eyes, and a bitter taste in the mouth. This pattern is sub-acute and is an interior excess heat pattern.

Pattern		Dryness Invading the Lung	Lung Yin Deficiency	Liver Fire Invading the Lung
Etiology		Exopathogenic dryness	Febrile disease, chronic illness, improper lifestyle	Emotional stress
Pathogenesis		Lung qi rebellion, failure in dispersing and descending		
		Dryness impairs Lung yin	Lung yin deficiency fails to nourish	Liver fire attacks the Lung and impairs the Lung yin
Characteristics		Distention or pain in the hypochondrium and chest, abnormal emotions, wiry pulse		
Symptoms	Common	Dry cough, cough with bleeding, thick yellow phlegm		
	Cough	Most occur in fall and winter, short course	Chronic cough, long course, worse at night	Cough induced or aggravated by emotional stress
	Sputum	White or slight yellow	Yellow	Yellow
	Other	Chills and fever, dry mouth and skin	Night sweats, five center heat, low-grade fever in the afternoon and evening	Irritability, anger, hypochondriac burning pain
Tongue		Dry, normal color, thin coating (may be slightly yellow)	Dry, red tongue, scanty coating, or no coating	Red tongue, thin yellow coating
Pulse		Superficial	Thin and rapid	Wiry and rapid
Treatment strategy		Expel wind, moisten dryness, stop cough	Nourish Lung yin, stop cough	Soothe Liver qi, clear heat from Liver, stop cough
Herbal formulas		Sang Xing Tang, Xing Su San, Qing Zao Jiu Fei Tang	Bai He Gu Jin Tang, Yang Yin Qing Fei Tang	Qing Jin Hua Tan Tang

Table 24.11.1 Comparison of Dryness Invading the Lung, Lung Yin Deficiency, and Liver Fire Invading the Lung

12. What is the pathogenesis of Liver Qi Stagnation and Liver Qi Rebellion? How are they different?

The Liver governs coursing and discharging (疏泄 shū xiè). Shū means to dredge while xiè means to release. When the Liver fails to course and discharge, there are two major pathological changes:
1) Liver qi stagnation (肝氣郁结 gān qì yù jié)
2) Liver qi rebellion, which includes:
   - Liver qi upward rebellion (肝氣上逆 gān qì shàng nì)
   - Liver qi transverse rebellion (肝氣横逆 gān qì héng nì)

The pathogenesis of Liver qi stagnation is the lack of coursing and discharging whereas for Liver qi rebellion it is a dysfunction of coursing and discharging that leads to abnormal circulation of the Liver qi. This may lead to its upward or transverse rebellion, which can 'assault' or impair the functions of other organs.

Although the pathogenesis for Liver qi stagnation and Liver qi rebellion are different, they have the same root, which is the Liver's failure to properly course and discharge. Thus they share many of the same clinical manifestations such as hypochondrium distention and pain, emotional abnormalities, and a wiry pulse.

Liver qi stagnation presents with depression, sluggishness, melancholy, frequent sighing, and distention and oppression in the hypochondrium and chest. Liver qi upward rebellion presents with vigor and hyperactivity, distending headache, eye pain, irritability, short temper, cough or even vomiting with blood, and syncope. As for Liver qi transverse rebellion, there are two resulting patterns. One is called Liver and Spleen disharmony, also known as Liver attacking the Spleen, which manifests with poor appetite, loose stools, and abdominal bloating and distention. The other is Liver and Stomach disharmony, also known as Liver attacking the Stomach, which exhibits epigastric distention, hiccups, nausea, vomiting, and belching.

Not many books discuss Liver qi upward rebellion, but it is commonly seen in clinical practice. *The Yellow Emperor's Inner Classic* (黃帝內經 huáng dì nèi jīng) first mentioned it in the *Spiritual Pivot* (靈樞 líng shū), Chapter 50, which states: "When angry, Liver qi will rush upward filling and expanding the chest. Meanwhile, the Gallbladder qi will transversely attack."

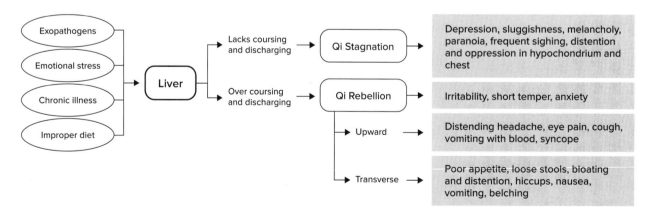

Chart 24.12.1 Etiology and pathogenesis of Liver Qi Stagnation and Liver Qi Rebellion

Pattern	Liver Qi Stagnation	Liver Qi Upward Rebellion	Liver Qi Transverse Rebellion
Pathogenesis	Dysfunction of Liver's coursing and discharging		
	Lack of coursing and discharging, leads to qi stagnation	Over coursing and discharging, leads qi to rebel upwards	Over coursing and discharging, disrupts qi movement, leads to qi rebellion that transversely attacks the Spleen or Stomach
Symptoms	Distention or pain in the hypochondrium and chest, abnormal emotions, wiry pulse		
	Distention or oppression in the hypochondrium and chest, depression, melancholy, frequent sighing, irregular menstrual cycle	Distending headache, eye pain, irritability, short temper, vomiting blood, fainting. If Lung is attacked: cough, dyspnea, or cough with blood	Attacks the Spleen / Attacks the Stomach; Depression or irritability; Poor appetite, loose stools, abdominal distention / Vomiting, nausea, belching, acid reflux, epigastric pain
Treatment strategy	Soothe Liver qi, relieve stagnation	Nourish and soften the Liver to restrain the Liver	Soothe the Liver qi, harmonize the Spleen and Stomach
Herbal formulas	Si Ni San, Xiao Yao San	Long Dan Xie Gan Tang, Zhen Gan Xi Feng Tang	Xiao Yao San / Chai Hu Shu Gan Wan

Table 24.12.1 Comparison of Liver Qi Stagnation and Liver Qi Rebellion

13. What is the clinical manifestation, etiology, and pathogenesis of Liver Fire?

'Liver fire' is a pathogenic factor but also the name of a pattern. It is a group of heat signs and symptoms that blazes upward due to the exuberance of the Liver's ministerial fire (相火 xiàng huǒ).

The etiology of this pattern includes Liver qi stagnation transforming into fire due to long-term emotional stress, overconsumption of alcohol and spicy foods, and exopathogenic invasions that transform into fire. The pathogenesis of this pattern involves the Liver's yang qi rising up excessively and the nature is interior excess heat. Pathological changes may include the generation of wind, bleeding, invasion of the Lung or Stomach, impairment of body fluids, and mixing with phlegm.

Thus Liver fire has different clinical manifestations in different people. The pattern can be subdivided into Liver fire blazing, Liver fire attacking the Lung, Liver fire attacking the Stomach, Liver fire with phlegm, and Liver fire impairing yin. The general clinical symptoms of Liver fire include red and swollen eyes, distention headache, flushed face, bitter taste in the mouth, irritability, short temper, sudden tinnitus and deafness, dry stools, yellow scanty urine, epistaxis or hematemesis, a red tongue with a dry yellow coating, and a rapid wiry pulse.

Liver fire blazing is a group of signs and symptoms caused by the flaring up of excess fire. When Liver fire flares up following the Liver channel, it passes through the hypochondrium and reaches the head, eyes, and ears, causing burning pain in the hypochondrium, a red face, and red eyes. When the fire disrupts the clear orifices, it leads to tinnitus, deafness, dizziness, and distending pain of the head. When Liver fire upwardly attacks the Lung, it impairs the Lung's dispersing and descending function, causing cough. When fire injures the Lung's blood vessels, it causes epistaxis or hemoptysis. When Liver fire transversely attacks the Stomach, it will impair the Stomach's transporting and descending function, injure its blood vessels, and cause Stomach qi rebellion and bleeding, manifesting with nausea, vomiting, acid reflux, or even hematemesis. When Liver fire scorches pathological fluids, it generates phlegm or mixes with pre-existing phlegm, and disturbs the 'clear orifices' (清竅 qīng qiào), causing dizziness and vertigo. It can also obstruct the throat, leading to 'plum-pit' syndrome. When Liver fire impairs yin fluids, it results in dry mouth and throat, thirst, dry stools, and scanty urine.

Pattern	Liver Fire				
	Blazing	Attacking the Lung	Attacking the Stomach	With Phlegm	Impairing Yin
Symptoms	Irritable, short temper, burning pain in the hypochondria and chest, bitter taste and dry mouth, dry stool, yellow scanty urine, a red tongue with dry yellow coating, a wiry rapid pulse				
	Conjunctivitis, red face, insomnia, sudden tinnitus or deafness, insomnia, distending headache	Cough, epistaxis, hemoptysis	Nausea, vomiting, hematemesis, acid reflux	Dizziness, plum-pit syndrome	Dry mouth and thirst, dry stools, scanty urine
Treatment strategy	Clear Liver heat				
	Drain fire	Stop cough, cool blood	Direct rebellious qi downward	Dissolve phlegm	Nourish yin, spread Liver qi
Herbal formulas	Long Dan Xie Gan Tang, Xie Qing Wan	Qing Jin Hua Tan Tang, Dai Ge San	Zuo Jin Wan, Chai Hu Qing Gan Tang	Ban Xia Hou Po Tang	Yi Guan Jian

Table 24.13.1 Comparison of the patterns related to Liver fire

14. What is the difference between Liver heat and Liver fire?

The nature of Liver heat (肝熱 *gān rè*) and Liver fire (肝火 *gān huǒ*) are the same, as they both are caused by an exuberance of yang, which may develop from Liver qi stagnation transforming into heat or fire, improper diet, overconsumption of alcohol or spicy foods, or exopathogenic invasions that transform into heat or fire. So both patterns present with yang excess signs and symptoms such as irritability, short temper, burning pain in the hypochondrium and chest, bitter taste, dry mouth, dry stools, yellow scanty urine, a red tongue with dry yellow coating, and a rapid wiry pulse.

Fire is stronger than heat and therefore Liver fire is more severe. It has a tendency to blaze upwards, causing various signs and symptoms that appear in the upper body, especially the head such as headache, dizziness, tinnitus, deafness, red and swollen eyes, and a flushed face.

The pathological changes of Liver fire include the generation of wind, bleeding due to blood vessel damage, attack of the Lung and Stomach, and mixing with phlegm. Thus Liver fire has symptoms of cough, epistaxis, hematemesis, acid reflux, dizziness, and plum-pit syndrome.

Liver heat is caused by Liver qi stagnation transforming into heat and is more local to the Liver. It presents more as a condition of 'constraint,' such as depression, distention or distress in the hypochondrium and chest, alternating chills and fever, or irregular menstruation. It may also affect its internally-externally paired organ, the Gallbladder, which can lead to a bitter taste in the mouth and jaundice.

Pattern	Liver Heat	Liver Fire
Etiology and pathogenesis	Emotional stress leads to Liver qi stagnation and generates heat	Overconsumption of alcohol or spicy foods, emotional stress leads to qi stagnation and transforms into fire
Characteristics	Milder, more localized	Stronger, upward, or attacking other organs
Symptoms	Irritability, short temper, burning pain in the hypochondrium and chest, bitter taste and dry mouth, dry stools, yellow scanty urine, a red tongue with dry yellow coating, a wiry and rapid pulse	
	Depression, distention or distress in the breasts and hypochondrium, alternating chills and fever, irregular menstruation	Conjunctivitis, red face, insomnia, sudden tinnitus or deafness, distending headache, epistaxis, hematemesis
Related patterns	Heat Congesting in the Liver and Gallbladder	Liver Fire Blazing, Liver Fire Attacking the Lung, Liver Fire Attacking the Stomach, Liver Fire with Yin Deficiency, Liver Fire with Phlegm
Treatment strategy	Spread Liver qi, clear heat	Clear Liver heat, drain fire
Herbal formulas	Jia Wei Xiao Yao San	Long Dan Xie Gan Tang, Xie Qing Wan

Table 24.14.1 Comparison of Liver Heat and Liver Fire

15. What are the pathological changes of the Liver?

The nature of the Liver is to grow and expand; it favors being soothed and dispersed, and disfavors depression and constraint. It is an unyielding organ, staunch and restless. Under normal circumstances, the Liver qi moves freely and is in charge of coursing and discharging. When there is emotional stress, sudden excessive emotional stimulus, or pathogenic factors invading the Liver, its coursing and discharging function can be disrupted and Liver qi circulation can become obstructed, resulting in pathological changes. The six major pathological changes of the Liver are as follows:

(1) Stagnation (郁結 *yù jié*): Emotional stress, worrying, or overthinking constrains qi, leading the Liver qi to become obstructed and manifests with depression, melancholy, worry, sadness, frequent sighing, breast distention and tenderness, and distress and distention in the chest or hypochondrium.

(2) Upward attack or 'upward disrupt' (上擾 *shàng rǎo*): Liver qi stagnation can transform into fire that flares up and disturbs the head and orifices (清竅 *qīng qiào*). Or, Liver yang excess due to yin deficiency may rise up to disturb the clear orifices of the head, resulting in dizziness, distention headache, flushed face, and red eyes.

(3) Downward attack or 'downward oppress' (下迫 *xià pò*): Liver yang deficiency with cold, cold obstruction in the Liver channel, or damp-heat following the Liver channel pours downward, resulting in lower abdominal pain that radiates to the genital area, vaginal pain, scrotum pain, inguinal hernia, or leukorrhea.

(4) Transverse attack or 'transverse rebellion' (橫逆 *héng nì*): Liver qi transversely attacks Spleen and Stomach, leading to Spleen and Stomach disharmony. The Stomach fails to descend and the Spleen fails to transform and transport, resulting in poor appetite, belching, nausea or vomiting, acid regurgitation, abdominal bloating or distention, abdominal pain, and loose stools or diarrhea.

(5) Random movement (竄行 *cuàn xíng*): Both Liver qi and Liver wind can move randomly. Liver qi may follow the Liver channel and move randomly upward to the top of the head or downward to the feet, causing pain that is unfixed in location, sometimes severe and sometimes mild. Liver wind can affect the entire body, causing symptoms such as dizziness, vertigo, tremors, spasms, convulsions, numbness, tingling, stiffness, shaking, or syncope.

(6) Syncope (厥脫 *jué tuō*): Extreme emotional stimulation disrupts Liver qi, preventing the Liver from moving qi smoothly. This can cause qi rebellion and obstruction, and a disconnect of yin and yang, resulting in fainting or syncope.

16. What is the clinical manifestation of internal wind?

Internal wind is a group of signs and symptoms induced by pathological changes of the Liver and the clinical manifestations are varied and complicated. However, ancient physicians summarized the symptoms in the following thirteen groups:

(1) Spasm (抽 *chōu*): A sudden, abnormal, involuntary muscle contraction. Tonic spasms consist of continued muscle contraction, while clonic spasms consist of a series of alternating muscle contractions and relaxations.

(2) Hand cramp (搦 *nuò*): Hands and fingers involuntarily open and close into tightly clenching fists.

(3) Jerk (挚 *zhì*): A quick, sharp pull, thrust, twist, throw, or the like. It usually occurs in the shoulders and arms, but can also occur in the entire body. It is a sudden, spasmodic, involuntary muscular movement like the reflex action of pulling the hand away from a flame.

(4) Tremor (颤 *chàn*): Rhythmic oscillations caused by intermittent muscle contractions. It is involuntary with quick, short movements, including trembling or shaking of the hands, the tongue, and lips. Muscles can quiver as if from fear, excitement, weakness, or cold.

(5) Opisthotonos (反 *fǎn*): Spasm of the muscles causing backward arching of the head, neck, and spine, as in severe tetanus, some types of meningitis, and strychnine poisoning.

(6) Bow (引 *yǐn*): Dystonia or muscle spasms of the hands and arms such that the arms are in flexion, resting against the body with the elbows bent and the forearms across the abdomen, wrists bent, and fingers closed; the posture is similar to a bow.

(7) Upward gaze (窜 *cuàn*): A condition in which both eyes stare upward and appear to roll backwards. It is commonly seen in febrile seizures.

(8) Sight (视 *shì*): Strabismus, exotropia, or esotropia. A condition in which the visual axes of the eyes are not parallel and the eyes appear to be looking in different directions.

(9) Dizziness or vertigo (晕 *yūn*): Feeling faint, dizzy, weak, unsteady, and lightheaded. Dizziness that creates the false sense that you or your surroundings are spinning is called vertigo.

(10) Numbness and tingling (麻 *má*): Numbness refers to a diminished sensation in feeling. Tingling is the sensation of neither pain nor itching, but rather, feels like insects crawling inside a muscle. This sensation is not alleviated by pressure and can become worse with scratching. Numbness is often accompanied with other changes in sensation such as the feeling of pins-and-needles, burning, or tingling.

(11) Itching (癢 *yǎng*): An irritating skin sensation that causes a desire to scratch. May feel like insects crawling.

(12) Shaking and swinging (動 *dòng*): Involuntary or uncontrollable movements such as involuntary shaking or nodding of the head, arrhythmic twitches, shaking or swinging of the extremities, grinding of teeth, clenching the jaw, or protruding and licking the tongue.

(13) Syncope (厥脫 *jué tuō*): Sudden fainting or loss of consciousness, tongue stiffness, difficulty speaking, deviated mouth and eyes, or hemiplegia.

When any one or more of the above arise, it can be diagnosed as Liver wind.

17. Does the pattern Liver Qi Deficiency exist?

Does Liver qi deficiency exist? Traditional Chinese medicine physicians and scholars have been debating this issue for centuries. Why is there a theory that the pattern Liver qi deficiency does not exist? There are a couple of reasons.

Zhu Danxi (朱丹溪, 1281-1358), one of the four great physicians of the Jin-Yuan dynasty, believed that the "surplus of qi forms fire" (氣有餘, 便是火 *qì yǒu yú, biàn shí huǒ*) and that in the human body, "yang is often excessive and yin is often inadequate" (陽常有餘, 陰常不足 *yáng cháng yǒu yú, yīn cháng bù zú*). Based on this belief, TCM physicians and scholars later developed the theory that "Liver qi and Liver yang are often excessive, while Liver blood and Liver yin are often inadequate."

Basic Questions (素問 *sù wèn*), Chapter 24, states that "Jueyin is a channel that contains more blood and less qi" (多血少氣 *duō xuè shǎo qì*). The volume of qi and blood are different in each organ and channel because of the differences between excess and deficiency of yin and yang. Liver qi regulates other *zàng fǔ* organs while Liver blood nourishes them. Thus sufficiency of Liver blood is a precondition for Liver qi to perform its function. Ancient books mostly recorded Liver blood deficiency, but not Liver qi deficiency in terms of pathology. They attribute the symptoms of Liver qi deficiency to the pathology of other *zàng fǔ* organs such as the Spleen, and attribute the 'yang hyperactivity' (陽亢 *yáng kàng*) of other organs to the pathology of the Liver. For instance, hyperactivity or *kàng* is usually blamed only on the Liver, while deficiency is blamed on the Spleen. However, the Spleen can *kàng* or overact on the Liver.

Liver qi is the active function, while Liver blood is the material basis; qi belongs to yang and blood belongs to yin. "The Liver takes blood as its body and qi as its function." According to yin and yang theory, Liver qi and Liver blood coexist inside the Liver in unity and interdependence. Physiologically, they coordinate and cooperate; pathologically, they mutually restrain and influence. Thus when there is a deficiency of the Liver, not only will the Liver blood and yin be deficient, but also the Liver qi and yang.

The *Yellow Emperor's Inner Classic* (黃帝內經 *huáng dì nèi jīng*) is the first book to document Liver qi deficiency. *Divine Pivot* (靈樞 *líng shū*), Chapter 54, states: "At fifty years old, Liver qi declines, the Liver lobe starts to thin, bile secretion decreases, and the eyes lose sharpness." *Basic Questions* (素問 *sù wèn*), Chapter

80, states: "When Liver qi is deficient, one dreams of fragrant grasses and trees." Liver qi deficiency was also mentioned in the *Treasury Classic* (中藏經 *zhōng cáng jīng*) and in Zhang Zhongjing's *Treatise on Cold Damage and Miscellaneous Diseases* (傷寒雜病論 *shāng hán zǎ bìng lùn*). Meanwhile, in the book *Records of Heartfelt Experiences in Medicine with Reference to the West* (醫學衷中參西錄 *yī xué zhōng zhōng cān xī lù*), Zhang Xichun introduced his treatment method for Liver qi deficiency. Thus it should not be denied that Liver qi deficiency exists.

The Liver has many different physiological functions. It stores blood, controls tendons and sinews, opens into the eyes, manifests on the nails, performs coursing and discharging, and is in charge of ascending and moving. The Liver channel passes through a large area. Starting at the lateral side of the big toe, it courses up the medial leg, encircles the external genitals, ascends the lower abdomen, connects with internal organs, and then distributes in the costal and hyphochondriac region, terminating at the top of the head. Thus the Liver has various kinds of pathological changes and covers many different specialties in the clinic. For instance, in gynecological diseases, the Liver is involved in irregular menstrual cycles, abnormal menstrual bleeding, infertility, and miscarriage. In andrological diseases, it is involved in ejaculation disorders, including premature ejaculation, retrograde ejaculation, delayed ejaculation, anejaculation, spermatorrhea, nocturnal emissions, and erectile dysfunction. In pediatric diseases, it is involved in 'five types of developmental delay' (五遲 *wǔ chí*) and 'five types of flaccidity' (五軟 *wǔ ruǎn*), infantile convulsions, and groin hernias. In internal diseases, it covers many illnesses from head to toe.

Taiping Holy Prescriptions for Universal Relief (太平聖惠方 *tài píng shèng huì fāng*) states: "When Liver function is impaired with qi and blood insufficiency, cold harms the interior, leading to fullness and distention in the hypochondrium, spasms of the tendons and sinews, cold limbs, abdominal pain, blurry vision, a blue-green color of the hands and feet, and an inability to sigh, all of which indicate Liver qi deficiency."

There are three special characteristics of Liver qi deficiency:
(1) Liver qi deficiency can induce a series of pathological changes in the upper body such as cerebral hypoxia, cerebral ischemia, and cerebral embolism. It has been said that "Liver qi deficiency harms the upper" (肝氣虛病損於上 *gān qì bìng sǔn yú shàng*). The Liver regulates blood volume and governs coursing and discharging, therefore deficient Liver qi is too weak to ascend the gathering qi and blood to nourish the Heart and brain. The brain is known as the 'sea of marrow,' and when the marrow fails to be nourished, there will be dizziness, vertigo, fainting, unconsciousness, tremor, hemiplegia, deviated eyes and mouth, and limb stiffness, atrophy, or flaccidity.
(2) Liver qi deficiency can affect the middle part of the body such as the Heart, Lung, and Spleen, causing a series of pathological changes called 'Liver qi deficiency harms the middle' (肝氣虛病損於中 *gān qì bìng sǔn yú zhōng*). The Liver not only governs coursing and discharging, but also stores blood, regulates emotions, plays a vital role in assisting the Spleen to transform food essence, and coordinates with the Lung for qi movement. Thus when Liver qi deficiency fails to course and discharge, there will be emotional or psychiatric disorders, qi and blood circulation issues, and gastrointestinal disorders. There may be depression, mental fatigue, anxiety, panic attacks, dream-disturbed sleep, sleepwalking, palpitations, spontaneous sweating, shortness of breath that is worse with exertion, cough

with a low volume, difficult breathing, panting or asthma, abdominal fullness and distention, poor appetite, loose stools, tenesmus, or even rectal prolapse, gastroptosis, and uterine prolapse.

(3) Liver qi deficiency can affect the lower part of the body such as the Gallbladder, the *fǔ* organs, and the Kidney, causing a series of pathological changes called 'Liver qi deficiency harms the lower' (肝氣虛病損於下 *gān qì bìng sǔn yú xià*). The Liver cooperates and coordinates with the Gallbladder and Kidney to assist their respective bile excretion and essence storing functions. Long-term emotional stress, emotional shock, chronic illness, and aging can all lead to Liver qi deficiency, and may result in 'Liver and Gallbladder qi deficiency' or 'Liver and Kidney qi deficiency.' Signs and symptoms include shortness of breath, an aversion to talking, fatigue, lethargy, spontaneous sweating, mental fatigue, depression, sadness, frequent sighing, fearfulness, vexation, insomnia, dizziness, vertigo, amenorrhea or infertility in women, 'five types of developmental delay' or 'five types of flaccidity' in children, and ejaculation disorders or impotency in men. The pulse will be deep and weak, and there may be yin jaundice.

Regarding treatment for Liver qi deficiency, the *Classic of Difficulties* (難經 *nán jīng*), 14th Difficulty, states: "When the Liver is deficient, use sweet-tasting herbs to nourish and tonify." *Criterion of Syndrome and Treatment* (證治準繩 *zhèng zhì zhǔn shéng*, 1602) recorded the physician Gu Bao-Ren's formula Tonify the Liver Powder (補肝散 *bǔ gān sǎn*) as the classic formula for treating Liver qi or Liver blood deficiency. And then in the 19th century, the physician Zhang Xi-Chun recorded the use of Huang Qi as the chief herb along with qi-regulating herbs as the deputy herbs for treating Liver qi deficiency.

Based on the physiological characteristics of the Liver, there are four aspects to pay attention to when formulating herbs to treat Liver qi deficiency:

(1) The pathogenesis of this pattern is the insufficiency of Liver qi, which impairs the Liver's function of coursing and discharging. Thus the primary task is to tonify Liver qi. The herbs include Huang Qi, Shan Zhu Yu, Yang Gan (lamb liver), Bai Zhu, Shan Yao, Gou Qi Zi, Da Zao, and Gan Cao, among others. Huang Qi has the function of tonifying and lifting qi, so it will always be the first choice. Shan Zhu Yu is sour and warm, and enters the Liver and Kidney channels with the function of replenishing yin and tonifying qi. It tonifies qi without dryness and is a major herb for tonifying Liver qi. Lamb liver nourishes Liver blood and tonifies Liver qi. It also nourishes and brightens the eyes, and is thus the best choice for eye diseases caused by Liver deficiency.

(2) Since the Liver stores blood and blood nourishes qi, when tonifying the Liver qi there must also be herbs that nourish the Liver blood. However, the purpose of nourishing the Liver blood is not only to generate Liver qi, but also to prevent warm and dry herbs from further damaging Liver blood. Dang Gui, Shu Di Huang, and Suan Zao Ren are the common herbs to use. Zhang Zhongjing used Dang Gui combined with Gui Zhi and Dang Gui combined with Wu Zhu Yu to treat Liver yang qi deficiency.

(3) The pathological tendency of Liver qi is to become constrained or depressed. Thus when tonifying Liver qi, herbs that soothe the Liver and move qi should be added such as Chai Hu and Bo He. This helps to prevent Liver qi stagnation due to Liver deficiency, and assists the Liver in recovering quicker.

This method is called 'following its nature to treat' (顺其性而治 shùn qí xìng ér zhì).

(4) Liver qi and Liver yang are closely related, as chronic qi deficiency will lead to yang deficiency, which appears with cold limbs, intolerance of cold, and a desire for warmth. Thus some yang tonics such as lamb, Lu Rong, Wu Zhu Yu, and Ba Ji Tian should be added.

18. What is the clinical manifestation, etiology, and pathogenesis of Liver Qi Deficiency?

Definition: A group of signs and symptoms caused by a deficiency in Liver qi that leads to hypoactive Liver function.

Clinical manifestation: Depression, melancholy, blurry or double vision, a stifling and sinking sensation in the hypochondrium, timidity, shortness of breath, listlessness, physical and mental fatigue, weakness or numbness of the limbs, spontaneous sweating, aversion to talking, a weak voice, internal organ prolapse, pale blue-green or dim facial complexion, a pale tongue, and a deep, weak, and wiry pulse.

Key points: Depression, melancholy, a stifling and sinking sensation in the hypochondrium, a wiry pulse, plus qi deficiency signs and symptoms.

Etiology and pathogenesis: This is a rare pattern since the Liver takes blood as its body and qi as its function, so pathological changes in the Liver are mostly due to qi excess or yang excess. However, Liver qi and Liver yang deficiency may occur under certain circumstances such as congenital deficiency, prolonged illness, or long-term Liver dysfunction.

The Liver is located under the right side of the rib cage and its channel passes through both sides of the hypochondrium. When Liver qi is insufficient, it lacks in discharging, causing a stifling and sinking sensation in the hypochondrium that is neither fullness, tightness, pulling, nor distention pain. It is also different from burning pain or a rushing sensation. This is the key point in distinguishing this pattern from other Liver patterns.

The Liver stores blood, anchors the ethereal soul (魂 hún), governs coursing and discharging, and regulates emotional activities. In Liver qi deficiency, the ethereal soul fails to anchor, affecting the Gallbladder's ability to make clear judgments and decisions, resulting in depression, melancholy, and timidity. This differs from patterns of Liver excess where the emotional aspect involves irritability and short temper.

The eyes are the orifices of the Liver: "When the Liver qi is harmonized, one can distinguish the five colors." Thus, in Liver qi deficiency, the eyes will lose nourishment, leading to diminished, blurry, cloudy, or distorted vision. The Liver also controls the tendons and sinews; therefore, in Liver qi deficiency, there is numbness and weakness of the limbs. Since tendons and sinews also include the connective tissues that hold organs in position, Liver qi deficiency can also involve internal organ prolapse. This is why in the clinic, Liver herbs such Chai Hu and Zhi Ke are used to treat organ prolapse. "The Liver is the origin of fatigue" (罷極之本 bà jí zhī běn): when the Liver qi is deficient, there will be extreme exhaustion and fatigue, which can appear with spontaneous sweating, aversion to talking, a low voice, a pale tongue, and a weak pulse.

294 Part 4 : Questions and Answers for Deeper Insight

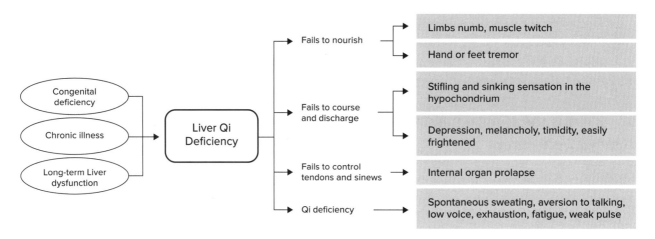

Chart 24.18.1 Etiology and pathogenesis of Liver Qi Deficiency

TCM Disease	Western Disease	Herbal Formulas		Acupuncture
Fatigue (虚劳)	Adrenal fatigue, CFS, Lyme disease, EBV, hypothyroidism, chronic hepatitis, anemia	Bu Gan Tang plus Huang Qi	Si Jun Zi Tang, Bu Gan Tang	CV-4, CV-6
Prolapse (下垂)	Anal prolapse, gastroptosis, uterine prolapse	Bu Zhong Yi Qi Tang, Sheng Xian Tang		GV-20, Ti Tuo
Numbness (麻木)	Peripheral neuropathy, diabetes, MS, Lyme disease, amyloidosis, Sjoren's syndrome, stroke	Bu Gan Tang		GB-34, GV-9, GV-14, Li-11, BL-14, BL-16, BL-60
Blurry vision (视物不清)	Night blindness, presbyopia, diabetes, glaucoma, cataract	Qi Ju Di Huang Wan		BL-1, BL-2, SP-10, ST-1
Irregular menses (月经不调)	Perimenopause, PCOS, anorexia, malnutrition, or caused by stress, D&C, miscarriage	Xiao Yao San		CV-4, CV-6, SP-10
Amenorrhea (闭经)	Anorexia, malnutrition, PCOS, hypothyroidism, bullimia	Ba Zhen Tang		

Acupuncture column also includes: LR-3, LR-8, SP-6, KI-3, BL-17, BL-18, BL-20, BL-23, ST-36

Table 24.18.1 Diseases and treatments related to Liver Qi Deficiency

19. Does the pattern Liver Yang Deficiency exist?

The Liver is an unyielding organ (剛臟 *gāng zàng*), staunch and restless; it "takes blood as its body and qi as its function" (體陰用陽 *tǐ yīn yòng yáng*); its nature is to grow and expand; it favors being softened and soothed, and disfavors oppression and constraint; and it holds the ministerial fire. These physiological characteristics of the Liver indicate that its pathological changes tend to be heat, yang excess, or blood deficiency, while deficiency cold is rare. In the 14th century, the physician Zhu Danxi proposed the theory "surplus of qi forms fire" (氣有余，便是火 *qì yǒu yú biàn shì huǒ*) and "yang is often excessive, yin is often inadequate" (陽常有余，陰常不足 *yáng cháng yǒu yú yīn cháng bù zú*). Under the influence of his theory, most physicians believed that "to treat the Liver, use a draining method only, not tonification" (肝有瀉無補 *gān yǒu xiè wú bǔ*). They emphasized the tendency of Liver yang to be hyperactive and rebellious, and the tendency of Liver blood and yin to be deficient. Furthermore, TCM medical literature rarely discussed Liver yang deficiency because its clinical manifestations are very complex, making it difficult to form a uniform diagnostic criteria.

Liver yang deficiency was documented in many classic texts such as in Zhang Zhongjing's *Treatise on Cold Damage Diseases* (傷寒論 *shāng hán lùn*), which discussed symptoms and treatments for Liver blood deficiency with Liver yang deficiency giving rise to deficiency cold that results in failure to warm the Jue Yin channel. This leads to cold limbs, groin hernia with abdominal cold pain, irregular menstruation, or abnormal menstrual bleeding. The recommended herbal formula is Tangkuei Ginger Lamb Soup (當歸生姜羊肉湯 *dāng guī shēng jiāng yáng ròu tāng*) or Sichuan Lovage Root, Tangkuei, Ass-Hide Gelatin, and Mugwort Decoction (芎歸膠艾湯 *xiōng guī jiāo ài tāng*). The major components of the formula function to nourish blood and warm the Liver yang.

Hua Tuo, in his book *Treasury Classic* (中藏經 *zhōng cáng jīng*), states: "When there is Liver deficiency cold, there is hypochondriac pain, blurry or double vision, arm pain, chills like in malaria, no desire for food, amenorrhea for women, shortness of breath, and a deep and weak pulse on the left middle position."

Sun Simiao was the first physician to mention the name of Liver deficiency cold in his book, *Important Formulas Worth a Thousand Gold Pieces* (千金要方 *qiān jīn yào fāng*), which states: "A deficient and deep pulse on the left middle position indicates foot Jue Yin Liver channel. When there is hypochondriac pain and distention, chills or fever, abdominal bloating and distention, no desire for food, melancholy, irregular menstruation for women with low back or abdominal pain, then this is Liver deficiency cold." He also formulated the Tonify Liver Decoction (補肝汤 *bǔ gān tāng*), Tonify Liver Powder (補肝散 *bǔ gān sǎn*), and Tonify Liver Liquor (補肝酒 *bǔ gān jiǔ*) for Liver yang deficiency.

Re-editing Yan's Formulary for Succoring the Sick (重輯嚴氏濟生方) includes a detailed description of Liver yang deficiency in which the physician Yan He says: "The Liver is Foot Jue Yin channel... [yang] deficiency will give rise to cold, resulting in hypochondriac pain and distention, alternating cold and fever, abdominal bloating, no desire for food, melancholy, timidity, paranoia, blurry or double vision, bitter taste in the mouth, headache, stiff joints, limb spasms or tremors, dry and brittle nails, a deep, thin, and slippery pulse. All are signs and symptoms of [Liver] deficiency cold." Furthermore, *Taiping Holy Prescriptions for Universal Relief* (太平聖惠方 *tài píng shèng huì fāng*) collects all the formulas prior to the Song dynasty for treating Liver yang deficiency.

The Liver 'takes blood as its body and qi as its function' (體陰用陽 *tǐ yīn yòng yáng*); therefore, the pathogenesis of Liver yang deficiency is different from that of other organs. Not only does Liver yang deficiency cause a failure to warm, but it is also paired with Liver blood deficiency, which fails to nourish, manifesting with symptoms such as blurry or double vision and dry brittle nails. The clinical manifestations of Liver yang deficiency are complex, but can be generalized into two groups:

(1) Liver organ signs and symptoms: These are the root signs and symptoms that usually appear in all manifestations of Liver yang deficiency. They include depression, melancholy, blurry or double vision, a stifling and sinking sensation in the hypochondrium, timidity, shortness of breath, listlessness, physical and mental fatigue, and cold limbs. The tongue is pale with a white coating, and the pulse is deep, feeble, and slow.

(2) Liver channel signs and symptoms: These appear on the Liver channel but can vary greatly, and the clinical manifestations are extremely complex and individualized. They include the following signs and symptoms.
   a. Headache that is dull and vague, felt on the top of the head. The headache has a sudden onset and is induced or worsened by exertion or cold, and may be accompanied with spitting of clear fluids.
   b. Deficiency cold in the Penetrating and Conception vessels exhibits cold pain in the lower abdomen with a preference for warmth and pressure. There is also scanty and pale menstrual bleeding or amenorrhea, infertility, and low libido.
   c. Liver channel deficiency cold: a sense of sinking and distention or cold pain in the lower abdomen; swelling, hardness, or pain in the testicles; tenderness, coldness, or clammy coldness in the scrotum; or impotency.
   d. Atrophy or weakness of tendons and sinews, joint stiffness, difficulty balancing or walking, difficulty holding or lifting, cold limbs, intolerance of cold, and backache or weakness with a cold sensation.
   e. Painful obstruction, chronic cold pain in the joints that are neither red nor swollen and become worse with cold and relieved by warmth; and weak limbs.

Warming and tonifying the Liver yang is the basic treatment principle for Liver yang deficiency. However, since the Liver 'takes blood as its body, and yang as its function,' its treatment strategies are different than those of other organs, requiring not only warming and tonifying Liver yang, but also nourishing Liver blood. Physician Qin Bo-Mo notes: "Using warming herbs combined with blood-nourishing herbs helps to replenish and regenerate, while using warming and hot herbs alone should be avoided" when treating Liver yang deficiency. The chief herb should be acrid, warm, and moist, to prevent impairing yin and blood. "It should also enter the Liver channel and into the blood to enable the regeneration of qi," according to Qin Bo-Mo's *Medical Collected Works* (秦伯末醫文集 *qín bó mò yī wén jí*, 1983). The common Liver yang tonics include Sheng Jiang, Xi Xin, Wu Zhu Yu, Yin Yang Huo, Ai Ye, Ba Ji Tian, Chuan Jiao, and Mu Gua.

Thus based on the clinical experiences of ancient physicians, the treatment principle for Liver yang deficiency is to nourish blood, regulate channels, and warm and tonify Liver yang. The basic herbal formula for this is the Warm the Liver Decoction (暖肝煎 *nuǎn gān jiān*). Clinical manifestations of Liver yang deficiency pattern vary due to different individual constitutions, and thus the herbal formula should be modified based on the chief complaints.

20. What is the clinical manifestation, etiology, and pathogenesis of Liver Yang Deficiency?

Definition: A group of signs and sympoms caused by Liver yang decline, resulting in Liver function hypoactivity.

Clinical manifestation: Depression, melancholy, blurry or double vision, a stifling and sinking sensation in the hypochondrium, timidity, shortness of breath, listlessness, physical and mental fatigue, tenseness or withering of the sinews, weakness of the hands and feet or an inability to make a fist or stretch the feet, a green-purple facial complexion, fear of cold, cold limbs, cold sensation in the genital area, low libido, impotence, testicular atrophy, or lower abdominal cold pain in women with irregular menstrual bleeding, or infertility. The tongue is pale with a white coating, and the pulse is deep, weak, and slow.

Key points: Depression, melancholy, a stifling and sinking sensation in the hypochondrium, blurry or double vision, symptoms involving the lack of nourishment to the tendons, plus yang deficiency signs and symptoms.

Etiology and pathogenesis: This is a rare pattern that can develop from Liver qi deficiency. Long-term suffering of emotional stress or panic and living in adverse environments all can lead to a decline of Liver yang qi. Pathogenic cold can also directly attack the Liver and, when untreated, can consume yang qi.

This pattern is substantially similar to Liver qi deficiency with the addition of cold symptoms, which are caused by yang deficiency failing to warm. The Liver channel starts at the inside of the big toe, courses up the inner leg, encircles the external genitals and bilateral lower abdomen, then distributes in the costal region and terminates at the top of the head. Liver yang deficiency fails to warm the Liver channel and cold causes constriction and spasming, resulting in a sense of sinking and distention or cold pain in the lower abdomen; swelling, hardness, or pain in the testicles; tenderness, cold, or clammy cold in the scrotum; or impotency. Liver yang deficiency fails to lift and ascend to the head, resulting in vertex headache, a cold sensation, and spitting of clear fluids. When Liver yang deficiency fails to control the tendons and sinews, there

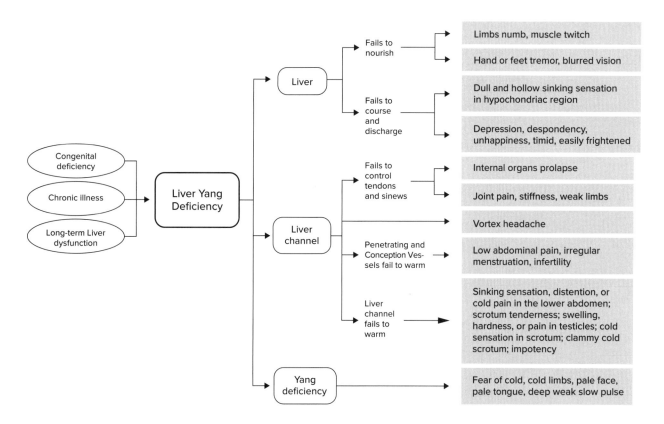

Chart 24.20.1 Etiology and pathogenesis of Liver Yang Deficiency

will be joint stiffness, weak limbs, and difficulty walking. Since the Penetrating vessel is the sea of blood, and the Liver stores blood, when Liver yang deficiency fails to promote, blood is unable to fill the Penetrating and Conception vessels, resulting in irregular menstruation or infertility.

TCM Disease	Western Disease	Herbal Formulas		Acupuncture	
Constraint (郁証)	Depression, anxiety, menopause syndrome, neurosis, hysteria, PMS	Gui Gan Long Mu Tang, plus Ying Yang Huo, Ba Ji Tian	Nuan Gan Jian	LR-3, LR-13, LR-14, LI-4, GB-34, TB-6, PC-6, GV-20	BL-18, BL-24, CV-4, CV-6, ST-36
Fatigue (虛勞)	Adrenal fatigue, hypothyroidism, CFS, Lyme disease, EBV	Ba Zhen Tang, plus Huang Qi		Moxa	
Impotence (陽痿)	Sexual neurosis, hormonal imbalance	You Gui Wan		SP-6, CV-2, BL-28, CV-4	
Infertility (不孕)	PCOS, hypothyroidism, LPD, POF	Wen Jing Tang		SP-6, KI-10	
Frigid extremities ()	Anemia, diabetic hypoglycemia, Raynaud's disease, scleroderma	Dang Gui Si Ni, plus Wu Zhu Yu Sheng Jiang Tang		LR-3, LI-4	
Headache (頭痛)	Hypertension, migraine or cluster headache, glaucoma, sinusitis, tension headache	Wu Zhu Yu Tang		GV-20, LI-4	
Hypochondriac pain (脇痛)	Hypochondriasis, costochondritis, pleurisy, arthritis, osteoporosis, intercostal neuralgia	Da Jian Zhong Tang		TB-5, GB-34, GB-40, LR-3, BL-19	
Irregular menstruation (月經失調)	Perimenopause, PCOS, anorexia, malnutrition, or caused by stress, D&C, hypothyroidism, bullimia	Wen Jing Tang, Xiong Jiao Ai Tang		SP-6, SP-10, CV-3	

Table 24.20.1 Diseases and treatments related to Liver Yang Deficiency

21. Why is Liver Qi Deficiency blamed on the Spleen? And how to distinguish Liver Qi Deficiency from Spleen Qi Deficiency?

Even though the term Liver qi deficiency was recorded early on in the *Yellow Emperor's Inner Classic* (黃帝內經 *huáng dì nèi jīng*), it never received much attention from ancient physicians. There are three main reasons for this:

(1) Liver qi deficiency is a very rare pattern because the Liver is considered an unyielding organ (剛臟 *gāng zàng*) — staunch and restless. It 'takes blood as its body and qi as its function' (體陰用陽 *tǐ yīn yòng yáng*). Moreover, Liver 'yang is often excessive, and yin is often inadequate' (陽常有餘，陰常不足 *yáng cháng yǒu yú, yīn cháng bù zú*); therefore, the Liver is more likely to be excessive than deficient.

(2) There are no records to be found in classic texts regarding diagnosis criteria, treatment principles, and herbal formulas for Liver qi deficiency.

(3) Pathologically, Liver qi deficiency will affect the Spleen, leading to Spleen qi deficiency, and therefore the clinical manifestation of Liver qi deficiency will be similar to Spleen qi deficiency. However, this means that the symptoms of Liver qi deficiency imposed on the Spleen are commonly seen in the clinic.

The Liver is in the hypochondrium, while the Spleen is in the abdomen. They are both located in the middle burner and have a close physiological relationship. The Liver governs coursing and discharging, while the Spleen controls transportation and transformation; they coordinate and cooperate to complete water and food metabolism. The Liver governs ascending, while the Spleen also performs lifting; both function to lift and hold organs in their position. The Liver governs the tendons and sinews, "it is the root of fatigue" (罷極之本 *bà jí zhī běn*), while the Spleen governs the limbs and is rooted in yang. Together, they are in charge of the movements of the extremities. However, these functions have traditionally been attributed only to the Spleen, ignoring the role of the Liver. Due to this one-sided understanding, the pattern of Liver qi deficiency has been neglected. In terms of atrophy or *wěi* syndrome (痿證 *wěi zhèng*), it has always been blamed on the Spleen, but actually any type of *wěi* syndrome, mild or extreme, involves both.

Congenital deficiency, prolonged illness, or long-term Liver dysfunction can all cause Liver qi deficiency. The clinical manifestation for Liver qi deficiency includes: depression, melancholy, blurry vision, a stifling and sinking sensation in the hypochondrium, timidity, shortness of breath, listlessness, physical and mental fatigue, weakness or numbness of the limbs, spontaneous sweating, aversion to talking, weak voice, internal organ prolapse, pale bluish-green or dim facial complexion, a pale tongue, and a deep, weak, and wiry pulse.

The Spleen governs transportation and transformation, and controls the muscles of the limbs. Thus symptoms such as poor appetite, bloating, fatigue, lassitude, weakness and atrophy of the limbs are mostly diagnosed as Spleen qi deficiency and treated by tonifying and strengthening the Spleen. However, the Liver is in charge of coursing and discharging, regulating the Spleen's ascending and the Stomach's descending digestive functions. *Basic Questions* (素問 *sù wèn*), Chapter 25, states that the "Earth receives Wood's help to achieve its function." When the Liver qi is deficient, it fails to assist the Spleen, leading to poor appetite and bloating, while also failing to nourish the tendons and sinews, resulting in lassitude, weakness, or atrophy of the limbs.

The key points to distinguish these two patterns are as follows:

(1) Key symptoms:
- Liver qi deficiency: Stifling or sinking sensation in the hypochondrium that is neither fullness, tightness, pulling, nor distention pain; nor is it burning pain or a rushing sensation. Depression, melancholy, timidity, blurry vision, and weakness and numbness of the limbs.

- Spleen qi deficiency: Poor appetite, bloating, and loose stools, edema, leukorrhea, obesity, weak muscles and emaciation, and sallow facial complexion.

(2) Liver qi deficiency symptoms are rare and usually appear in those with weak constitutions or in the later stage of an illness, while Spleen qi deficiency is mild and is commonly seen in the clinic.

Pattern		Liver Qi Deficiency	Spleen Qi Deficiency
Etiology		Congenital weakness, chronic illness	
		Long-term Liver dysfunction	Improper diet, physical or emotional overstrain, aging, improper care
Pathogenesis		Diminished coursing and discharging leads to qi stagnation, which fails to assist the Spleen	Spleen's failure to transport and transform leads to qi deficiency and dampness accumulation
Characteristics		Rare, severe, later stage of illness	Mild, can appear at any stage of illness, commonly seen in the clinic
Symptoms	Common	Shortness of breath, listlessness, lassitude, physical and mental fatigue, spontaneous sweating, weak or atrophied limbs, aversion to talking, weak voice, internal organ prolapse, pale or dim facial complexion, a pale tongue, and a deep weak pulse	
	Different	Depression, melancholy, timidity, blurry or double vision, stifling and sinking sensation in the hypochondrium, limb weakness or numbness, pale bluish-green facial complexion	Poor appetite, bloating, loose stools, obesity, edema, vaginal discharge, weak muscles and emaciation, pale or sallow facial complexion
Tongue & pulse		Pale tongue and a deep weak pulse	
		Pale-bluish tongue and a wiry pulse	Teeth marks on tongue and a soft pulse
Treatment strategy		Tonify and nourish the Liver, soothe and replenish the Liver qi	Tonify and strengthen the Spleen
Herbal formulas		Sheng Xian Tang, Bu Gan San, plus Huang Qi, Shan Zhu Yu	Si Jun Zi Tang, Bu Zhong Yi Qi Tang, Shen Ling Bai Zhu San

Table 24.21.1 Comparison of Liver Qi Deficiency and Spleen Qi Deficiency

Tonifying the qi is the major treatment method for both Liver qi deficiency and Spleen qi deficiency. The herbs of choice would be Huang Qi, Bai Zhu, Ren Shen, Dang Shen, Da Zao, and Gan Cao. Huang Qi tonifies and lifts qi, which is suitable for Liver qi deficiency, while Bai Zhu tonifies qi and dries dampness, which is more suitable for Spleen qi deficiency. Since there are differences in physiological and pathological characteristics between the Liver and Spleen, the selection of chief herbs will also be different. The Liver favors being softened and soothed and disfavors oppression; thus, when tonifying the Liver qi, formulas should be combined with yin and blood tonics, as well as qi-regulating herbs that release constraints. Meanwhile, the Spleen favors dryness and disfavors dampness; therefore, when tonifying the Spleen, formulas should incorporate herbs that dry dampness.

22. What are the similarities and differences between the patterns Liver Qi Stagnation, Liver Fire Blazing, and Liver Yang Rising?

The relationship among these three patterns is that of reciprocal causation. For instance, Liver qi stagnation can develop into Liver fire blazing if qi stagnation transforms into fire. Liver fire blazing can develop into Liver yang rising if heat consumes the yin, which then fails to constrain the yang. Liver fire can also develop into Liver qi stagnation if heat impairs the yin, which fails to nourish the Liver, resulting in coursing and discharging dysfunction that leads to qi stagnation. Thus these three patterns can transform into each other, combine, or co-exist such as Liver qi stagnation with heat, Liver yang rising with heat, or all three patterns may appear simultaneously. Thus, these patterns must be identified carefully.

Constraint (郁 *yù*) is the major clinical symptom of Liver qi stagnation, which manifests as depression, melancholy, an unpleasant fullness in the chest and hypochondrium, breast distention, frequent sighing, and poor appetite. There are no obvious signs of heat or cold, but emotional stress is clearly involved. The Liver qi fails to discharge and course, leading to constraint within. This pattern is considered to be one of internal excess manifesting as external deficiency, or true excess with false deficiency, where internal excess presents as an unpleasant fullness in the chest and hypochondrium, while external deficiency presents as dizziness, irregular menstrual cycle, and melancholy that improves with exercise. The treatment principle for this pattern should be to soothe the Liver and release constraint.

Fire (火 *huǒ*) is the main symptom in the pattern of Liver fire blazing, which presents with fever, thirst, desire for cold drinks, red face and eyes, bitter taste in the mouth, burning pain in the chest and hypochondrium, irritability, short temper, constipation, yellow urine, a red tongue, and a rapid pulse. It is an excess heat condition without clear signs of yin deficiency. Fire flaring upward disturbs the head, causing headaches, irritability, and a red face. This pattern usually has an acute onset with severe symptoms, but is short course. The treatment strategy for this pattern is to clear and drain fire.

In Liver yang rising, which is essentially Liver excess with Kidney deficiency, the major symptoms show excess above (上亢 *shàng kàng*) and deficiency below. The Liver 'takes blood (yin) as its body and qi (yang) as its function' (體陰用陽 *tǐ yīn yòng yáng*). When there is excessive yang, or insufficient yin or blood to restrain the yang, the Liver yang can become hyperactive. When the upbearing of Liver yang is excessive, qi and blood surge upward, disrupting the clear orifices (清窍 *qīng qiào*). Symptoms of excess above include dizziness, vertigo, tinnitus, distending headache, distention pain around the eyes, a flushed face, a 'top-heavy' sensation, irritability, short temper, and a wiry forceful pulse. Symptoms of deficiency below include weakness and aching in the lower extremities and the lower back. This pattern is usually chronic with milder symptoms and a longer course. Not clearly present in this pattern are heat signs and symptoms such as thirst, desire for cold water, fever, yellow urine, and a red tongue. The treatment method for this pattern is to calm the Liver and subdue the yang.

Pattern		Liver Qi Stagnation	Liver Fire Blazing	Liver Yang Rising
Relationship		Reciprocal causation: develop and transform into each other, combine and co-exist		
Characteristic		Gradual onset, long course	Acute onset, short course	Gradual or sub-acute onset, long course
Eight principles		True excess, false deficiency	Excess, heat	Excess above, deficiency below, heat
Emotion		Depression, melancholy	Irritability, short temper, agitation, anxiety	
Symptoms	Common	Distress in the chest and hypochondrium		
Symptoms	Different	An unpleasant fullness in the chest and hypochondrium, poor appetite, breast distention, irregular menstrual cycle	Dizziness, tinnitus, distending pain in the head and eyes, red face and eyes	
Symptoms	Different		Thirst, bitter taste in the mouth, yellow urine, burning pain in the hypochondrium, constipation	Top-heavy feeling, tendency to fall, weakness in the lower back and knees
Tongue		Dusky	Red with yellow coating	Red with thin yellow coating or dry coating
Pulse		Wiry	Wiry, rapid, forceful	Wiry, thin
Treatment strategy		Soothe the Liver, release constraint	Clear Liver heat	Calm the Liver, subdue the yang
Herbal formulas		Xiao Yao San, Si Ni San, Su Gan San	Zuo Jin Wan, Chai Hu Qing Gan Tang	Tian Ma Gou Teng Yin

Table 24.22.1 Comparison of Liver Qi Stagnation, Liver Fire Blazing, and Liver Yang Rising

23. What are the similarities and differences between the patterns Liver and Gallbladder Damp-Heat and Damp-Heat Encumbering the Spleen?

Both patterns can be caused by exopathogenic damp-heat invasion or improper diet such as the overconsumption of greasy, sweet, or spicy foods, dairy, and alcohol. Thus both present with damp-heat signs and symptoms such as nausea, poor appetite, thirst with no desire to drink, distress and discomfort in the chest and epigastrium, heaviness, fever, thick yellow vaginal discharge, yang-type jaundice with bright yellow skin, yellow urine, loose and sticky stools, a yellow greasy tongue coating, and a rapid slippery pulse.

However, the location and pathogenesis of these two patterns are different, and consequently the clinical manifestations are different. The pattern Liver and Gallbladder damp-heat involves more heat than dampness, and is characterized by the accumulation of damp-heat that steams the Liver and Gallbladder, causing a bitter taste in the mouth, bright yellow eyes or skin, and distention pain in the hypochondrium. When damp-heat obstructs the Liver and Gallbladder channels, it can result in vaginal discharge or itching and scrotal itching or swelling. If damp-heat follows the channel, attacking upward, it can cause red swollen eyes or ear pain with yellow discharge. Since the Gallbladder channel runs along the side of the body, located between the exterior and interior of the body, when exopathogenic damp-heat invades, antipathogenic qi (正氣 zhèng qì) and pathogenic qi (邪氣 xié qì) will lock up and lead to alternating chills and fever.

In contrast, the pattern damp-heat encumbering the Spleen involves more dampness than heat, and is characterized by damp-heat stagnation that causes the Spleen's failure to properly transport and transform, leading to fullness, distention, bloating, poor appetite, nausea, vomiting, and diarrhea with sticky loose stools. Since this pattern involves more dampness than heat, the accumulation of dampness traps heat inside, resulting in unsurfaced fever that does not decline after sweating.

The key points to distinguish these two patterns are as follows:
(1) Pathological location: Liver and Gallbladder vs. Spleen and Stomach
(2) Fever: alternating chills and fever vs. unsurfaced fever
(3) Pulse: wiry pulse vs. soft pulse

Pattern		Liver and Gallbladder Damp-Heat	Damp-Heat Encumbering the Spleen
Etiology		Exopathogenic damp-heat directly invades the organ (Liver, Gallbladder, or Spleen), improper diet, overconsumption of sweet, greasy, spicy food, dairy, and alcohol	
		Damp-heat transfers from Spleen and Stomach	
Pathogenesis		Damp-heat leads to Liver and Gallbladder dysfunction, or damp-heat becomes obstructed in their channels	Damp-heat accumulation in the Spleen, disrupts Spleen and Stomach function
Location		Liver and Gallbladder organs and channels	Spleen and Stomach
Symptoms	Common	Nausea, poor appetite, thirst with no desire to drink, heavy sensation, yellow urine, loose and sticky stools, jaundice with bright yellow skin	
	Different	Fullness and pain in the hypochondria, bitter taste, jaundice, vaginal discharge or itching, scrotal itching or swelling, red and swollen eyes	Epigastric and abdominal distress and discomfort, loose stools with foul odor, no appetite
	Fever	Alternating chills and fever	Unsurfaced fever
Tongue		Red with yellow greasy coating	
Pulse		Slippery, rapid, wiry	Slippery, rapid, or soggy
Treatment strategy		Drain excess fire from the Liver and Gallbladder, clear and drain damp-heat from the lower burner	Clear heat, transform damp, regulate qi, harmonize the Spleen and Stomach
Herbal formulas		Yin Chen Hao Tang, Long Dan Xie Gan Tang	Yin Chen Wu Ling San, Huo Xiang Zheng Qi San

Table 24.23.1 Comparison of Liver and Gallbladder Damp-Heat and Damp-Heat Encumbering the Spleen

24. Why is Liver Yang Deficiency commonly blamed on the Kidney? How is Liver Yang Deficiency distinguished from Kidney Yang Deficiency?

Liver is an unyielding organ (剛臟 *gāng zàng*), staunch and restless; 'it takes blood as its body and qi as its function' (體陰用陽 *tǐ yīn yòng yáng*). Over hundreds of years, ancient physicians, influenced by the theory that Liver 'yang is often excessive, and yin is often inadequate' (陽常有餘，陰常不足 *yáng cháng yǒu yú yīn cháng bù zú*), have ignored the existence of Liver yang deficiency. And thus there are very few records in classic texts regarding diagnosis criteria, treatment principles, and herbal formulas for Liver yang deficiency.

Physiologically, the Liver and Kidney have a mutually generating and controlling relationship, and hence it is said that the 'Liver and Kidney are homologous (肝腎同源 *gān shèn tóng yuán*)'. They store essence and blood, coordinate conducting and storage, and control yin and yang. Pathologically, they also affect each other and both belong to the lower burner. These two patterns share many signs and symptoms such as listlessness, physical and mental fatigue, pale complexion, aversion to cold, cold limbs, or sexual dysfunction in men, or lower abdominal cold pain with menstruation disorder or infertility in women, a pale tongue with white coating, and a deep, feeble, and slow pulse. Thus it is very easy to misdiagnose these two patterns. Furthermore, since Liver yang deficiency is considered rare and often neglected, its symptoms are commonly blamed on Kidney yang deficiency instead.

Even though Liver yang deficiency and Kidney yang deficiency share many similar signs and symptoms, they are indeed different. Pathological changes for Kidney yang deficiency are located in the Kidney, which is the 'powerful official' (作強之官 *zuò qiáng zhī guān*) in charge of the body's strength and intelligence. It stores essence, governs the bones, generates marrow, opens to the ears, and is internally-externally connected with the Urinary Bladder. The lumbar area is known as the 'residence of the Kidney.' Signs and symptoms of Kidney yang deficiency include premature ejaculation, weakness or aching in the lumbar, groin, or knees, tinnitus, hearing loss, copious clear and frequent urination, frequent nighttime urination, or difficult urination, and a weak pulse on the proximal position.

Pathological changes for Liver yang deficiency are to be found in the Liver. The Liver is the 'general in charge of strategies' (將軍之官 *jiāng jūn zhī guān*). It stores blood, governs tendons and sinews, opens to the eyes, is internally-externally connected with the Gallbladder, and its channel passes through the costal area. Signs and symptoms of Liver yang deficiency include blurry or double vision, floaters or dark spots in front of the eyes, a stifling and sinking sensation in the hypochondrium, head or body numbness, spasms or stiffness in the extremities due to tendon or sinew constriction caused by cold, and a deep wiry and weak pulse in the left middle position.

Cold extremities, erectile dysfunction and impotence, and abdominal cold pain can all appear in both patterns; however, the clinical manifestations are not exactly same.

(1) For cold extremities: Kidney yang deficiency presents with a cold sensation that extends above the elbow or knee and is difficult to warm up. There may also be fatigue and lassitude combined with a pale white complexion, facial edema or puffiness, weakness or aching in the lumbar, groin, or knees, and stupor and daze. Liver yang deficiency presents with cold extremities that are felt more on the fingers or toes, no facial puffiness, and a pale bluish-green complexion. There may also be timidity, depression, and unhappiness.

(2) For erectile dysfunction and impotence: Kidney yang deficiency fails to warm and store essence, and fails to control the anterior and posterior yin orifices. Thus signs and symptoms usually begin with a failure to maintain an erection, later developing into spermatorrhea or premature ejaculation, and

then impotence. For Liver yang deficiency, the Liver fails to course and discharge and fails to nourish the tendons and sinews. Deficiency cold obstructs the Liver channel, resulting in incomplete erection or difficult ejaculation, a cold and clammy scrotum, and impotence. Thus Liver yang deficiency does not have leakage symptoms such as premature ejaculation, which is caused by Kidney qi failing to secure.

(3) For abdominal cold pain: Kidney yang deficiency fails to warm and transform, resulting in water and dampness accumulation that obstructs qi movement. This leads to abdominal cold pain without affecting appetite. In contrast, Liver yang deficiency fails to course and discharge, which overacts on the Spleen. This results in abdominal cold pain with bloating and poor appetite.

	Pattern		Liver Yang Deficiency	Kidney Yang Deficiency
Etiology			Congenital weakness, chronic illness	
			Develops from Liver qi deficiency	Aging, physical or sexual overstrain, improper diet or treatment
Pathogenesis			Liver lacks coursing and discharging due to yang and blood insufficiency	Kidney yang fails to warm and promote
Characteristics			Rare or ignored, develops from Liver qi deficiency	Appears in any stage of illness, commonly seen in the clinic
Symptoms	Common		Listlessness, physical and mental fatigue, pale complexion, fear of cold, cold limbs, erectile dysfunction or impotence in men, lower abdominal cold pain with abnormal menstruation in women	
	Different	Cold limbs	Cold extremities, which is more on finger and toes	Cold sensation extending above elbow or knee, and difficulty warming up
		ED or impotence	Starts with incomplete erection or difficult ejaculation, cold wet sensation in scrotum, then impotency	Starts with failure to maintain erection, later develops into spermatorrhea or premature ejaculation, then impotence
		Abdominal pain	Abdominal cold pain, bloating, poor appetite	Abdominal cold pain
		Others	Depression, despondency, unhappiness, timidity, blurry or double vision, hollow and falling downward sensation in the hypochondria, weakness or numbness of limbs, pale greenish facial complexion	Pale whitish facial complexion, facial edema or puffiness, weakness or aching in the lumbar or knees, tinnitus, impaired hearing, clear copious and frequent urination, frequent nighttime urination, difficult or dripping urination
Tongue & pulse			Pale tongue with a white coating; a deep, weak, and slow pulse	
			Pale bluish tongue, wiry pulse	Thick tongue coating
Treatment strategy			Tonify and warm Liver yang, nourish the Liver blood	Tonify and warm Kidney yang
Herbal formulas			Nuan Gan Jian, You Gui Wan	You Gui Wan, Jin Gui Shen Qi Wan

Table 24.24.1 Comparison of Liver Yang Deficiency and Kidney Yang Deficiency

25. What are the different types of fever and their associated pathogenesis and *zàng fǔ* patterns?

Fever can manifest as an abnormally high body temperature or as a subjective sensation of heat or warmth in the body. Fever is a result of antipathogenic qi resisting pathogens, and is essentially an excess state of yang arising from either exposure to pathogenic factors or a *zàng fǔ* organ disorder.

Pathogenic factors such as heat, cold, dryness, or damp-heat can enter from the exterior; or they can arise from a *zàng fǔ* organ disorder such as blood stasis, phlegm, or food stagnation. Generally speaking, pathogenic factors from the exterior lead to acute high fevers, while pathogenic factors associated with internal disorders cause chronic low-grade fevers. *Zàng fǔ* organ disorders can cause a deficiency of yin, blood, or qi, any of which can cause a relative excess of yang, giving rise to either a chronic low-grade fever or feverish sensations.

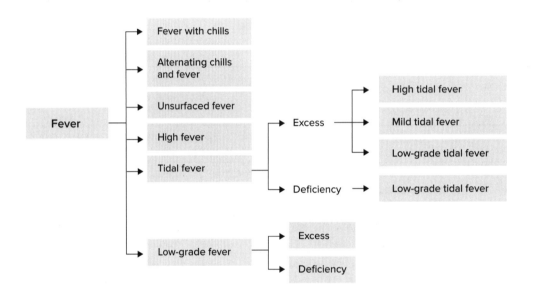

Chart 24.25.1 Fever types

Fever with chills or simultaneous chills and fever (惡寒發熱 *wù hán fā rè*): A sensation of chills while body temperature has increased above a normal level. It is seen in the initial stage of an exterior pattern caused by exogenous pathogens. It reflects the struggle between protective qi (衛氣 *wèi qì*) and pathogenic qi (邪氣 *xié qì*). Fever with chills as the main symptom usually appears in the following patterns: wind-cold invading the Lung, wind-heat invading the Lung, dryness invading the Lung, or early stage of wind-water invading the Lung. Fever and chills may also appear in the early stage of certain patterns not due to the invasion of exopathogenic factors such as cold-water shooting into the Lung, Small Intestine excess fire, Large Intestine cold-dampness, Large Intestine damp-heat, Liver and Gallbladder damp-heat, and Urinary Bladder damp-heat.

Alternating chills and fever (寒熱往來 *hán rè wǎng lái*): Chills and fever that occur one after the other. The Gallbladder channel runs along the side of the body and is located between the exterior and interior.

When pathogens invade this channel, they become locked between the exterior and interior in a struggle with antipathogenic qi (正氣 *zhèng qì*). When antipathogenic qi is stronger than the pathogens or the pathogens decline, the yang will dominate and the body temperature will rise; when the pathogens predominate or antipathogenic qi is weaker, yin will dominate and there will be chills. This type of fever is usually seen in the patterns Gallbladder heat or Liver and Gallbladder damp-heat.

Unsurfaced fever (身熱不揚 *shēn rè bù yáng*): The patient feels hot, but their skin feels sticky and not hot with initial touch, or the skin feels warmer only with prolonged pressure. When heat and dampness accumulate, the heavy and sticky nature of dampness traps heat within, blocking it from surfacing. Heat builds up inside and does not reduce after sweating. This type of fever is usually seen in the pattern damp-heat encumbering the Spleen.

High fever (高燒 *gāo shāo*): Body temperature that rises above 102° F (38.8° C) and persists without aversion to cold. High fever is a symptom of antipathogenic qi resisting pathogens. The fever's severity depends on the strength of both the antipathogenic qi and the pathogens. The more intense the struggle, the higher the body temperature. Thus high fever indicates an excess heat condition and hyperactive yang qi. This type of fever is usually the main symptom in the patterns heat congesting the Lung, Large Intestine heat accumulation, Stomach and Large Intestine heat accumulation (*yáng míng fǔ* pattern), heat invading the Pericardium, and extreme heat generating wind. High fever may also appear in phlegm-fire harassing the Heart, Liver fire blazing, Heart fire blazing, Urinary Bladder damp-heat, and Stomach fire.

Tidal fever (潮熱 *cháo rè*): Fever occurs or worsens at a fixed hour of the day, just like the regular rise and fall of the tides. Tidal fever can also include a patient's subjective sensation of heat without any measurable increase in body temperature. Tidal fever can be caused by excess such as with stagnation and accumulation, or by deficiency related to disharmony of yin and yang.

Tidal fever caused by excess conditions of obstruction or pathogen stagnation can be seen in the following patterns: (1) Stomach and Large Intestine heat accumulation (*yáng míng fǔ* pattern): high fever that is worse in the afternoon around 3 p.m. to 5 p.m. with severe constipation and abdominal pain. (2) Damp-heat encumbering the Spleen: unsurfaced fever that is worse in the afternoon or evening. (3) Blood stagnation: fever worse in the evening.

Tidal fever caused by deficiency conditions are low-grade fevers or feverish sensations and can be seen in the following patterns: (1) Spleen and Stomach qi deficiency: fever or feverish sensation that appears in the morning. (2) Yin deficiency (Kidney yin deficiency, Heart yin deficiency, Lung yin deficiency, Liver yin deficiency, Liver and Kidney yin deficiency, Spleen yin deficiency, and yin deficiency generating wind): fever or feverish sensation that is worse in the late afternoon or evening.

Low-grade fever (低燒 *dī shāo*): Body temperature that is consistently between 98.6° and 100.4° F (37°-38° C) over a period of at least two weeks. Low-grade fever can also include a patient's subjective sensation of heat without any measurable increase in body temperature. Most low-grade fevers are caused by deficiency, and are commonly seen in the following patterns: (1) yin deficiency (Kidney yin deficiency, Lung yin deficiency, Liver yin deficiency, Heart yin deficiency, Spleen yin deficiency, Stomach yin deficiency, Lung and Kidney yin deficiency, Liver and Kidney yin deficiency, Heart and Kidney disharmony, or yin deficiency generating wind): low-grade fever that appears in the late afternoon or evening. (2) Spleen and Stomach qi deficiency: low-grade fever that appears in the morning. (3) Blood deficiency and yang deficiency: rare.

Low-grade fevers can also be caused by excess conditions of stagnation and accumulation, as in the following patterns: (1) Liver qi stagnation: low-grade fever or afternoon tidal fever that changes with shifts in emotions and moods. (2) Food stagnation: low-grade fever that is worse in the afternoon along with abdominal pain and distention. (3) Blood stagnation: low-grade fever in the afternoon or evening, or heat sensations in the local area with fixed sharp pain.

Fever	Pathogenesis	Zàng Fǔ Pattern	Treatment Strategy	Herbal Formulas
Fever with chills	Initial stagnation of exopathogens invading, struggle between protective qi and pathogens	Wind-cold invading the Lung	Diaphoresis, release the exterior	Ma Huang Tang, Gui Zhi Tang, Xing Su San
		Wind-heat invading the Lung		Yin Qiao San, Sang Ju Yin
		Dryness invading the Lung		Qing Zao Jiu Fei Tang, Bai He Gu Jin Tang, Sha Shen Mai Men Dong Tang
		Wind-water invading the Lung		Yue Bi Tang, Xiao Qing Long Tang
Alternating chills and fever	Antipathogenic qi and pathogens locked between exterior and interior	Gallbladder heat	Harmonize shào yáng, drain heat, clear dampness from the Liver and Gallbladder	Da Chai Hu Tang, Xiao Chai Hu Tang
		Liver and Gallbladder damp-heat		Yin Chen Hao Tang, Long Dan Xie Gan Tang
Unsurfaced fever	Heat and dampness accumulation, dampness traps heat inside	Damp-heat encumbering the Spleen	Drain dampness, clear heat, strengthen the Speen	Yin Chen Wu Ling San
High fever	Antipathogenic qi excess, fiercely fighting pathogens	Heat congesting the Lung	Clear excess heat	Bai Hu Tang, Xie Bai San
		Heat invading the Pericardium	Clear heat from Ying	Qing Ying Tang, Xi Jiao Di Huang Tang
		Extreme heat generating wind	Cool the Liver, extinguish wind	Ling Jiao Gou Teng Tang
Tidal fever	Excess pathogens accumulate, generating heat	Stomach and Large Intestine heat accumulation	Strongly purge heat accumulation	Da Cheng Qi Tang, Xiao Cheng Qi Tang, Tiao Wei Cheng Qi Tang
		Damp-heat encumbering the Spleen	Drain dampness, clear heat	Yin Chen Wu Ling San
	Qi deficiency leads to stagnation, generating heat	Spleen qi deficiency	Tonify qi	Bu Zhong Yi Qi Tang
Low-grade fever	Yin deficiency leads to relative yang excess	Kidney yin deficiency	Nourish yin	Zhi Bai Di Huang Wan
		Lung yin deficiency		Bai He Gu Jin Tang, Sha Shen Mai Men Dong Tang
		Liver yin deficiency		Yi Guan Jian
		Heart yin deficiency		Huang Lian E Jiao Tang, Bu Xin Tang
		Spleen yin deficiency		Zhong He Li Yin Tang, Sha Shen Mai Men Dong Tang
		Stomach yin deficiency		Yi Wei Tang, Sha Shen Mai Men Dong Tang
		Lung and Kidney yin deficiency		Bai He Gu Jin Tang, Qi Wei Du Qi Wan
		Liver and Kidney yin deficiency		Yi Guan Jian, Zuo Gui Wan
		Heart and Kidney disharmony		Tian Wang Bu Xin Dan, Jiao Tai Wan
	Stagnation generating heat	Liver qi stagnation	Soothe Liver qi, clear heat	Jia Wei Xiao Yao San
		Food stagnation	Disperse food, clear heat	Bao He Wan, Xiao Pi Wan

Table 24.25.1 Fever: common patterns and treatments

26. What is Stomach Qi Deficiency?

Definition: A group of signs and symptoms involving the failure of Stomach qi to descend due to hypofunction.

Clinical manifestation: Dull or faint epigastric pain that is relieved by warmth and pressure, worse with an empty stomach; aversion to food with no desire to eat due to discomfort after eating, even vomiting immediately after eating; vomiting with clear fluids; sensitivity to many different kinds of food; frequent belching without foul odor; epigastric fullness and distention (心下痞滿 *xīn xià pǐ mǎn*); low and inconsistent hiccups; nausea; lack of appetite; indefinable epigastric discomfort (嘈雜 *cáo zá*); fatigue; lassitude; shortness of breath; aversion to talking; low voice; sallow complexion; a pale tongue with a white coating; and a weak deficient pulse.

Key points: Dull or faint epigastric pain that is relieved by pressure, lack of appetite plus qi deficiency signs and symptoms.

Etiology and pathogenesis: The Stomach is the organ with abundant qi and blood, thus Stomach qi deficiency is rare and not mentioned in most TCM textbooks. However, Stomach qi deficiency can occur when there is a failure to generate qi to replenish the Stomach due to long-term improper diet, aging, chronic illness, or physical overstrain. Severe diarrhea or vomiting can also impair Stomach qi.

When Stomach qi is insufficient, it fails to move and promote, leading to qi stagnation, which manifests as a dull and faint epigastric pain that can be relieved by pressure or warmth. This pain can also be relieved or aggravated by eating. Food is the source of nutritive qi (谷氣 *gǔ qì*) and helps generate Stomach qi to relieve pain; however, deficient Stomach qi is unable to properly digest food and therefore eating will lead to pain or vomiting immediately afterwards.

Indefinable epigastric discomfort (嘈雜 *cáo zá*) is an uncomfortable feeling that is neither pain nor nausea but rather an empty, burning, and uneasy sensation in the epigastric region. It is caused by Stomach qi deficiency combined with turbid waste and phlegm accumulation in the middle burner.

When the Stomach is deficient, it fails to receive and decompose food, and therefore qi and blood production decreases. Since qi is the motive force of the human body, when qi is deficient, it fails to push and promote. The lack of qi manifests as shortness of breath, fatigue, aversion to talking, weak limbs, low voice, sallow complexion, a pale tongue, and a weak pulse.

When qi deficiency disrupts the Stomach's descending function, there will be qi rebellion. This presents as belching without foul odor, epigastric fullness and distention (心下痞滿 *xīn xià pǐ mǎn*), low and inconsistent hiccups, nausea, and vomiting with clear fluids.

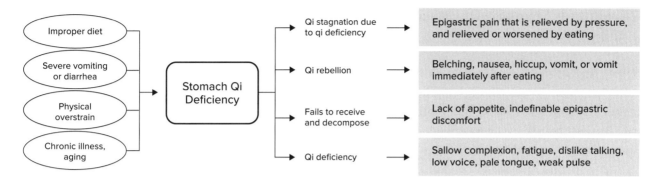

Chart 24.26.1 Etiology and pathogenesis of Stomach Qi Deficiency

TCM Disease	Western Disease	Herbal Formulas		Acupuncture
Epigastric pain (胃痛)	Atrophic gastritis, gastric neurosis, peptic ulcer, GERD, gastric carcinoma, acid reflux, esophagitis	Huang Qi Jian Zhong Tang	Huang Qi Jian Zhong Tang	ST-25, SP-4, CV-14
Indefinable epigastric discomfort (嘈雜)	GERD, peptic ulcer, acid reflux, gastritis, esophagitis, hiatal hernia, SIBO, esophagitis	Yi Gong San		ST-10
Hiccups (呃逆)	GERD, alcoholism, diabetes, stroke, MS, tumors, steroid or tranquilizer use	Liu Jun Zi Tang	ST-36, CV-12, BL-21, CV-6	BL-17
Belching (噯氣)	GERD, lactose intolerance, IBS, aerophagia	Xuan Fu Dai Zhe Tang		TB-6, CV-10, ST-44
Vomiting (嘔吐)	Motion sickness, gastroenteritis, pregnancy, stomach flu	Li Zhong Wan		SP-6, LI-4, PC-6
Fatigue (虛勞)	Adrenal fatigue, hypothyroidism, CFS Lyme disease, EBV	Si Jun Zi Tang		CV-4, GV-4, BL-23, BL-24, BL-26
Morning sickness (妊娠惡阻)	Hyperemesis, gravidarum, morning sickness	Xiang Sha Liu Jun Zi Tang		PC-6

Table 24.26.1 Diseases and treatments related to Stomach Qi Deficiency

27. What is Middle Qi Insufficiency (中氣不足 zhōng qì bù zú)? How does Stomach Qi Deficiency compare with Spleen Qi Deficiency?

Both the Spleen and Stomach are located in the middle burner and are inter-connected by a membrane in the abdomen, forming an interior and exterior relationship. They coordinate and cooperate to maintain normal digestive function. The Spleen governs transportation and transformation, belongs to yin earth, ascends, favors dryness and disfavors dampness. The Stomach governs reception and decomposition, belongs to yang earth, descends, favors moisture, and disfavors dryness. The Stomach prepares the food for the Spleen to transport and transform, while the Spleen sends body fluids to the Stomach to support its proper function. If the Stomach is unable to receive and decompose food, it will affect the Spleen's transportation and transformation function; likewise, if the Spleen fails to transport and transform, it will affect the Stomach's receiving and decomposition function. Thus qi deficiency often occurs in both organs at the same time and is called Spleen and Stomach qi deficiency (脾胃氣虛 pí wèi qì xū). Since the Spleen and

Stomach are both located in the middle burner, this pattern is also called middle qi insufficiency (中氣不足 *zhōng qì bù zú*).

Spleen qi deficiency and Stomach qi deficiency share many common signs and symptoms such as sallow complexion, fatigue, lassitude, weak limbs, shortness of breath, aversion to talking, low voice, reduced appetite, a pale tongue with a white coating, and a weak or soft pulse. However, the pathogenesis and clinical manifestation of the two patterns are different. Dysfunction of the Stomach in reception and decomposition will lead to a dull or faint epigastric pain, lack of appetite or an aversion to food, and indefinable epigastric discomfort (嘈雜 *cáo zá*) that is an uneasy sensation that is neither pain nor hunger. Dysfunction of the Spleen in transportation and transformation will lead to abdominal distention or bloating after eating and loose stools.

The Stomach governs descending and the Spleen governs ascending. If the Stomach qi rebels and ascends rather than descends, there may be nausea, vomiting, hiccups, or belching. If the Spleen qi descends rather than ascends, there may be diarrhea, loose stools, rectal prolapse, or dizziness due to clear yang qi not rising to nourish the brain. Furthermore, the Spleen is one of the most important organs responsible for water metabolism; thus when Spleen qi deficiency fails to transport and transform, the accumulation of water or dampness results in edema and a flabby tongue. The Spleen is also the organ that keeps blood inside the vessels, and therefore bleeding or easy bruising is one of the major symptoms seen in Spleen qi deficiency.

The key points to distinguish these two patterns are as follows:
(1) Etiology: severe diarrhea or vomiting vs. long-term worry or overthinking
(2) Location: epigastric vs. abdominal
(3) Symptoms: bleeding, organ prolapse, and edema can appear in Spleen qi deficiency

Pattern		Stomach Qi Deficiency	Spleen Qi Deficiency
Etiology		Constitutional deficiency, improper diet, physical overstrain, aging, severe illness, improper care	
		Severe vomiting or diarrhea	Long-term worrying or overthinking
Pathogenesis		Fails to receive and decompose; fails to descend	Fails to transport and transform; fails to ascend and control blood
Characteristics		Sub-chronic, milder	Chronic, more severe
Symptoms	Common	Sallow complexion, fatigue, lassitude, weak limbs, shortness of breath, aversion to talking, low voice, reduced appetite, bloating and distention, a pale tongue with a white coating, and a weak or soft pulse	
	Different	Lack of appetite or aversion to food, epigastric bloating and distention	No hunger, no desire to eat, abdominal bloating and distention, a pale and flabby tongue
	Main symptoms	Dull or faint epigastric pain, hiccups, belching, nausea or vomiting	Abdominal bloating and distention, loose stools after eating
	Other symptoms	Indefinable epigastric discomfort	Edema, bleeding, organ prolapse
Treatment strategy		Tonify Stomach qi	Tonify Spleen qi
Herbal formulas		Huang Qi Jian Zhong Tang	Si Jun Zi Tang, Bu Zhong Yi Qi Tang

Table 24.27.1 Comparison of Stomach Qi Deficiency and Spleen Qi Deficiency

28. Since the Spleen favors dryness and disfavors dampness, does the pattern of Spleen Yin Deficiency exist?

To answer this question, the concepts of yin and dampness must first be differentiated. According to Chinese medicine theory, the human body is an organic unity based on the opposing and complementary relationships of yin and yang. The body's organs and tissues can be classified according to yin-yang theory based on their functions and locations. Each organ can also be further divided into yin and yang aspects. The body's physical form belongs to yin while the body's activities or functions belong to yang. Both the body's physical form and functions are dynamically balanced, mutually restricting and supporting of one another. When yin and yang are in harmony, health is achieved. *Basic Questions* (素問 *sù wèn*), Chapter 3, states: "Calm yin and steady yang means good vitality and spirit. Separation of yin and yang means vitality and spirit are failing."

The physical forms of organs and tissues belong to yin, while their functions belong to yang. However, the physical forms can be further divided such that solid materials like muscles, bones, or membranes belong to yang and liquid materials like blood, body fluids, and essence belong to yin. Yin fluids (阴液 *yīn yè*) is the general term for all kinds of liquid material, and this is what we usually refer to as 'yin.' They are the basic physiological products of the body. They nourish and moisten the body to support physical activities and functions.

In contrast to yin, dampness is the pathological product of water metabolism, which requires the cooperation of the Lung, Spleen, Kidney and Triple Burner in order to function properly. The Lung governs dispersing and descending, regulates the water passages, and is responsible for the distribution of fluids to the entire body, while the Spleen is in charge of transportation and transformation of water into body fluids. The Kidney transforms qi, provides energy to all the organs for water metabolism, distributes body fluids, reabsorbs clear water essence, and expels turbid water waste. Furthermore, the Kidney controls the opening and closing of the two yin orifices, which regulates urinary functions.

When Lung, Spleen, or Kidney function is compromised, water cannot be transformed into body fluids, and waste fluids cannot be expelled, leading to the accumulation of dampness. Thus dampness is a pathological product that most affects the Spleen.

The concept of 'Spleen yin deficiency' began to attract attention after Li Dong-Yuan (李東垣, 1180-1251) expounded on his theory about 'middle qi sinking' (中氣下陷 *zhōng qì xià xiàn*) and 'fever due to qi deficiency' (氣虛發熱 *qì xū fā rè*). Zhu Dan-Xi (朱丹溪, 1281-1358) added the physiological and pathological theory about 'Spleen yin deficiency' and 'Stomach yin deficiency,' which gradually developed and matured through the Ming and Qing dynasties. The essence of Spleen yin deficiency is that 'yin deficiency leads to yang hyperactivity'. Qin Jing-Min, in his book *Pattern, Cause, Pulse and Treatment* (証因脈治 *zhèng yīn mài zhì*), said: "There are two kinds of Spleen deficiency: yin deficiency and yang deficiency. When Spleen yin is deficient, Spleen blood will be consumed, and Spleen fire will flare up. When the Spleen is deficient but still has heat, the use of warming and tonifying treatment methods may increase heat and further impair yin. Thus in this case Spleen yin must be nourished and replenished, increasing the yin to reduce the yang and thereby balancing yin and yang."

There is no precise definition of Spleen yin at present, but there are generally two opinions. The first is that Spleen yin refers to the essence of water and food, yin fluids, or nutritive fluids (營陰 *yíng yīn*) that exist in the Spleen. The second is that Spleen yin is a term defined by its relationship to Spleen yang, and refers to substances in the Spleen that have calming, inhibiting, and astringent effects; these substances are in between blood and qi in that they are like blood but not blood, and like qi but not qi.

There are three major physiological functions of Spleen yin:

(1) Transform and transport: This function relies on the collective effect of Spleen yin and Spleen yang. Tang Zong-Hai (唐宗海, 1851-1908) in his book *Treatise on Blood Syndromes* (血証論, 1884) states: "When Spleen yang is insufficient, water and grain cannot be transformed; when Spleen yin is insufficient, water and grain also cannot be transformed. Similar to cooking rice, when there is no fire under the pot, the rice cannot be cooked, and when there is no water in the pot, the rice also cannot be cooked." Only when Spleen yin and Spleen yang are sufficient can digestion and absorption be normal, and the water and grain essences be dispersed throughout the body to nourish and moisten the *zàng fǔ* organs, limbs, muscles, and bones, enabling normal physiological functions.

(2) Control and generate blood: Blood circulation relies on the Spleen, both Spleen yang and Spleen yin. Tang Zong-Hai (唐宗海, 1851-1908) in his book *Treatise on Blood Syndromes* (血証論, 1884) states: "Deficient Spleen yang cannot control the blood, and deficient Spleen yin cannot nourish and generate the blood." This is the most accurate description of the Spleen's function in controlling blood.

(3) Nourish and moisten: According to TCM theory, the Spleen is the acquired root of humans, the source of qi and blood. The Spleen generates the qi and blood that is needed to nourish and moisten the *zàng fǔ* organs, limbs, muscles, and bones, enabling them to perform their physiological functions. Thus is it said that the Spleen controls the muscles. However, the Spleen's nourishing and moistening function relies on the adequacy of Spleen yin. As Zhang Xi-Chun (張錫純, 1860-1933) quoted Chen Xiu-Yan (陳修園, 1753-1823) in his book *Records of Traditional Chinese in Combination with Western Medicine* (醫學衷中參西錄 *yī xué zhōng zhōng cān xī lù*, 1909): "The Spleen is *tài yín*; it is the first in three yin *zàng* organs. When treating Spleen yin deficiency, mainly nourish the Spleen yin. When the Spleen yin is adequate, it can irrigate the other *zàng fǔ* organs and the entire body naturally." This is also the best interpretation of the concept that "The Spleen is a solitary *zàng* organ, belonging to earth, and located at the center; all other *zàng fǔ* organs depend on the Spleen for irrigation," as stated in the *The Yellow Emperor's Internal Classic* (黃帝內經 *huáng dì nèi jīng*, c. 200).

Common factors that can lead to Spleen yin deficiency include improper diet, emotional stress, and improper treatment such as the overuse of warm or hot herbs, emetics, purgatives, or diuretics that impair yin and throw yin and yang out of balance.

There are three major aspects to the clinical manifestation of Spleen yin deficiency:

(1) Failure to transform and transport, manifesting in poor appetite, abdominal bloating and loose stools after meals, or defecation with stools that start off dry and then become loose.

(2) Failure to nourish and moisten, manifesting in a sallow and pale complexion, tiredness, lassitude, emaciation, lack of strength, weak limbs, *wěi* syndrome (痿証 *wěi zhèng*), dry skin, and keratinization around the nails.

(3) Deficient heat manifesting with dry mouth and lips, chapped lips, thirst with no desire to drink much fluid, low-grade fever or feverish sensation, five center heat, a dry red tongue with a scanty or peeling coating, and a soft, faint, and rapid pulse. Spleen yin deficiency is usually combined with yin deficiency of other organs such as Spleen and Lung yin deficiency, Heart and Spleen yin deficiency, Kidney and Spleen yin deficiency, and Spleen and Stomach yin deficiency.

Treatment strategies for Spleen yin deficiency generally follow the principles of *The Yellow Emperor's Internal Classic* (黃帝內經 *huáng dì nèi jīng*, c. 200), which states: "To strengthen the Spleen, use sweet and bland taste [herbs]." *Basic Questions* (素問 *sù wèn*), Chapter 72, states: "Use sweet tasting [herbs] to relieve the Spleen; use bitter tasting [herbs] to clear and use sweet [herbs] to nourish."

Thus the treatment of Spleen yin deficiency is based on sweet and cool herbs such as Shan Yao, Bai Bian Dou, Lian Zi Rou, Yi Yi Ren, Fu Ling, Qian Shi, Yu Zhu, Huang Jing, Gan Cao, Tai Zi Shen, Bai Zhu, Shi Hu, Gou Qi Zi, Shan Zha, Wu Mai, and Bai Shao.

29. What is Stomach Excess with Spleen Deficiency? How to distinguish this pattern from Stomach Fire?

Definition: 'Stomach excess with Spleen deficiency' (胃強脾弱 *wèi qiáng pí ruò*) means the rotting and ripening function of the Stomach has become hyperactive, while the Spleen's transportation and transformation function has declined, manifesting clinically as Stomach heat with Spleen deficiency (胃熱脾虛 *wèi rè pí xū*).

Clinical manifestation: Excessive appetite, feeling hungry even after abundant food intake, emaciation, indefinable epigastric discomfort (嘈雜 *cáo zá*), bad breath and lack of taste, thirst, abdominal bloating and distention after meals, loose stools or diarrhea with undigested food or dry stools first then loose stools, irritability, dizziness, jaundice, pica disorder, malnutrition or obesity, a red flabby tongue with a yellow coating, and a thin, rapid, and wiry pulse.

Key points: Excessive appetite, feeling hungry even after abundant food intake, emaciation, and loose stools or diarrhea.

Etiology and pathogenesis: This pattern is usually caused by improper diet such as overconsumption of alcohol and greasy, sweet, or spicy foods that increase heat in the Stomach, or overconsumption of cold foods that impair Spleen qi. Parasites may also consume and deplete qi and blood, cause malnutrition, and lead to Spleen qi deficiency. Meanwhile the Stomach will be in a state of compensatory hyperactivity, resulting in Stomach fire.

The Stomach is the organ that is abundant in qi and blood, and is prone to excess conditions. When excess heat invades the Stomach, it will speed up decomposition and transportation, which increases peristalsis, and results in the patient feeling hungry even after abundant food intake, as well as indefinable epigastric discomfort. Heat consumes body fluids, causing thirst. Heat can also steam the odor of rottened and ripened food up from the Stomach, causing bad breath.

The Spleen is in charge of transportation and transformation and cooperates with the Stomach to generate qi, blood, and body fluids for distribution to the entire body. When Spleen qi is insufficient, qi, blood and body fluids cannot be generated and distributed, resulting in emaciation. Spleen qi deficiency can also lead to accumulation of water or dampness, which pours down to the Large Intestine, causing loose stools or diarrhea. When dampness accumulates in the tongue, it become flabby. If the condition is caused by parasites, it may present as pica disorder.

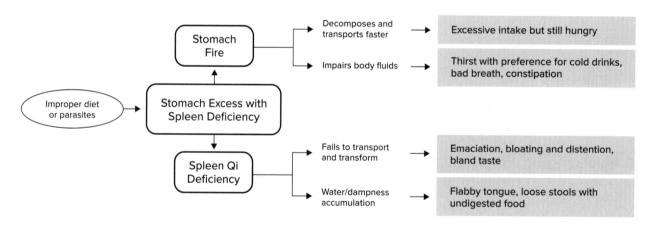

Chart 24.29.1 Etiology and pathogenesis of Stomach Excess with Spleen Deficiency

The clinical manifestations for this pattern vary and it can appear in different kinds of diseases such as jaundice, child malnutrition, pica disorder, diabetes, 'wasting and thirsting' syndrome (消渴証 *xiāo kě zhèng*), or obesity.

Stomach excess with Spleen deficiency and Stomach fire are two different patterns. Stomach fire only has excess heat in the Stomach and manifests as hyperactive function with symptoms including epigastric burning pain that resists pressure, thirst with desire to drink cold water, excessive appetite, insatiable hunger, bad breath, painful and swollen bleeding gums, sores in the mouth, vomiting with a sour or bitter taste, acid regurgitation, constipation with dry stools, scanty yellow urine, a red tongue with a yellow coating, and a slippery and rapid pulse.

Stomach excess with Spleen deficiency is Stomach fire with Spleen qi deficiency. Besides the Stomach fire signs and symptoms mentioned above, this pattern also presents those of Spleen qi deficiency such as abdominal bloating and distention, emaciation, loose stools or diarrhea, and a flabby tongue.

<table>
<tr><th>TCM Disease</th><th>Western Disease</th><th colspan="2">Herbal Formulas</th><th colspan="2">Acupuncture</th></tr>
<tr><td>Wasting and thirsting (消渴)</td><td>Diabetes, hyperthyroidism, binge-eating disorder</td><td rowspan="4">Yu Nu Jian, Jian Pi Wan</td><td>Xiao Ke Fang</td><td rowspan="4">ST-44, CV-12, LI-14, LI-11, ST-36, CV-4, CV-6, SP-3, SP-6, BL-20, BL-21</td><td>Yi Shu (胰腧)</td></tr>
<tr><td>Childhood nutritional impairment (疳積)</td><td>Child malnutrition, parasites</td><td>Gan Ji San</td><td>Si Feng (四縫)</td></tr>
<tr><td>Jaundice (黃疸)</td><td>Cholecystitis, gallstones, hepatitis</td><td>Xiao Chai Hu Tang</td><td>BL-18, BL-19, GB-34, SI-4, SP-9</td></tr>
<tr><td>Obesity (肥胖)</td><td>Diabetes, binge-eating disorder, PCOS, Cushing's syndrome</td><td>Shen Ling Bai Zhu San</td><td>ST-25, ST-35, ST-40, SP-9</td></tr>
</table>

Table 24.29.1 Diseases and treatments related to Stomach Excess with Spleen Deficiency

30. Is the pattern Stomach Excess with Spleen Deficiency the same as Constrained Spleen? If not, how are they different?

The 'constrained Spleen' pattern (脾約証 *pí yuē zhèng*) is a term from the *Yáng Míng* chapter of the *Treatise on Cold Damage* (傷寒論 *shāng hán lùn*) and has also been called 'Stomach excess with Spleen deficiency' in some textbooks. However, the deficiency in this pattern refers to Spleen yin deficiency and thus the pathogenesis of this pattern is excess fire in the Stomach with Spleen yin deficiency, whereby Spleen function is 'constrained' by Stomach fire.

When the Spleen cooperates and coordinates with the Stomach to transport and transform body fluids, there are two major functions it performs. One is to absorb the excess of food and body fluids for distribution to the entire body, while the other is to transform water into body fluids for distribution to the gastrointestinal tract to moisten food residue, waste, and stool so that they move downward smoothly. In modern medicine, these processes are similar to intestinal absorption and secretory functions.

Stomach heat with Spleen yin deficiency can result from the invasion of exopathogens that transform into heat and then impair the body fluids. Other etiological factors include aging, constitution, chronic illness, or an improper diet that impairs yin.

When Stomach yang is in excess, yin fluids will be impaired by Stomach fire and the Spleen will use up all the fluids. The Stomach and Intestines cannot be moistened, leading to dryness in the intestinal tract and constipation. Due to Spleen deficiency, water that is consumed cannot be transformed into body fluids.

Stomach yang excess damages the body fluids, leading to dry stools that block the intestines, causing abdominal bloating and distention or abdominal pain. Excess heat in the Stomach will manifest with dry mouth and thirst with a preference for cold water, bad breath, irritability, a red tongue with a yellow coating, and a slippery and rapid pulse.

Thus even though many textbooks use 'Stomach excess with Spleen deficiency' to describe the 'constrained Spleen' pattern, they are indeed different patterns. Both of them have the signs and symptoms of excess heat in the Stomach; however, in Stomach excess with Spleen deficiency, the 'Spleen deficiency' is Spleen qi deficiency, which manifests with loose stools or diarrhea, abdominal bloating and distention after eating, and emaciation. In contrast, the Spleen deficiency in the 'constrained Spleen' pattern is Spleen yin deficiency, which mainly presents with dry stools.

The key points to distinguish these two patterns are as follows:
(1) Etiology: improper diet vs. febrile disease or aging, constitution, and chronic illness
(2) Main symptoms: Excessive appetite, feeling hungry even after abundant food intake, emaciation, loose stools or diarrhea vs. constipation

Pattern		Stomach Excess with Spleen Deficiency	Constrained Spleen
Etiology		Improper diet (overconsumption of alcohol, spicy, greasy, sweet, or cold foods), or parasites	Exopathogens invade, transform into heat, and impair body fluids; aging, constitution, chronic illness, improper diet
Pathogenesis		Stomach heat with Spleen qi deficiency	Stomach heat with Spleen yin deficiency
Symptoms	Common	Abdominal bloating and distention, dry mouth and thirst with preference for cold water, bad breath, irritability, red tongue with yellow coating, a slippery and rapid pulse	
	Main	Excessive appetite, feeling hungry even after abundant food intake, emaciation	Constipation with dry stools, frequent urination
	Different	Loose stools or diarrhea, or dry stools first then loose stools	Constipation with frequent urination
Treatment strategy		Clear Stomach heat, strengthen the Spleen	Clear heat, move qi, lubricate and moisten the intestines
Herbal formulas		Yu Nu Jian, Jian Pi Wan	Ma Zi Ren Wan

Table 24.30.1 Comparison of Stomach Excess with Spleen Deficiency and Constrained Spleen

31. How does Damp-Heat in the Spleen and Stomach compare with Damp-Heat in the middle burner?

Damp-heat in the Spleen and Stomach and damp-heat in the middle burner have the same pathological location and etiological factors. They share many clinical symptoms including nausea, poor appetite, thirst with no desire to drink, distention and discomfort in the epigastrium and abdomen, lassitude and body heaviness, yellow scanty urine, loose and sticky stools with foul odor, a red tongue with a yellow greasy tongue coating, and a rapid slippery pulse. However, these two patterns are from different pattern identification systems, one is 'zàng fǔ pattern identification' and the other is 'Triple Burner pattern identification.'

Zàng fǔ pattern identification is a method used to analyze signs and symptoms of disease according to the physiological functions and pathological characteristics of the zàng fǔ organs. This helps to infer etiopathology, to determine location, and to judge the nature of the pathological change as well as the condition of the body's antipathogenic qi. Zàng fǔ pattern identification is one of the core methods in TCM diagnosis and the foundation for clinical analysis and differentiation of every disease, particularly for interior and chronic conditions.

Triple Burner pattern identification comes from the 'warm diseases' (温病 wēn bìng) school of TCM theory. It is used to analyze signs and symptoms of disease according to the Triple Burner categories, which can be separated into upper, middle, and lower functional groups of zàng fǔ organs and associated etiology, pathogenesis, onset, stage, location, progression, treatment method, and prognosis. It is used to differentiate exogenous febrile diseases according to the characteristics of its contraction.

The main differences between these two patterns are:

(1) Etiology: Damp-heat in the Spleen and Stomach is mostly due to improper diet such as the overconsumption of sweet greasy foods and alcohol; Spleen and Stomach deficiency failing to transport and transform, resulting in accumulation of dampness that generates heat; or exopathogenic damp-heat invasion, although this pattern is mainly an endogenous damp-heat condition. In contrast, damp-heat in the middle burner is more due to exopathogenic damp-heat, summer-dampness invasion, or damp-heat transferred from the upper burner. Thus it is an exogenous disease.

(2) Type of disease: Damp-heat in the Spleen and Stomach is considered an endogenous disease, while damp-heat in the middle burner is considered an exogenous febrile disease.

(3) Pathogenesis: Damp-heat in the Spleen and Stomach is a condition in which internal damp-heat accumulation hinders transportation and transformation. In contrast, damp-heat in the middle burner is considered one stage of exogenous febrile disease development.

(4) Clinical manifestation: Since the location and etiology are the same, the two patterns share many symptoms such as nausea, poor appetite, thirst with no desire to drink, distention and discomfort in the epigastrium and abdomen, lassitude and body heaviness,

yellow scanty urine, loose and sticky stools with foul odor, a red tongue with a yellow greasy tongue coating, and a rapid slippery pulse. However, damp-heat in the middle burner further presents with unsurfaced fever (身熱不揚 shēn rè bù yáng), which is a fever that subsides after sweating but recurs quickly, and is worse in the afternoon.

Pattern		Spleen and Stomach Damp-Heat	Damp-Heat in the Middle Burner
Etiology		Improper diet, exopathogenic damp-heat invasion	Exopathogenic damp-heat or summer-dampness invasion
Pathogenesis		Endogenous disease	Exogenous febrile disease
		Damp-heat disrupts the transporting and transforming function of the Spleen and Stomach	
Symptoms	Common	Nausea, poor appetite, thirst with no desire to drink, distention and discomfort in the epigastrium and abdomen, lassitude and body heaviness, yellow scanty urine, loose and sticky stools with foul odor, a red tongue with a yellow greasy coating, a slippery rapid pulse	
	Different		Unsurfaced fever, fever that subsides after sweating, but recurs quickly, worse in the afternoon, profuse sweating, thirst
	Fever	No fever	High fever, unsurfaced fever, worse in the afternoon
Tongue & pulse		Red tongue with a yellow greasy coating, a slippery and rapid pulse	
		Soggy pulse	Surging or forceful pulse
Treatment strategy		Clear heat, transform dampness, regulate qi, harmonize the Spleen and Stomach	Clear heat and dry dampness
Herbal formulas		Yin Chen Wu Ling San, Huo Xiang Zheng San	Bai Huang Jia Cang Zhu Tang, Lian Pu Yin

Table 24.31.1 Comparison of Spleen and Stomach Damp-Heat and Damp-Heat in the Middle Burner

32. What is Kidney essence and Kidney qi? What are Kidney yin, Kidney yang, true yin, true yang, primary yin, primary yang, *mìng mén* fire, and *mìng mén* water? How are they all related to each other?

Essence (精 jīng) is one of the most valuable fluid materials of the human body. It is the basic material and the nutritional composition that forms the *zàng fǔ* organs, tissues, skin, hair, tendons, and muscles. It is responsible for the growth and development of embryos and how life comes into being, and it is essential for maintaining the various physiological activities of the human body.

Essence can be divided into two main categories: congenital or pre-natal essence and acquired or post-natal essence. Congenital essence is inherited from the parents and is fundamental in the creation of life. It forms the *zàng fǔ* organs, tissues, skin, hair, tendons, and muscles, and promotes the growth and development of the embryo. On the other hand, acquired essence, also known as water and food essence (水谷之精 shuǐ gǔ zhī jīng), is generated by the Spleen and Stomach. It is the material basis for post-natal growth and development and enables the body's various physiological functions.

Depending on the function and location, essence can be further divided into reproductive essence (生殖之精 *shēng zhí zhī jīng*), and *zàng fǔ* essence (臟腑之精 *zàng fǔ zhī jīng*). Reproductive essence is stored inside the Kidney, is derived from congenital essence, is nourished and assisted by acquired essence, and has the function of procreation. *Zàng fǔ* essence is stored inside the different *zàng fǔ* organs, and maintains their physiological activities.

Starting from the fetal stage, congenital essence is stored inside the Kidney and is a major component of Kidney essence. During growth and development, it can be allocated to other organs to assist in their functions. Acquired essence is stored in all the organs and is the primary substance and energy that enables all their functions. Any surplus in acquired essence is transported to the Kidney for storage and for nourishing congenital essence. Thus Kidney essence is a general term for the essence stored in the Kidney that contains both congenital and acquired essence.

Kidney essence and Kidney qi are the same substance, but in different forms. Kidney essence is the liquid state while Kidney qi is the gaseous state. Depending on the circumstances, they may transform into each other or supplement each other. Together they are called essence qi (精氣 *jīng qì*). Essence qi provides the motive force for the body's metabolic and physiological functions. Kidney essence transforms into Kidney qi, which can be further divided into Kidney yin and Kidney yang. The Kidney is called the 'root of yin and yang' (陰陽之根 *yīn yáng zhī gēn*) and the 'house of water and fire' (水火之宅 *shuǐ huǒ zhī zhái*) because Kidney yin and Kidney yang are the root of the entire body's yin and yang.

Kidney yang is also called primary yang (原陽 *yuán yáng*), true yang (真陽 *zhēn yáng*), true fire (真火 *zhēn huǒ*), and *mìng mén* fire (命門之火 *mìng mén zhī huǒ*). It has the functions of warming, promoting, stimulating, and transforming qi. Kidney yin is also called primary yin (原陰 *yuán yīn*), true yin (真陰 *zhēn yīn*), true water (真水 *zhēn shuǐ*), and *mìng mén* water (命門之水 *mìng mén zhī shuǐ*). It has the functions of nourishing, moistening, restraining, and gathering. Kidney yin and Kidney yang are mutually dependent, promoting, and restraining. The dynamic interaction between the two maintains the normal activities of life, leading to an internal harmony of yin and yang, and a healthy functioning of the body's organs.

33. What is the concept of *mìng mén*? Where is it located and what is its form and function?

Mìng mén (命門 *mìng mén*) is often translated as 'gate of vitality' or 'gate of life.' This term can be traced back 2,500 years, when it was first mentioned in the *Divine Pivot* (靈樞 *líng shū*), Chapter 5: "*Mìng mén*, is eye." About this discourse, there are many interpretations, but overall, *mìng mén* is only a term of location during that period of time. The *Classic of Difficulties* (難經 *nán jīng*) was the first to indicate that *mìng mén* is the storage place for congenital qi, and the root of human life. Since then, *mìng mén* has taken on the meaning of 'gate of vitality' and has drawn a lot of attention, becoming one of the most important parts for *zàng fǔ* study.

There is a lot of controversy regarding *mìng mén*'s location, which can be summed up in the following discussion:

(1) One theory is that the right side Kidney is *mìng mén*. This point first appeared in the *Classic of Difficulties* (難經 *nán jīng*), 36th question: "There are two Kidneys, the one on the left side is the Kidney and the one on the right side is *mìng mén*. *Mìng mén* is the house of the essence and *shén*, and the storage place for primary qi (原氣 *yuán qì*). Thus it stores the essence and sperm in men, and is connected with the womb in women." This interpretation is followed by Wang Shu-He (王叔和, 210-280) in the *Pulse Classic* (脈經 *mài jīng*), Chen Wu-Ze (陳無擇, 1131-1189) in *Three Reason Formula* (三因方 *sān yīn fāng*), Yan Yong-He (顏用和, 1199-1267) in *Formula for Succoring the Sick* (濟生方 *jǐ shēng fāng*), and Li Chan (李梴, 1575) in *Introduction to Medicine* (醫學入門 *yī xué rù mén*). All follow this theory.

(2) Another theory is that *mìng mén* is a general term for both Kidneys. The Ming dynasty physician Yu Tuan (虞摶, 1438-1517) rejected the theory that the left side is the Kidney and the right side is *mìng mén*. In his book *Medical Story* (醫學正傳 *yī xué zhèng zhuàn*), Yu wrote that "both Kidneys are the root of primary qi, the fundamental element of life, even though it is a water organ, it stores the ministerial fire; therefore, both Kidneys should be called *mìng mén*." Zhang Jing-Yue (張景岳, 1563-1640) also pointed out in *Systemic Compilation of the Internal Clinic* (類經附翼 *lèi jīng fù yì*), Vol. 3: "Both Kidneys are *mìng mén*. *Mìng mén* is the house for water and fire, root of the yin and yang, sea of the essence, and is the place for life or death."

(3) Another theory is that *mìng mén* is located between the Kidneys, independent from and outside of the Kidneys. This theory was introduced by Zhao Xian-Ke (趙獻可, 1573-1664), and is based on *Basic Questions* (素問 *shù wèn*), Chapter 52, which states: "next to the 7th vertebrae, there is a small 'heart' in between," which he believes to be *mìng mén* between the two Kidneys. He discussed this idea in his book *Key Link of Medicine* (醫貫 *yī guàn*): "These two Kidneys, left side belonging to yin water and right side belonging to yang water. Moving 1.5 cun towards the center from each side arrives at the house of *mìng mén*. Its right side is ministerial fire, its left side is primary water." This argument influenced TCM theory in the Qing Dynasty, as can be seen in the books *Medical Three Character Classic* (醫學三字經 *yī xué sān zì jīng*) by Chen Xiu-Yan (陳修園, 1753-1823), *Judgment and Treatment for Similar Patterns* (類証治裁) by Lin Pei-Qin (林佩琴, 1771-1839), *Origin of Materia Medica* (本經逢原 *běn jīng féng yuán*) by Zhang Lu (張璐, 1617-1700), and *New Compilation of Materia Medica* (本草求真 *běn cǎo qiú zhēn*) by Huang Gong-Xiu (黃宮繡, 1720-1817). These books all share a similar view of *mìng mén*.

(4) There is saying that *mìng mén* is a motive force between the Kidneys. This theory believes that *mìng mén* is located between the two Kidneys, but that it is neither water nor fire; it is only the place for primary qi. Moreover, this theory suggests that *mìng mén* is a formless organ. Sun Yi-Kui (孫一奎, 1522-1619) put forward this view in his book *Medical Purpose Thread* (醫旨緒餘 *yī zhǐ xù yú*), stating: "*Mìng mén* is the motive qi in between the Kidneys, it is neither water nor fire, it is the essential element for human procreation, it is the root of yin and yang, it is the prenatal Taiji, and the movement of the five phases starts from here to form *zàng fǔ* organs."

Despite the differing theories about the location and form of *mìng mén*, they all agree on its main physiological functions. *Mìng mén* is yang and possesses fire, while the Kidney belongs to water. *Mìng mén* fire is the fire within the water, and generates primary qi. It is the root and basic element of human life. The physiological functions of *mìng mén* can be summarized as follows:

(1) It is the root of primary qi, and the origin of the motive force and thermal energy that carries out body metabolism.
(2) It provides thermal energy to the Triple Burner, assisting its function of qi transformation.
(3) *Mìng mén* fire warms the Spleen and Stomach, assisting their function of transformation and transportation.
(4) It stores essence in the Kidney, stimulates development of secondary sexual characteristics and maturation of sexual instincts during puberty, and maintains healthy sexual capacity.
(5) It receives qi to assist the Lung in respiration, receiving oxygen to provide energy to the entire body.
(6) It supplies ministerial fire to the Liver, assisting its function of coursing and discharging.

Ancient physicians agree that the physiological function of *mìng mén* and the Kidney are closely related. *Mìng mén* fire is Kidney yang, primary yang (原陽 *yuán yáng*), and true yang (真陽 *zhēn yáng*); while *mìng mén* water is Kidney yin, primary yin (原陰 *yuán yīn*), and true yin (真陰 *zhēn yīn*). Through discourse on this concept of *mìng mén*, ancient physicians brought attention to this significant aspect of the Kidney's physiological function.

34. What is the difference between Kidney Yang Deficiency (腎陽虛) and *mìng mén* Fire Decline (命門火衰)?

As noted above, the concept of *mìng mén*, its location, form, and function, has been debated for millenia by ancient physicians, and even today there are still differing opinions. There are two views regarding its form: tangible or visible vs. intangible or invisible; and three views about its location: right side Kidney, both Kidneys, or in between the two Kidneys. However, when it comes to the physiological function of *mìng mén* and the Kidney, there is general agreement that Kidney yang is the same as *mìng mén* fire, while Kidney yin is the same as *mìng mén* water. Zhang Jing-Yue (張景岳, 1563-1640), in *Appendices to the Classified Classic* (類經附翼 *lèi jīng fù yì*, 1624), said: "*Mìng mén* fire is called primary qi (原氣 *yuán qì*). *Mìng mén* water is called primary essence (原精 *yuán jīng*)." This thesis established the foundation for *mìng mén* fire being the same as Kidney yang. Zhao Xian-Ke (趙獻可, 1573-1664) also noted: "*Mìng mén*, king fire, is fire within the water; they are interdependent and never separate."

The clinical manifestations of *mìng mén* fire decline (命門火衰 *mìng mén huǒ shuāi*) are the same as what is seen in Kidney yang deficiency including lower back pain, soreness and weakness in the knees, dark facial complexion, impotency or premature ejaculation in men, infertility in women, cold limbs, fatigue, and melancholy. The herbal formula for *mìng mén* fire decline also has the function of replenishing Kidney yang. Thus *mìng mén* fire decline is basically the same as Kidney yang deficiency. The reason it is called '*mìng mén* fire decline' is simply to emphasize the importance of this aspect of Kidney yang.

35. What is the basis for the saying that Kidney disease only has deficiency patterns?

Northern Song dynasty physician Qian Yi (錢乙, 1032-1113) in *Craft of Medicines and Patterns for Children* (小兒藥証直訣 *xiǎo èr yào zhèng zhí jué*) stated that "Kidney disease mainly has deficiency patterns, no excess patterns." He was the first person to propose this theory, which gradually emerged in the medical field and has greatly influenced later generations of physicians. It is still maintained that the replenishing or tonifying method is the universal treatment principle for Kidney disease.

Zhang Yuan-Su (張元素, 1131-1234) in *Origin of Medicine* (醫學啟源 *yī xué qǐ yuán*) stated: "The Kidney does not have an excess pattern, therefore purging or reducing treatments should not be used. There are only herbs to tonify the Kidney in Dr. Qian's formula, and no herbs to drain the Kidney." Liu Chun (劉純, 1363-1489) in *Primary Study Medical Classic* (醫經小學 *yī jīng xiǎo xué*) compared the Liver and Kidney to prove that there is no statement of Kidney excess pattern. He said: "The Kidney governs sealing and storing, while the Liver governs coursing and discharging; the Kidney belongs to primary water, and should only be replenished without purging; while the Liver belongs to ministerial fire, and should only be purged without tonifying." There are many other books such as *Medical Story* (醫學正傳 *yī xué zhèng zhuàn*, 1515) by Yu Tuan (虞摶), *Medical Checklist* (醫學綱目 *yī xué gāng mù*, 1565) by Lou Ying (樓英), *Medical Notes* (醫林繩墨 *yī lín shéng mò*, 1584) by Fang Yu (方隅), *Required Book for Grandmaster* (醫宗必讀, 1637) by Li Zhong-Zi (李中梓), *Lantai Criterion* (蘭臺軌範, 1764) by Xu Ling-Tai (許靈胎), and *Wondrous Lantern for Peering into the Origin and Development of Miscellaneous Disease* (雜病源流犀燭, 1773) by Shen Jin-Ao (瀋金鰲), that are unanimous in stating that Kidney disease is without excess patterns.

Even today's national textbook for TCM universities in China still agree that "Kidney disease is without excess patterns, and should not be drained, purged, or reduced." The textbook *Chinese Internal Medicine* (中醫內科學 *zhōng yī nèi kē xué*) states: "Generally speaking, Kidney disease is without excess patterns and exterior patterns. Kidney heat pattern belongs to pathological changes of the Kidney yin, while Kidney cold pattern belongs to pathological changes of the Kidney yang." This means there are heat and cold conditions in Kidney disease, but they are deficiency heat and deficiency cold, not excess heat and excess cold. The general treatment principle for Kidney disease is to 'replenish its deficiency, not reduce its excess.' *Textbook TCM Diagnosis* (中醫診斷學 *zhōng yī zhěn duàn xué*) only lists the patterns Kidney qi deficiency, Kidney yang deficiency, Kidney essence deficiency, Kidney yin deficiency, Kidney qi failing to secure, and Kidney failing to grasp qi. There are no Kidney excess patterns mentioned in this book.

There are three major reasons why many physicians today believe that Kidney disease does not have excess patterns, and therefore purging and reducing treatment methods should not be used for Kidney disease.

(1) The Kidney is prone to deficiency. The Kidney is the organ that stores essence. The nature of the Kidney is "storing and sealing without releasing, fulfilling without overage." *Basic Questions* (素問 *sù wèn*), Chapter 6, states: "The Kidney takes charge of hibernation, and is responsible for storing and sealing." The Kidney stores 'congenital essence,' which is the basis of yin and yang, and the root of human life. Thus the Kidney has been called the 'congenital root.' Kidney essence has the function of promoting growth, development, and

reproduction, Kidney essence transforms into primary yin and primary yang, which are the root of the entire body. Thus if Kidney essence is impaired or consumed, it can affect the whole body or involve other organs. By the same token, pathological changes in other organs can readily affect the Kidney, leading to Kidney deficiency. That is why Kidney disease is commonly seen as essence qi insufficiency (精氣奪 *jīng qì duó*).

(2) Influence of ancient physicians. There are many ancient physicians such as Qian Yi (錢乙), Zhao Xian-Ke (趙獻可), and Zhang Jing-Yue (張景岳), who hold the view that "Kidney disease is without excess patterns" and treatment methods for Kidney disease should "tonify and replenish." There are many herbal formulas based on this theory still widely used today, imperceptibly influencing modern physicians.

(3) Influenced by the theory that states: "Excess is *tài yáng* disease, while deficiency is *shào yīn* disease." This theory indicates the regular pattern of pathological change, and was proposed by Ke Yun-Bo (柯韻伯, 1662-1735), a well-known classics scholar in the Qing dynasty. For pathological changes in the *tài yáng* and *shào yīn*, deficiency patterns are attributed to the Kidney, while excess patterns are attributed to its internally-externally related organ, the Urinary Bladder. An example of such an excess pattern would be damp-heat in the Urinary Bladder.

36. Do Kidney excess patterns exist and why?

Qian Yi (錢乙, 1032-1113), in his book *Craft of Medicines and Patterns for Children* (小兒藥証直訣 *xiǎo èr yào zhèng zhí jué*), advanced the theory that Kidney disease only has deficiency patterns. His theory had a great impact on subsequent generations of physicians, causing many to ignore the patterns and pathological changes of of Kidney excess.

Records of the existence of Kidney excess can be traced back to the *Yellow Emperor's Internal Classic* (黃帝內經 *nèi jīng*) such as this passage in *Divine Pivot* (靈樞 *líng shū*), Chapter 18: "When the Kidney is deficient, there are cold limbs; when the Kidney is excessive, there is abdominal distention or bloating." *Divine Pivot*, Chapter 35, further mentions Kidney excess signs and symptoms: "Kidney distention, manifesting with abdominal distention and bloating that radiates to the back with aching and pain in the lower back, loins, and thighs." Sun Si-Miao (孫思邈, 581-682), in *Thousand Ducat Formulas* (備急千金要方 *bèi jí qiān jīn yào fāng*, 652), Vol. 19, Chapter 2, discusses both Kidney deficiency and excess patterns. At the end of the chapter, there are treatment strategies and herbal formulas for Kidney excess patterns such as Drain Kidney Decoction (瀉腎湯 *xiè shèn tāng*) and Glans Pain Decoction (莖頭痛方 *jīng tǒu tòng fāng*). Zhang Jing-Yue (張景岳, 1563-1640), in *Collected Treaties of Jing-Yue* (景岳全書 *jīng yuè quán shū*, 1624), states: "Kidney excess is mostly caused by stagnation or obstruction in the lower burner and manifests as pain, distention, burning urination, or burning defecation."

Overall, there are many other books that document the existence of Kidney excess along with its patterns and treatments. These books include the *Treasury Classic* (中藏經 *zhōng zàng jīng*, 184-220), *Sacred and Favorite Formulas from Tai Ping Era* (太平聖惠方 *tài píng sh`eng huì fāng*, 978-992), *Comprehensive Re-*

cording of Sage-like Benefit from the Zheng He Era (聖濟總錄 *shèng jí zǒng lù*, 1122), and *Precious Mirror of Oriental Medicine* (東醫寶鑑 *dōng yī bǎo jiàn*, 1611). Thus many physicians do believe that Kidney excess patterns clinically exist.

The idea that Kidney disease does not have excess patterns is incompatible with the foundational theories of TCM. First of all, *zàng fǔ* theory uses the five *zàng* organs as a unit to study physiological activities and pathological changes of the human body. Pathological change in the internal organs is either excess or deficiency. Suggesting that the Heart, Lung, Spleen, and Liver all have excess and deficiency patterns, but the Kidney does not, is contrary to *zàng fǔ* theory.

The TCM university textbook *Traditional Chinese Medicine Fundamental Theory* (中醫基礎理論 *zhōng yī jī chǔ lǐ lùn*) states: "Excess patterns mainly refer to the hyperactivity of pathogenic factors or pathogenic qi (邪氣 *xié qì*). In the early stages of illness, it is common to see exogenous diseases caused by the six exopathogenic factors; in the mid-stage of illness, it is common to see pathological changes caused by phlegm, food, blood stagnation, or water retention." Since the Kidney is connected with all other organs, why can other organs be invaded by pathogenic factors but not the Kidney? Moreover, phlegm, dampness, and water can invade any area of the body, from the body's surface to the internal organs. Thus the Kidney would be no exception.

Furthermore, the dynamic of opposites is fundamental to the theory of yin and yang. Deficiency patterns are associated with yin, while excess patterns are associated with yang. From a clinical treatment perspective, when addressing the pathological changes of any organ, there are opposing methods. For instance, if there is tonifying, then there is reducing, if there is binding, then there is purging, and if there is warming, then there is cooling. The notion that Kidney disease only has deficiency patterns would suggest that the Kidney is an independent unit from all other organs and is contrary to the theory of yin and yang. Thus the concept that Kidney disease is without excess patterns is inconsistent with the theories of Chinese medicine.

The pathogenesis of Kidney excess patterns can be summed up in three aspects: exopathogenic invasion of the Kidney; pathological changes of other organs affecting the Kidney; and internal injury of the Kidney, leading to an excess of pathogenic factors. The most common Kidney excess patterns seen in the clinic are the following:

(1) Fixed Kidney disorder (腎著 *shèn zhuó*): Wind, cold, and dampness invading the Kidney channel and manifesting with aching or pain in the lower back, loins, and knees, abdominal pain that is resistant to pressure, lower abdominal spasms, constipation, difficult urination, dysmenorrhea, or amenorrhea. The pulse is deep and forceful.

(2) Turbid dampness encumbering the Kidney (濕濁困腎 *shī zhuó kùn shèn*): Long-term accumulation of turbid dampness that encumbers the Kidney, leading to uremia or an increased concentration of waste products in the blood. It is a critical condition and manifests with scanty urine or anuria, headache with dizziness, blurry vision, tinnitus, deafness, or even coma, loss of consciousness, or convulsions.

(3) Damp-heat accumulating in the Kidney (濕熱蘊腎 *shī rè yùn shèn*): Damp-heat accumulation that impairs the qi transformation function of the Kidney, manifesting with yellow or cloudy urine, hematuria, and urination that is urgent, frequent, burning, or painful. The pain may radiate to the lower back, and there may be dry mouth or a bitter taste in the mouth, facial or entire body edema, or even symptoms of urinary calculi. The pulse is wiry and rapid.

(4) Blood stagnation in the Kidney (淤血阻腎 *yū xuě zú shèn*): Blood stasis obstruction in the Kidney or the Kidney channel, blocking qi and blood circulation, and manifesting with severe lower back pain or pain with pressure, limited and difficult movement, impotency, or erectile dysfunction.

37. In which conditions do we see the pattern Kidney Qi Failing to Secure (腎氣不固)?

The Kidney is the prenatal root; it stores essence, possesses the primary yang, and governs hibernation. *Basic Questions* (素問 *sù wèn*), Chapter 9, states: "The Kidney governs hibernation; it is the root of storage and sealing." When Kidney qi is deficient, the Kidney cannot store and seal properly, resulting in 'leakage,' which can be seen in the following five conditions:

(1) Anterior yin orifice failing to secure, leading to Urinary Bladder dysfunction, which results in frequent urination, nocturnal urination, enuresis, oliguria, anuria, incontinence of urine, dribbling after urination, or bedwetting.
(2) Posterior yin orifice failing to secure, leading to Large Intestine dysfunction, which results in loose stools or chronic diarrhea.
(3) 'Essence gate' (精關 *jīng guān*) failing to secure, leading to seminal emission, impotence, premature ejaculation, copious clear vaginal discharge, and habitual miscarriage.
(4) Penetrating vessel and Conception vessel (衝任 *chōng rèn*) failing to secure, leading to irregular uterine bleeding such as spotting, menorrhagia, or metrorrhagia.
(5) Fetus failing to be secure, leading to miscarriage

Other related symptoms include aching, soreness, and weakness in the lower back and knees, physical and mental fatigue, hearing loss, tinnitus, a pale tongue with a white coating, and a deep weak pulse.

38. Kidney yin deficiency can cause both amenorrhea and menorrhagia. What is the pathogenesis of these conditions?

Menses occurs in the uterus but is closely related to the function of the Kidney, which stores prenatal and postnatal essence. The physiology of puberty, fertility, conception, pregnancy, and menopause are greatly influenced by the condition of Kidney essence. *Basic Questions* (素問 *sù wèn*), Chapter 1, states: "For a female, the Kidney qi prevails, the teeth change, and the hair grows when seven years old. When she is fourteen years old, the heavenly dew appears, the Conception vessel opens, the Penetrating vessel becomes exuberant, and menstruation begins to regularly occur so that she can become pregnant and bear children. At the age of forty-nine, the Conception vessel becomes debilitated, and the qi and blood of the Penetrating vessel declines and becomes scanty. The heavenly dew is exhausted, and the menstrual tunnel becomes obstructed. Her physique becomes old and feeble, and she can conceive no more."

Heavenly dew (天癸 tiān guǐ) is an invisible liquid that helps in the development of the human body, sexual functions, and in women, the ability to produce offspring. It is a type of yin essence and part of congenital essence that is derived from the parents at conception and is stored inside the Kidney after birth. It is nourished and replenished by post-natal essence and is stimulated by Kidney qi to develop and mature, increasing and decreasing with Kidney qi. Furthermore, Kidney essence transforms into blood, which is the primary ingredient of menses. Thus Kidney essence is one of the most fundamental substances in the formation of menstrual blood.

When Kidney yin is deficient, Kidney essence will lose nourishment and be consumed. Heavenly dew decreases as well. With the lack of blood being generated, the Penetrating and Conception vessels cannot be filled, resulting in scanty menses or amenorrhea. The book *True Lineage of Medicine* (醫學正傳 yī xué zhèng zhuàn, 1515) states: "Menstruation depends on Kidney essence to nourish and fertilize; if Kidney essence is insufficient, then menses will be dry and exhausted."

When Kidney yin is insufficient, it cannot anchor yang. This leads to a relative excess of yang, which generates deficiency fire. Deficiency fire disturbs the Penetrating and Conception vessels, pushing blood outward, resulting in menorrhagia and metrostaxis. As the *Ten Books of Dong Yuan, Blue Room Secret Treasures* (東垣十書, 蘭室密藏 dōng yuán shí shū, lán shì mì zàng) states: "Women who have excessive menstrual bleeding (崩漏 bēng lòu, menorrhagia, and metrostaxis) have insufficient Kidney liquid (yin) that cannot hold the fire of the uterus and the Penetrating and Conception vessels. This fire pushes the blood, resulting in profuse bleeding."

In summary, Kidney yin deficiency can lead to two opposite symptoms: amenorrhea or menorrhagia/metrostaxis. This is due to a difference in pathogenesis. Amenorrhea is due to Kidney yin insufficiency, resulting in Kidney essence and blood deficiency that cannot fill the Penetrating and Conception vessels, while menorrhagia or metrostaxis is due to yin deficiency fire that pushes the blood, resulting in heavy bleeding.

39. What is the history and development of *zàng fǔ* pattern identification?

Zàng fǔ pattern identification (臟腑辯證 *zàng fǔ biàn zhèng*) is based on the understanding of the physiological functions and pathological characteristics of the *zàng fǔ* organs, a comprehensive analysis of the symptoms, signs, and related disease data collected by the four examination techniques to determine the location of the disease and its pathological characteristics. This means that *zàng fǔ* pattern identification uses the location and pathological characteristics of the *zàng fǔ* organs as a guideline to classifying disease patterns.

The significance of *zàng fǔ* pattern identification is the ability to more accurately identify the location of disease, and is therefore the most common pattern differentiation method used in clinical practice. It is the most important system of traditional Chinese medicine pattern identification with a wide range of applications and is especially suitable for the differentiation of internal diseases, gynecological conditions, and pediatric issues.

The establishment, development, and completion of the *zàng fǔ* pattern identification system progressed over several dynasties from the contributions of many medical experts who analyzed and summarized the clinical experience and theories of their predecessors. This is a process of inheritance and development, including the four most important stages below:

(1) Theory gestation or embryonic stage (萌芽時期 *méng yá shí qī*)

The origin of pattern identification can be traced back to the *Yellow Emperor's Inner Classic* (黃帝內經 *huáng dì nèi jīng*, c. 200). The book records the names of many disease patterns and their clinical manifestations. For example, *Basic Questions* (素問 *sù wèn*), Chapter 29, points out that "Spleen qi deficiency can manifest as weakness in the limbs and can involve other *zàng fǔ* organs." *Divine Pivot* (靈樞 *líng shū*), Chapter 8, specifically describes the clinical manifestations of qi deficiency syndrome in the five *zàng* organs, and points out the importance of examining the signs and symptoms in order to judge the state of qi (excess or deficiency) and decide the appropriate treatment method. *Basic Questions*, Chapter 19, expounds on the pathogenesis of different clinical manifestations from the perspective of location (*zàng fǔ* organ), etiology, and nature of the disease, along with principles of treatment.

Although a system of pattern identification and treatment strategies (辯證論治 *biàn zhèng lùn zhì*) was not in the *Yellow Emperor's Inner Classic*, it did contain theories about the physiology and pathology of the *zàng fǔ* organs, channels, qi, blood, and body fluids; theories on the etiology of the six exopathogens, seven emotions, diet, physical overstrain; theories on the pathogenesis of the battle between antipathogenic qi and pathogenic qi (正邪相爭 *zhèng xié xiāng zhēng*); mechanisms of ascending and descending qi (氣機升降 *qì jī shēng jiàng*); yin and yang disharmony; the diagnostic methods of combining observation (望 *wàng*), listening and smelling (聞 *wén*), inquiry (問 *wèn*), and palpation (切 *qiè*); as well as the basic principles of treatment and herbal prescription. All the above has become the theoretical foundation in forming the pattern identification and treatment system.

During the Eastern Han Dynasty (20-220), Zhang Zhong-Jing's (張仲景, 150-215) *Discussion of Cold Damage and Miscellaneous Diseases* (傷寒雜病論 *shāng hán zá bìng lùn*) was the first book to more clearly present the concept of pattern identification and treatment, and established a relatively complete system. 'Normal pulse' (平脈 *píng mài*) pattern identification in the *Discussion of Cold Damage* (傷寒論 *shāng hán lùn*) is the earliest record of pattern identification. Moreover, both *Discussion of Cold Damage* and *Essentials from the Golden Cabinet* (金匱要略 *jīn guì yào luè*) include the titles "Differentiation of Taiyang disease and Treatment Strategies," establishing both the six channels pattern identification system and the *zàng fǔ* pattern identification system. They also pointed out the need to observe and analyze the pulse and symptoms, judge the development and change of the disease, and determine the treatment principle according to different patterns, which reflects the basic idea of pattern identification. In *Discussion of Cold Damage and Miscellaneous Diseases*, concepts such as the exterior, interior, cold, heat, deficiency, excess, yin, yang, *zàng fǔ* organs, qi, and blood are widely used as the basic content of pattern identification, aiming to target different pathogeneses and patterns with corresponding treatment principles and prescriptions. Since then, physicians in subsequent dynasties have greatly enriched and developed the content of pattern identification and treatment from many different angles. Thus the *Yellow Emperor's Inner Classic* and *Discussion of Cold Damage* form the foundation of the embryonic period of *zàng fǔ* pattern identification.

(2) The first systematic organization and development

Treasury Classic (中藏經 *zhōng cáng jīng*), published in the Han Dynasty (202 BCE–220 CE), pioneered the eight principles of *zàng fǔ* organ pattern identification, namely the indicators of deficiency, excess, cold, heat, life, death, smooth flow (順 *shùn*), and reversed flow (逆 *nì*), and was the first to summarize and organize the scattered *zàng fǔ* organs theory mentioned in the *Yellow Emperor's Inner Classic*. The first and middle volume of the book are divided into eleven chapters that comprehensively discuss each *zàng fǔ* organ from the aspects of deficiency, excess, cold, heat, life, and death. This book basically combines the previous literature on *zàng fǔ* organ disease patterns, but offers more in-depth development of the basic conceptual relationships. The book takes deficiency, excess, cold, and heat as the main points of pattern differentiation, and establishes treatment strategies for *zàng fǔ* disease patterns, stating: "If deficient, then replenish and tonify; if excessive, then relieve and purge; if cold, then warm; if hot, then cool; if neither deficiency nor excess, then adjust the channels." Furthermore, this book included discussion of the *fǔ* organs and marks the initial formation of a true system of *zàng fǔ* pattern identification.

(3) The second systematic organization and improvement

Following the *Treasury Classic*, many other works helped to further develop *zàng fǔ* pattern identification such as the *Pulse Classic* (脈經 *mài jīng*) by Wang Shu-He (王叔和, 220-581) and *Treatise on Causes and Symptoms of Diseases* (諸病源候論 *zhū bìng yuán hòu lùn*) by Chao Yuan-Fang (巢元方, 610). However, what can be deemed the second time that the *zàng fǔ* pattern identification system was comprehensively re-organized is in the *Emergency Formulas Worth a Thousand Gold Pieces* (備急千金要方 *bèi jí qiān jīn yào fang*, 652) by Sun Si-Miao (孫思邈, 581-682). This book was not limited to theory, it also supplemented the content of prescriptions, using deficiency and excess as guidelines for treatment, and adding corresponding pulse images as the basis for judging disease location and nature. In addition, it added the passageways of *zàng fǔ* channels, expanded on the pathological characteristics of *zàng fǔ* organs, and opened up new ideas for determining the location and nature of the pathogeneses involving *zàng fǔ* organs. Overall, this book showed a deeper understanding of the physiology, pathology, diagnosis, and treatment of *zàng fǔ* organs, and presented a more systematic discussion and narrative.

Craft of Medicines and Patterns for Children (小兒藥証直訣 *xiǎo ér yào zhèng zhí jué*), written by Qian Yi (錢乙, 1032-1113) and compiled by Yan Xiao-Zhong (閻孝忠, 1119), was the first major breakthrough of *zàng fǔ* pattern identification in the field of pediatrics. It provided a concise summary of pediatric physiology, pathology, five *zàng* organ patterns, their treatment principles, and the scope of application. Qian Yi believed that physically, a child's "five *zàng* organs and six *fǔ* organs are formed, but not completely developed; or completely developed, but not strong." Thus pathologically, a child's *zàng fǔ* organs are weak in function, prone to deficiency or excess, and readily develop heat or cold conditions. This theory became his guiding principle in the clinic. His book systematically presented the pattern identification theory of the five *zàng* organs in the field of pediatrics, listing the main syndromes, treatment strategies, and prescriptions. He also believed that the five *zàng* organs are connected as a whole, and that they are closely related to the natural environment.

(4) The third systematic organization and maturation

Liu Wan-Su (劉完素, 1110-1200), in *Basic Questions: Discourse on Mechanisms for Preserving Life* (素問病機氣宜保命集 *sù wèn bìng jī qì yí bǎo mìng jí*), put forward the theory involving the pathogenesis of the six qi in relation to the *zàng fǔ* organs. The core content for his theory was that all illnesses originate from the dysfunction of the internal *zàng fǔ* organs or the channels and collaterals. He emphasized that the internal organs correspond to "the heavens and the earth," referring to the natural environment. When the internal organs are deficient or excessive, syndromes similar to wind, cold, dampness, fire, dryness, and heat may appear. However, he also emphasized that changes in the body's own qi are involved with the development of the disease.

In the book *Medical Origin* (醫學啟源 *yī xué qí yuán*, 1186), Zhang Yuan-Su (張元素) comprehensively explained the physiology of the *zàng fǔ* organs, patterns and symptoms, pulse conditions, prognosis, treatment strategies and methods, herbal formulas, and individual herbs. His greatest contribution to the pattern identification of *zàng fǔ* organs was putting forward the theory relating herbs to channels, specifically the concepts of attributive channels (歸經 *guī jīng*) and guiding channels (引經

yīn jīng), which marked a significant advance in the developoment of the theory of herbal pharmacology. He pointed out the corresponding relationships between specific herbs and *zàng fǔ* organs, making a huge impact on *zàng fǔ* pattern identification for later generations.

(5) Promotion and widespread usage

In recent decades, ancient medical records have been continuously sorted and summarized, and a relatively complete system of *zàng fǔ* pattern identification theory has been consolidated. In the middle of the 20th century, *zàng fǔ* pattern identification was incorporated into the textbooks of colleges and universities of TCM, and since then, has quickly spread and become widely used in clinical practice.

Zàng fǔ pattern identification is the core of TCM pattern identification theory. It has formed through many generations of practitioners over a period of more than two thousand years of clinical practice, continually revised, developed, improved, and supplemented. The *zàng fǔ* organs are the main basis for clinical disease and syndrome positioning, and *zàng fǔ* pattern identification is the foundation for other pattern identification methods. Its precise concept, specific content, clear outline, and complete systemization, makes it easier to fit into clinical practice, resulting in widespread usage.

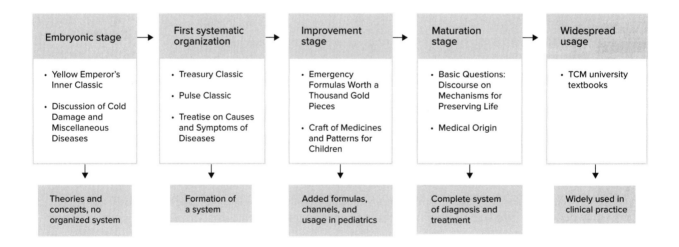

Chart 24.39.1 History and development of pattern identification in TCM diagnosis

40. What are the pattern identification methods and their relationships?

A pattern (證 *zhèng*) can also be referred to as a syndrome, which is a combination of signs and symptoms that form a distinct clinical picture indicative of a particular disorder. It is the summary of the environment, pathogens, pathological location, pathogenesis, condition of the antipathogenic qi (正氣 *zhèng qì*) and pathogenic qi (邪氣 *xié qì*), signs and symptoms, and the constitution of the patient. The pattern comprehensively and concretely reflects the nature and features of a disease at a given stage. Thus, the pattern reflects the essence of a disease at the moment of the assessment.

Pattern identification (辯證 *biàn zhèng*), also known as pattern classification or syndrome differentiation, is the most critical component of traditional Chinese medicine diagnosis. It is the process by which clinical information obtained from examination through observation (望 *wàng*), listening and smelling (聞 *wén*), inquiry (問 *wèn*), and palpation (切 *qiè*) is analyzed, synthesized, and inferred, leading to a clear representation of a particular phase of a TCM disease pattern.

I. Basic principles of TCM pattern identification

Pattern identification is one of the most important and unique diagnosis methods in TCM. Only on the basis of pattern identification can the treatment method be determined. Pattern identification has been established and developed based on the following TCM theories:

(1) Holistic approach

Holism is a fundamental concept of TCM. The holistic approach in diagnosis refers to the comprehensive consideration of the human body and its natural surroundings. This has two aspects. First, the human body is viewed as an organic whole, the internal *zàng fǔ* organs are the center of the body, and the outer parts such as the limbs, five sensory organs, nine orifices, skin, muscles, vessels, tendons, and bones, are all linked to the *zàng fǔ* organs through channels and collaterals. During the diagnostic process, special attention is paid to the interrelation and interaction between local pathological changes and the maladjustment of the whole body. Local pathological changes may affect the whole body and pathological changes of the whole body may, in turn, be reflected locally. External disorders may penetrate into the interior or pathological changes of the internal organs may manifest externally.

Second, is the aspect of the unification of the human body and its surroundings. Human beings are affected by such natural conditions as weather and other environmental influences. When there are abnormal changes in the natural environment, or when the human body fails to adapt itself to such changes, pathological change will certainly occur in the body.

(2) Dynamic approach

One of the key characteristics of TCM is to study the human body as a dynamic equilibrium that can self-adjust to maintain its own stability within certain limits. TCM theory states that there is a normal state of relative equilibrium between the human body and the external environment, as well as among the *zàng fǔ* organs within the body. This balance is dynamic and constantly self-adjusting to sustain normal physiological activity in the human body. If this dynamic balance is broken to the extent that it cannot immediately be restored through self-adjustment, then the disease process will occur.

Disease represents the entire course of pathological changes associated with an illness. Over the course of the disease, pathogenic qi battles with antipathogenic qi in a process that is dynamic; the presentation will therefore undergo continuing changes in accordance with certain rules. By contrast, the pattern describes the pathology at a particular stage of the disease, where there is a certain configuration in the battle between the pathogenic qi and antipathogenic qi. A single disease can evolve through multiple patterns, and the same pattern can be found in multiple diseases.

II. Characteristics of the pattern identification method

Pattern identification is an important way of clinical thinking. It involves a comprehensive inspection of all aspects of a patient's situation beyond current signs and symptoms, including etiology, disease onset, pathogenesis, medical history, environmental factors, and the strength of a patient's antipathogenic qi in relation to the invading pathogenic qi. Differences in individual factors (因人 *yīn rén*), geographical factors (因地 *yīn dì*), and seasonal or climatic factors (因時 *yīn shí*) are also taken into consideration. In TCM, the "same disease can have a different pattern" (同病異証 *tong bìng yì zhèng*) and a "different disease can have the same pattern" (異病同証 *yì bìng tong zhèng*). Thus pattern identification aims to determine the appropriate treatment strategy for a specific pattern or presentation of a disease in an individual, rather than for a disease in general.

Pattern identification searches for the root of a disease and can determine cause and effect (因果 *yīn guǒ*), primary and secondary issues, priority of issues, the main signs and symptoms, and the nature of a disease at a specific stage. Thus it is very good at highlighting key points of a disease, providing a guideline for appropriate treatment choices, and emphasizing the dynamic changes in the course of disease and treatment.

III. Different pattern identification methods, applications, and relationships

The history of pattern identification can be traced back to the *Yellow Emperor's Internal Classic*. This book records many disease patterns and their clinical manifestations. Over thousands of years of clinical practice, many pattern identification methods were developed such as eight principles pattern identification, six channels pattern identification, four levels pattern identification, and etiology pattern identification, among others. These methods summarize pathological tendencies and the understanding of patterns from different perspectives. Each method has its special emphasis and they are mutually related and supplemental. The following eight pattern identification methods are the most commonly used.

(1) Eight principles pattern identification (八綱辯證 *bā gāng biàn zhèng*)

The eight principles (八綱 *bā gāng*) refers to the four complimentary pairs of indications: exterior and interior, heat and cold, excess and deficiency, and yin and yang. The eight principles pattern identification organizes the clinical manifestations of disease into the general categories of yin and yang, classifying the disease location as exterior or interior, the thermal nature of the pathogen as cold or hot, and the strength of the antipathogenic qi against the pathogenic qi as deficient or excessive.

Eight principles pattern identification helps in understanding the location and nature of pathological changes, the course of the disease, and the condition and strength of the antipathogenic qi against the pathogenic qi. It also helps in predicting disease development and directing treatment. Thus the eight principles guides all pattern identification methods, and the specifics of each method can be summarized in the eight principles.

Eight principles pattern identification is closely related and complementary to *zàng fǔ* pattern identification. Whereas the former summarizes a disease condition into four indications that provides general treatment guidance, the latter delves into more specifics that are especially useful in the diagnosis of miscellaneous diseases such as in internal medicine, gynecology, or pediatrics.

(2) Qi, blood, and body fluid pattern identification (氣血津液辯證 *qì xuě jīn yè biàn zhèng*)

This method analyzes and summarizes clinical manifestations using the theory of qi, blood, and body fluids along with the theory of *zàng fǔ*. Qi, blood, and body fluids are the fundamental materials in the composition of the human body as well as the motive force for maintaining the body's physiological activities. The production and proper usage of qi, blood, and body fluids depends on the proper functioning of the *zàng fǔ* organs.

When there is dysfunction of the *zàng fǔ* organs, there must also be a pathological change in qi, blood, and body fluids, while dysfunction of qi, blood, and body fluids, in turn, indicates abnormal function of the *zàng fǔ* organs. Physiologically, they coexist and are interdependent; pathologically, they influence and affect each other. Thus it is commonly seen in clinic for *zàng fǔ* pattern identification to be combined with qi, blood, and body fluids pattern identification.

(3) Etiology pattern identification (病因辯證 *bìng yīn biàn zhèng*)

This method analyzes the signs and symptoms with bodily evidence of the disease in order to grasp the cause of disease, differentiate the nature of the pattern, and determine the treatment method. The purpose is to eliminate pathogenic factors in order to heal the disease.

TCM theory states that there is a normal state of relative equilibrium between the human body and the external environment, as well as among the *zàng fǔ* organs within the body. This balance is dynamic and constantly self-adjusting in order to sustain normal physiological activity in the human body. If this dynamic balance is broken such as by a pathogenic invasion, and cannot immediately be restored through self-adjustment, the disease process will then occur.

The signs and symptoms of any disease reflect the pathological reactions of the body to certain pathogenic factors. The pathogenic factors are therefore studied as the objective causes of disease, and examined for how they affect the body. On the basis of this understanding, TCM is able to identify pathogenic factors of disease by analyzing clinical manifestations. This is known as 'finding the pathogenic factors by pattern differentiation' (辨證求因 *biàn zhèng qiú yīn*). As such, TCM etiology not only studies the properties and pathogenic characteristics of given pathogenic factors, it also studies the clinical manifestations of the patterns and diseases caused by these various pathogenic factors in order to direct clinical diagnosis and treatment.

Pathogenic factors invade the *zàng fǔ* organs, breaking up their state of relative balance, which leads to *zàng fǔ* organ dysfunction and disease development. Thus *zàng fǔ* pattern identification has to be integrated with etiology pattern identification in order to establish proper treatment strategies to eliminate the pathogens.

(4) *Zàng fǔ* pattern identification (臟腑辯證 *zàng fǔ biàn zhèng*)

This method is used to analyze and generalize signs and symptoms of disease according to the physiological functions and pathological characteristics of the *zàng fǔ* organs, in order to infer etiopathology, to determine the location, and judge the nature of pathological changes as well as the state of body's antipathogenic qi against pathogenic factors.

All physiological functions and pathologic changes are related to the *zàng fǔ* organs. Most often times, the occurrence and development of diseases are the result of *zàng fǔ* organ dysfunction. Thus *zàng fǔ* pattern identification is one of the core fundamental methods in TCM diagnosis and the foundation for clinical analysis and differentiation of every disease, particularly for interior and chronic conditions.

(5) Channel pattern identification (經絡辯證 *jīng luò biàn zhèng*)

This method analyzes the clinical manifestation of a disease based on the physiological and pathological characteristics of the twelve channels, the eight extraordinary channels, and its related *zàng fǔ* organ, to determine which channels the disease belongs to.

The channels and collaterals are the pathways that direct the body's qi and blood; connect the *zàng fǔ* organs, joints, and limbs; and facilitate the communication of the upper, lower, interior, and exterior areas of the body. When exopathogens invade the body and disrupt qi function in the channels, they inhibit the body's ability to guard, nourish, and regulate, allowing the pathogens to gradually spread into the *zàng fǔ* organs through the channels and collaterals. Conversely, if the pathological changes first appear in the *zàng fǔ* organs, they can also be reflected on the body's surface along the channels and collaterals. Each channel and collateral has its pathway and connection to a *zàng fǔ* organ. Thus the channels and collaterals can regularly reflect related signs and symptoms, which is helpful in determining the channel and organ affected by the disease as well as the nature and development of the disease.

Since channels and collaterals connect *zàng fǔ* organs and direct qi and blood, their pathological changes will affect each other. Thus channel pattern identification should be combined with *zàng fǔ* pattern identification and qi, blood, and body fluids pattern identification.

(6) Six channels pattern identification (六經辯證 *liù jīng biàn zhèng*)

This method is for the pattern identification of exogenous febrile diseases caused by cold pathogens (傷寒病 *shāng hán zhèng*). This theoretical system was expounded in *Discussion of Cold Damage and Miscellaneous Diseases* (傷寒雜病論 *shāng hán zá bìng lùn*) written by Zhang Zhong-Jing (張仲景, 150-219). This was the first clinical book to systematically describe the pathology and treatment of disease caused by the invasion of external pathogenic factors, and was developed from a theory analyzed in the *Yellow Emperor's Inner Classic* (黃帝內經 *huáng dì nèi jīng*). It is the first clinical pattern identification method in the history of Chinese medicine, and laid the foundation for the various pattern identification methods that followed.

Based on the clinical characteristics, exogenous diseases can be classified into six patterns during their development: *tài yáng, yáng míng, shào yáng, tài yīn, shào yīn,* and *jué yīn*. The first three are known as the 'three yang patterns' and reflect pathological changes in the *fǔ* organs, while the latter three are referred to as the 'three yin patterns' and reflect pathological changes in the *zàng* organs. The six patterns also reflect the pathogenesis of their corresponding channels. Thus six channels pattern identification is related to and inseparable from *zàng fǔ* pattern identification and channel pattern identification.

(7) Four levels pattern identification (衛氣營血辯證 *wèi qì yíng xuè biàn zhèng*)

This method is mainly used for the pattern identification of exogenous febrile diseases caused by warm pathogens (溫病 *wēn bìng*), and was established by Ye Tian-Shi (葉天士, 1666-1745) during the Qing Dynasty. It analyzes and summarizes the clinical manifestations, pathological characteristics, and pathogenesis, using *wèi, qì, yìng, xuè* as the guideline for differentiating patterns, distinguishing the location of pathological change, classifying the pattern type, judging the nature of the pathology, predicting the prognosis, and determining the treatment principle.

338 Part 4 : Questions and Answers for Deeper Insight

(8) Triple Burner pattern identification (三焦辯證 *sān jiāo biàn zhèng*)

This method is mainly used for the pattern identification of warm febrile diseases (溫病 *wēn bìng*), and was established by Wu Ju-Tong (吳鞠通, 1758-1836) during the Qing Dynasty. It comprehensively analyzes and summarizes various clinical manifestations in the development of febrile disease, using the upper, middle, and lower burners as a guideline in determining the disease location, pathological stage, pattern type, treatment principle, and prognosis.

IV. Pattern identification applications and relationships

The pattern identification methods of eight principles; etiology; qi, blood, and body fluids; channel; and *zàng fǔ* summarize pathological change from different perspectives. Each method has its special emphasis, character, and focus, but they are all related. The first four methods are the basis for *zàng fǔ* pattern identification, while *zàng fǔ* pattern identification is also the basis of all the other methods. Tang Rong-Chuan (唐容川, 1846-1897) noted: "If a doctor doesn't know *zàng fǔ* pattern identification, he cannot identify location and cause of the disease nor establish the proper treatment principle." The following chart summarizes the most commonly used methods of differentiation and their relationships.

The six channel, four level, and Triple Burner pattern identification methods are used for exogenous febrile diseases. Although six channel pattern identification is applicable to all types of exogenous diseases, it is

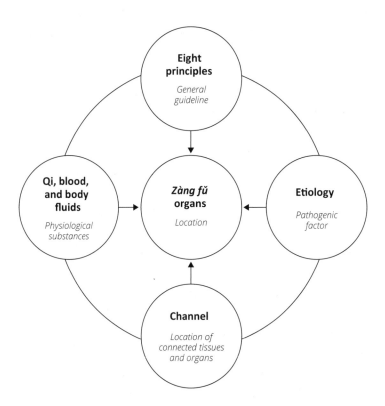

Chart 24.40.1 Most common pattern identification methods and their relationships

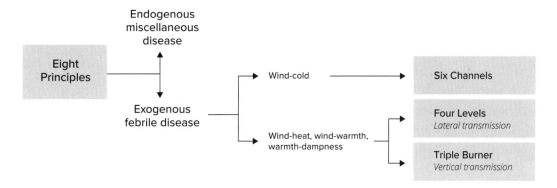

Chart 24.40.2 Pattern identification methods for exogenous febrile disease

mainly used for those caused by cold pathogens. Four level and Triple Burner pattern identification methods are mainly used for exogenous diseases caused by heat pathogens. Four level pattern identification is more suitable in cases where a warm exopathogen attacks and transforms from the exterior to the interior, from shallow to deep, or has a lateral development of pathological changes. Meanwhile, Triple Burner pattern identification is more suitable in cases where a warm exopathogen attacks and transforms from the upper body to the lower body, or has a vertical development of pathological change.

Part 5

COMPREHENSIVE EXAMINATION

CONTENTS

CHAPTER 25: EXAM QUESTIONS AND ANSWER KEY, 338

ANSWER KEY, 404

Chapter 25
Exam Questions and Answer Key

1. What are the most common symptoms of Heart disease?

   a. Chest pain
   b. Panting and wheezing
   c. Palpitations
   d. Depression

2. Which of the following signs and symptoms can appear in both Lung yin deficiency and dryness invading the Lung?

   a. Dry cough with blood-stained sputum and difficult expectoration
   b. Slight chills, fever, and a superficial rapid pulse
   c. Night sweats and low-grade fever in the afternoon or evening
   d. A red and cracked tongue with scanty yellow coating

3. What pattern is indicated by the following signs and symptoms: palpitations, shortness of breath, oppression in the chest that is aggravated by exertion, spontaneous sweating, a pale tongue with a white coating, and a weak and knotted pulse?

   a. Heart blood deficiency
   b. Heart qi deficiency
   c. Heart yang deficiency
   d. Heart yin deficiency

4. Dry cough, scanty sticky phlegm, difficult expectoration, dry mouth and throat, five center heat, night sweats, a dry red tongue, and a thin rapid pulse, indicate which of the following patterns?

   a. Dryness invading the Lung
   b. Lung yin deficiency
   c. Heat congesting the Lung
   d. Phlegm-dryness obstructing the Lung

5. Which of the following is NOT commonly seen in Heart disease patterns?

   a. Insomnia, dream-disturbed sleep
   b. Heartburn
   c. Canker sores
   d. Coma, delirium

6. All of the following symptoms are manifestations of Heart blood deficiency, EXCEPT:

   a. Continuous or fright palpitations
   b. Insomnia, dream-disturbed sleep
   c. Dizziness, blurry vision
   d. Night sweats, vexation

7. What pattern is indicated by the following signs and symptoms: depression, apathy, dementia, lethargic stupor, aphasia or soliloquy, laughing or crying, and a greasy tongue coating?

   a. Phlegm misting the Heart
   b. Phlegm-fire harassing the Heart
   c. Phlegm obstructing the Heart vessels
   d. Gallbladder stagnation with phlegm disturbance

8. All of the following signs and symptoms can appear in Heart fire blazing, EXCEPT:

   a. Vexation and hot sensation in the chest
   b. Apathy, lethargic stupor, aphasia or soliloquy
   c. Tongue ulcers
   d. Hematemesis and epistaxis

9. Which of the following signs and symptoms can appear in both Heart blood deficiency and Heart yin deficiency?

   a. Dizziness, blurry vision, pale dull complexion
   b. Five center heat, low-grade fever in the afternoon and evening, night sweats
   c. Palpitations, insomnia, dream-disturbed sleep
   d. Pale tongue and lips, thin pulse

10. Feeble cough and dyspnea, shortness of breath that is worse with exertion, low voice, fatigue, spontaneous sweating, aversion to wind, easy to catch colds, and pale complexion, indicate which of the following patterns?

   a. Heart qi deficiency
   b. Lung yin deficiency
   c. Kidney qi deficiency
   d. Lung qi deficiency

11. Which of the following pathogens may cause Heart vessels obstruction?

    a. Phlegm
    b. Blood stasis
    c. Cold
    d. All of the above

12. Which of the following is the key symptom for Lung diseases?

    a. Fatigue
    b. Cough
    c. Oppression in chest
    d. Phlegm

13. Which of the following is rarely seen in Lung diseases?

    a. Hematemesis
    b. Asthma or wheezing
    c. Chest pain
    d. Hemoptysis

14. What pattern is indicated by the following signs and symptoms: cough with thick yellow phlegm, sore throat, slight aversion to cold, fever, red tongue tip, thin yellow tongue and coating, a superficial rapid pulse?

    a. Heat congesting the Lung
    b. Heat-phlegm in the Lung
    c. Dryness invading the Lung
    d. Wind-heat invading the Lung

15. All of the following signs and symptoms can appear in Lung qi deficiency, EXCEPT:

    a. Feeble cough
    b. Clear thin phlegm
    c. Spontaneous sweating, aversion to wind
    d. Thin and rapid pulse

16. Which of the following symptoms are NOT associated with dryness invading the Lung?

    a. Dry cough with scanty sticky phlegm that is difficult to expectorate
    b. Shortness of breath
    c. Dry mouth, nose, and throat
    d. Slight chills and fever

17. Which of the following symptoms or signs does NOT appear in the small intestine pattern?

    a. Copious or scanty urination
    b. Abdominal distention or pain
    c. Constipation with dry stool
    d. Diarrhea or loose stool

18. Which of the following is the main symptom for Large Intestine damp-heat?

    a. Constipation
    b. Dark brown urination
    c. Diarrhea or dysentery
    d. Anus prolapse

19. What type of cough is characteristic of phlegm-dampness obstructing the Lung?

    a. Feeble cough that is worse with exertion
    b. Cough without phlegm or with a small amount of sticky phlegm
    c. Chronic cough coming in bouts with profuse white sticky phlegm that is easy to expectorate
    d. Barking cough with profuse sticky yellow or green phlegm, difficult to expectorate

20. Which of the following is NOT associated with phlegm misting the Heart?

    a. Yin mania
    b. Epilepsy
    c. Syncope due to phlegm
    d. Dizziness and vertigo

21. The symptom of having a bitter taste in the mouth might appear in which of the following patterns?

    a. Gallbladder heat
    b. Liver fire blazing
    c. Phlegm-fire harassing the Heart
    d. All of the above

22. Which of the following signs and symptoms can appear in both Large Intestine damp-heat and Large Intestine heat accumulation?

    a. Fever, thirst with a desire to drink cold water, and abdominal pain
    b. Constipation
    c. Tidal fever
    d. Watery stools with blood and pus

23. Cough with scanty white or blood-stained sputum that is difficult to expectorate indicates Lung obstructed by which of the following?

    a. Heat-phlegm
    b. Phlegm-dampness
    c. Phlegm-dryness
    d. Wind-phlegm

24. Which of the following signs and symptoms is NOT associated with Liver and Gallbladder damp-heat?

    a. Bitter taste in the mouth
    b. Edema
    c. Alternating chills and fever
    d. Jaundice

25. What is the primary manifestation of Gallbladder stagnation with phlegm disturbance?

    a. Jaundice, yellow skin and sclera
    b. Alternating chills and fever
    c. Scanty and dark yellow urine
    d. Timidity, easily startled, and insomnia

26. What pattern is indicated by the following signs and symptoms: dizziness, vertigo, tinnitus, muscle twitching and trembling, pale and withered nails, scanty menstrual bleeding or amenorrhea, a pale tongue, and a thin pulse?

    a. Liver blood deficiency
    b. Liver yang rising with Kidney yin deficiency
    c. Extreme heat generating wind
    d. Liver fire blazing

27. Liver qi stagnation often causes which of the following symptoms?

    a. Headache
    b. Hypochondrium pain
    c. Lumbar pain
    d. Abdominal pain

28. Which of the following are main clinical manifestations of cold stagnation in the Liver channel?

    a. Distention pain in the hypochondrium
    b. Numbness and trembling in the hands and feet
    c. Cold contracture pain of the scrotum
    d. Swollen, hot, and painful scrotum

29. Which of the following is NOT a symptom of Liver blood deficiency?

   a. Joint stiffness
   b. Limb numbness
   c. Lower backache
   d. Trembling hands and feet

30. Which of the following symptoms is NOT a clinical manifestation of Liver qi stagnation?

   a. Mental depression, short temper
   b. Irregular menstrual cycle
   c. Blurry vision
   d. Plum-pit syndrome (globus hystericus)

31. Liver wind can be caused by all of the following, EXCEPT:

   a. Yang deficiency
   b. Liver yang rising
   c. Extreme heat
   d. Blood deficiency

32. Which of the following types of abnormal loose stools or diarrhea is caused by Spleen and Kidney yang deficiency?

   a. Chronic loose stools with Borborygmus
   b. Early morning diarrhea
   c. Acute diarrhea with foul odor
   d. Dry stools first and then loose watery stools

33. Which of the following signs and symptoms can appear in both Kidney yin deficiency and Kidney essence deficiency?

   a. Soreness and weakness in the lower back and knees
   b. Poor development and growth in children
   c. Night sweats, tidal fever
   d. A red and cracked tongue with little yellow coating

34. Which of the following signs and symptoms can appear in both Kidney yang deficiency and Kidney qi failing to consolidate?

   a. Intolerance of cold, cold limbs
   b. Pale face, frequent copious urination
   c. Edema below the waist
   d. Habitual miscarriage

35. What pattern is indicated by the following signs and symptoms: soreness and weakness in the lower back and knees, frequent and copious urination, incontinence of urine, a pale tongue, and a weak pulse?

    a. Kidney yang deficiency
    b. Kidney qi failing to consolidate
    c. Kidney essence insufficient
    d. Kidney yin deficiency

36. Which of the following is NOT commonly seen in Kidney disease?

    a. Soreness and weakness in the lower back and knee
    b. Tinnitus or deafness
    c. Oppression in the chest
    d. Edema, abnormal urination or bowel movements

37. Which of the following is the main symptom for Kidney failing to grasp qi?

    a. Wheezing and asthma with difficult inhalation
    b. Wheezing and asthma with difficult exhalation
    c. Cough with copious clear sputum
    d. Incontinence of urine

38. All of the following types of abnormal urination can appear in Kidney yang deficiency, EXCEPT:

    a. Difficult and scanty urine
    b. Copious and clear urine
    c. Scanty and yellow urine
    d. Frequent nocturnal urination

39. All of the following signs and symptoms can appear in Kidney essence deficiency, EXCEPT:

    a. Loose hair and teeth
    b. Dizziness and deafness
    c. Short stature
    d. Constipation

40. Which of the following signs and symptoms are NOT associated with Kidney essence deficiency?

    a. Amenorrhea or infertility for women
    b. Frequent copious clear urination
    c. Mentally and physically delayed development
    d. Delay in closing of fontanel

41. All of the following signs and symptoms can appear in Urinary Bladder damp-heat, EXCEPT:

    a. Frequent urination
    b. Urgent and burning urination
    c. Yellow urination
    d. Enuresis or bed-wetting

42. Which of the following is NOT commonly seen in Spleen diseases?

    a. Abdominal bloating and distention
    b. Belching and hiccups
    c. Loose stools
    d. Chronic bleeding

43. Which of the following is the characteristic of Stomach yin deficiency?

    a. Belching and acid regurgitation
    b. Vomiting immediately after eating
    c. Hungry but no desire to eat
    d. Slippery and rapid pulse

44. Severe constipation with dry and difficult bowel movements a few times a week, epigastric discomfort and burning pain, acid regurgitation, bad breath, thirst, a preference for cold drinks, a red tongue with a yellow coating, and a slippery and rapid pulse indicate which of the following patterns?

    a. Large intestine dryness
    b. Food stagnation
    c. Damp-heat encumbering the Spleen
    d. Stomach fire

45. Which of the following are the common signs and symptoms of Spleen qi deficiency, Spleen yang deficiency, and Spleen qi sinking?

    a. Weakness of limbs
    b. Heaviness of limbs
    c. Edema of limbs
    d. Stiffness of limbs

46. Which of the following is NOT associated with cold invading the Stomach?

    a. Cold pain in the epigastrium
    b. Chronic loose and watery stools
    c. Vomiting after eating, pain relieved after vomiting
    d. Deep and tight pulse

47. Which of the following signs and symptoms are common between cold-dampness encumbering the Spleen and damp-heat encumbering the Spleen?

   a. Yellow tint of the skin, eyes, and face
   b. Pale tongue with a white greasy coating
   c. Loose and foul-smelling stools
   d. A soft and rapid pulse

48. What is the primary manifestation of Stomach fire?

   a. Hunger but no desire to eat
   b. Vomiting immediately after eating
   c. Excessive appetite, eats a lot but still feels hungry
   d. Poor appetite, aversion to food

49. Which of the following signs and symptoms are NOT associated with Spleen qi deficiency?

   a. Poor appetite, abdominal distention, and loose stools
   b. Chronic bleeding
   c. Weak and heavy limbs
   d. Dysentery, stools with blood and pus

50. What pattern is indicated by the following signs and symptoms: epigastric distending pain, acid regurgitation, fetid belching, aversion to food, nausea, and pain that is relieved after vomiting or defecating?

   a. Food stagnation
   b. Excess Stomach fire
   c. Stomach yin deficiency
   d. Damp-heat encumbering the Spleen

51. What pattern is indicated by the following signs and symptoms: chronic loose stools or diarrhea, and anal prolapse?

   a. Spleen yang deficiency
   b. Kidney qi deficiency
   c. Spleen qi sinking
   d. Large Intestine deficiency cold

52. Besides insomnia, which of the following are key symptoms for Heart and Kidney disharmony pattern?

   a. Palpitations, irritability, and a red tongue with little coating
   b. Irritability, poor memory, and a thin rapid pulse
   c. Palpitations, ankle swelling, and scanty urination
   d. Irritability, seminal emissions, hot flashes, and lower backache

53. Which of the following are key symptoms for Heart and Kidney yang deficiency pattern?

   a. Palpitations, pale face, and fatigue
   b. Lower backache, intolerance of cold, and cold limbs
   c. Palpitations, intolerance of cold, and edema of the limbs
   d. Distress and fullness in the chest and a dim purple tongue

54. Cough, wheezing, palpitations, distress and fullness in the chest, pale face, fatigue, and a pale tongue indicate which of the following patterns?

   a. Lung qi deficiency
   b. Cold-phlegm obstructing the Lung
   c. Blood stagnation in the Heart
   d. Lung and Heart qi deficiency

55. Besides insomnia, which of the following are key symptoms for Heart and Spleen deficiency?

   a. Palpitations, pale face, and fatigue
   b. Irritability, palpitations, and a thin rapid pulse
   c. Poor memory, poor appetite, bloating, and a pale tongue
   d. Palpitations, irritability, dream-disturbed sleep

56. Which of the following are key symptoms for Heart and Liver blood deficiency?

   a. Dizziness, vertigo, and trembling hands and feet
   b. Insomnia, dream-disturbed sleep, numbness in the limbs, and a thin pulse
   c. Dizziness, vertigo, and amenorrhea
   d. Blurry vision and dry withered nails

57. Cough with thin sputum, panting, shortness of breath, pale face, fatigue, poor appetite, bloating, a pale tongue, and a weak pulse indicate which of the following patterns?

   a. Cold-phlegm obstructing the Lung
   b. Spleen and Lung qi deficiency
   c. Heart and Lung qi deficiency
   d. Lung and Kidney qi deficiency

58. Acute jaundice is usually caused by:

   a. Urinary Bladder damp-heat
   b. Liver and Gallbladder damp-heat
   c. Liver qi stagnation with heat flaring up
   d. Large Intestine damp-heat

59. Which of the following are key symptoms for Lung and Kidney yin deficiency?

    a. Cough with scanty sputum, hoarse voice
    b. Soreness and weakness in the lower back and knees, hot flashes, and steaming bone disorder
    c. Cough with scanty blood-stained sputum, night sweats, and seminal emissions
    d. Red tongue with little coating and a thin rapid pulse

60. Chronic cough, panting, shortness of breath, fatigue, spontaneous sweating, tinnitus, a pale tongue, and a weak pulse indicate which of the following patterns?

    a. Lung qi deficiency
    b. Kidney qi deficiency
    c. Spleen and Lung qi deficiency
    d. Lung and Kidney qi deficiency

61. A female patient complains of having scanty menstruation for three months. The menstrual blood is very thin and light. Other symptoms include a pale face, fatigue, dizziness, blurry vision, nervousness, easily startled, paranoia, shortness of breath, insomnia, and a pale tongue. What is the pattern identification for her?

    a. Liver blood and Gallbladder qi deficiency
    b. Qi deficiency failing to control the blood in the vessels
    c. Heart and Liver blood deficiency
    d. Liver and Kidney yin deficiency

62. A patient suffers from loose stools for over one year accompanied by a pale face, cold limbs, lower backache, cold pain in the lower abdomen, a pale and flabby tongue body with a white slippery coating, and a deep and thin pulse. What is the pattern?

    a. Spleen and Kidney yang deficiency
    b. Cold-dampness encumbering the Spleen
    c. Kidney qi deficiency
    d. Spleen yang deficiency

63. Which of the following are the key symptoms for Liver fire invading the Lung?

    a. Red tongue with a yellow coating
    b. Cough with yellow sticky sputum that may contain blood
    c. Burning pain in the hypochondrium and cough with sputum and blood
    d. Dizziness, headache, irritability, and a short temper

64. Yin deficiency commonly appears in all of the following pairs of organs, EXCEPT

    a. Heart and Kidney
    b. Liver and Kidney
    c. Lung and Kidney
    d. Spleen and Kidney

65. Stomach discomfort, acid regurgitation, hypochondriac pain, irritability, short temper, no desire to eat, and a wiry rapid pulse indicate which of the following patterns?

   a. Excess heat in the Stomach
   b. Liver overacting on the Stomach
   c. Liver and Spleen disharmony
   d. Food stagnation

66. Dizziness, vertigo, tinnitus, poor memory, a dry mouth and throat, insomnia, dream-disturbed sleep, hypochondriac pain, soreness and weakness in the lower back and knees, five center heat, and nocturnal emissions indicate which of the following patterns?

   a. Liver yang rising
   b. Kidney yin deficiency
   c. Liver and Kidney yin deficiency
   d. Heart and Liver fire blazing

67. All of the following signs and symptoms belong to Liver wind, EXCEPT:

   a. Dizziness and vertigo
   b. Convulsions and paralysis
   c. Tingling or numbness of the limbs
   d. Irritability and anxiousness

68. Severe watery diarrhea with paroxysmal cold pain of the umbilicus, borborygmus, a thick white tongue coating, and a tight wiry pulse, indicate which of the following patterns?

   a. Spleen yang deficiency
   b. Kidney yang deficiency
   c. Large Intestine cold-dampness
   d. Small Intestine deficiency cold

69. Which of the following signs and symptoms indicate a disharmony between the Liver and Spleen?

   a. Loose stools induced or aggravated by stress
   b. Depression, frequent sighing
   c. Watery stools, bloating
   d. Acid regurgitation, irritability, short temper

70. Which of the following signs and symptoms can distinguish Liver blood deficiency from Heart blood deficiency?

   a. Pale face and lips
   b. Deep and thin pulse
   c. Light and scanty menstruation
   d. Dizziness and fatigue

71. Which kind of headache is caused by Liver yang rising?

   a. Heavy pain
   b. Dull pain
   c. Moving pain
   d. Distending pain

72. Alternating chills and fever, thirst, and a desire to drink water are the primary symptoms of which of the following patterns?

   a. Liver and Gallbladder damp-heat
   b. Liver fire blazing
   c. Gallbladder heat
   d. Gallbladder stagnation with phlegm disturbance

73. Extreme heat in the Liver generating wind can be differentiated from other wind patterns by the presence of which of the following signs and symptoms?

   a. Numbness and tingling of the limbs
   b. Difficulty speaking due to tongue stiffness
   c. Dizziness and vertigo
   d. High fever

74. Which of the following signs and symptoms would distinguish Liver yang rising from Liver fire blazing?

   a. Dizziness and vertigo
   b. Top-heavy sensation, tendency to fall
   c. Tinnitus
   d. Headache

75. Which of the following types of diarrhea or loose stool is caused by Large Intestine deficiency cold?

   a. Early morning diarrhea with undigested food
   b. Intermittent soft and loose stools worse with the intake of greasy or cold foods
   c. Loose stools like duck droppings, light-colored without strong odor
   d. Acute watery diarrhea

76. Which of the following signs and symptoms would distinguish Heart fire blazing from phlegm-fire harassing the Heart?

   a. Irritability and restlessness
   b. Normal mental behavior
   c. Constipation
   d. Red tongue and rapid pulse

77. Which of the following signs and symptoms is key to distinguishing wind-heat invading the Lung from wind-cold invading the Lung?

   a. Sweating
   b. Shortness of breath
   c. Sore throat
   d. Cough

78. Intermittent soft and loose stools, worse with the intake of greasy or cold foods, indicate which of the following patterns?

   a. Large Intestine deficiency cold
   b. Spleen yang deficiency
   c. Kidney yang deficiency
   d. Cold-dampness in the Large Intestine

79. A 28-year-old male patient suffers from violent twisting pain in his left lower abdomen that radiates to his groin and testicles. He also complains of borborygmus, abdominal bloating and distention, and pain relief after passing gas. His tongue is normal with a thin white coating, and his pulse is deep and wiry. His abdominal pain is caused by which of the following patterns?

   a. Cold stagnation in the Liver channel
   b. Blood stagnation in the Stomach
   c. Small Intestine qi stagnation
   d. Large Intestine heat accumulation

80. Ellen, a 45-year-old female, suffers from insomnia and dream-disturbed sleep for over a year. Other symptoms include poor memory, dry eyes, dry skin, blurry vision, irritability, fatigue, and frequent dizziness. She complains that in the past year her menstruation has been very scanty and lasts only two days. Her nails are also easily broken. Upon examination you find that her face is pale, her tongue is pale and thin, and her pulse is thin and weak. Which of the following patterns matches her condition?

   a. Liver overacting on Spleen
   b. Heart and Kidney disharmony
   c. Heart and Liver blood deficiency
   d. Liver and Kidney yin deficiency

81. A 34-year-old female patient was diagnosed with Dumping syndrome after she had weight loss surgery five years ago. Her symptoms include epigastric cramps or burning pain, nausea, vomiting, sweating, feeling flushed, dizziness, low energy, feeling full after eating a small amount, loose stools, gas, and bloating. She drinks a lot of water because she always feels thirsty. She has a red tongue with a crack in the middle, a scanty tongue coating, and a weak pulse. What is the pattern identification for her?

a. Food stagnation
b. Spleen and Kidney yang deficiency
c. Spleen and Stomach disharmony
d. Stomach yin and Spleen qi deficiency

82. A 56-year-old male patient said that three years ago he noticed his ankles became swollen and puffy. It gradually got worse, but he didn't receive any treatments. Two months ago, he started experiencing palpitations, lethargy, weakness, fatigue, shortness of breath, pitting edema of his legs, and puffiness around his eyes. He also complains of cold limbs, scanty urine, and dribbling. His tongue is pale and flabby with a white moist coating. His pulse is deep, thin, and slow. Western diagnosis for him is chronic renal failure. What is the pattern identification for him?

a. Kidney and Spleen yang deficiency
b. Kidney and Heart yang deficiency
c. Kidney and Heart disharmony
d. Lung and Kidney qi deficiency

83. A 51-year-old female patient has been diagnosed with postmenopausal syndrome. Symptoms include mood swings, irritability, depression, worrying, distress and distention in the chest and hypochondrium, lower backache and weakness, hot flashes, night sweats, low sex drive, dizziness, blurry vision, tinnitus, poor memory, and a dry mouth and throat. Her tongue is red and cracked with a scanty coating, and her pulse is thin and wiry. The diagnosis for her is menopause syndrome due to which of the following patterns?

a. Heart and Kidney disharmony
b. Liver and Kidney yin deficiency
c. Heart and Spleen deficiency
d. Heart and Liver blood deficiency

84. A 49-year-old female patient has been suffering from menopausal syndrome for over a year. She complains of palpitations, insomnia, and vexation. Other symptoms include dry mouth, hot flashes, five center heat, night sweats, and weakness of the knees. She has a red tongue with little coating, and a thin rapid pulse. The diagnosis for her is menopause syndrome due to which of the following patterns?

a. Heart and Kidney disharmony
b. Liver and Kidney yin deficiency
c. Heart and Spleen deficiency
d. Heart and Liver blood deficiency

85. A 84-year-old male suffers from chronic obstructive pulmonary disease (COPD) due to emphysema, which was diagnosed 15 years ago. He complains of cough with profuse white sputum, wheezing, and shortness of breath. He feels tired all the time, chest oppression and distress, and palpitations that are aggravated by exertion and exposure to cold. He has also been diagnosed with benign prostatic hyperplasia (BPH) and experiences frequent dribbling urine and nocturia.

His face is pale and his tongue is pale with a white coating. He has a deep weak pulse. What is the pattern identification for him?

   a. Heart and Kidney yang deficiency with Lung qi deficiency
   b. Heart blood and Spleen qi deficiency with Liver blood deficiency
   c. Heart and Kidney yin deficiency with cold-phlegm obstructing the Lung
   d. Heart and Liver blood deficiency with Lung qi deficiency

86. A 54-year-old female patient has been suffering from chronic colitis, which was diagnosed three years ago. She complains of loose stools 5-8 times per day. The stool is watery and contains undigested food. Other symptoms include cold limbs and body, lassitude, fatigue, shortness of breath, and chronic cold sensations in the lower back. Her face is pale, and she has a pale and flabby tongue with a white slippery coating. Her pulse is deep, weak, and slow. Which of the following patterns matches her condition?

   a. Food stagnation
   b. Spleen and Kidney yang deficiency
   c. Spleen and Stomach disharmony
   d. Damp-heat in the lower burner

87. Bette, a 40-year-old female, suffers from perimenopausal syndrome. Her periods have increased from 4-5 days of flow to 7-8 days. Her periods are now more frequent; often the cycle is as short as 21 or 22 days from day one to day one. She also experiences easy bruising and lower backache with her period. She received IVF treatments five times without success, and her OBGYN told her that she is no longer ovulating. She has a pale tongue and a thin and deficient pulse. Her condition belongs to which of the following patterns?

   a. Kidney and Spleen qi deficiency
   b. Heart and Spleen deficiency
   c. Liver qi stagnation and Spleen qi deficiency
   d. Liver qi stagnation and Liver blood deficiency

88. Which of the following signs or symptoms would distinguish Gallbladder heat from Liver fire blazing?

   a. Bitter taste in the mouth
   b. Dizziness
   c. Red eyes or tongue
   d. Jaundice

89. Jerome, 30, has been trying to have a baby with his wife for the past five years. He has been diagnosed with impotence and azoospermia. All neurological tests are negative, but microscopic examination of seminal fluid shows an absence of sperm. Bilateral biopsy of the testes shows moderate atrophy. He complains that his erection is weak and can't be sustained. He also suffers from dizziness, blurry vision, disturbed sleep, soreness and weakness in the lower back and

knees, and occasional involuntary nocturnal emissions. You also find that his hair is very thin with lots of graying hairs. He has a pale face and a small tongue. His pulse is deep and thin. Which of the following patterns matches his condition?

   a. Kidney yang deficiency
   b. Kidney essence deficiency
   c. Kidney yin deficiency
   d. Kidney qi failing to consolidate

90. A 55-year-old male was diagnosed with atrophic gastritis over two years ago. His symptoms include an uncomfortable feeling in the epigastrium, poor appetite, loss of taste, and loose stools. He always feels tired, especially in the mornings. He has a pale tongue with a thin white coating, and his pulse is deficient, especially on the right middle position. What is the pattern identification for him?

   a. Spleen yang deficiency
   b. Spleen qi deficiency
   c. Stomach qi deficiency
   d. Stomach yin deficiency

91. A 35-year-old female has been trying to get pregnant for over two years without success. She tells you that she always has scanty and light menstrual flow and a long menstrual cycle of 30-35 days. She was diagnosed with premature ovary failure (POF) one year ago. Other signs and symptoms include tiredness, dizziness, poor concentration, decreased sex drive, vaginal dryness, blurry vision, and numbness and tingling of the limbs. Upon examination, you find that she has a sallow complexion and a pale tongue that is paler on the sides. Her pulse is weak and thin. The diagnosis for her is infertility due to which of the following patterns?

   a. Kidney essence deficiency with Liver blood deficiency
   b. Spleen qi and Liver blood deficiency
   c. Spleen qi deficiency with dampness accumulation
   d. Liver and Kidney yin deficiency

92. Charles has chronic nephritis (diffuse glomerular and tubular stage) manifesting with severe protracted edema that is worse below the loins, scanty urine, distended abdomen, pallor, anorexia, bloating sensation after meals, loose stools, aching loins and legs, intolerance of cold, cold limbs, a flabby tongue with teeth marks, a white tongue coating, and a weak pulse. What is the pattern identification for him?

   a. Spleen yang deficiency
   b. Kidney yang deficiency
   c. Spleen and Kidney yang deficiency
   d. Heart and Kidney yang deficiency

93. John, 10 years old, reports that an hour after his dinner last night he began feeling discomfort and pain in the epigastrium, belching with foul odor, acid regurgitation, and abdominal fullness and distention. This morning the symptoms were reduced after having diarrhea. Upon closer examination you find that his tongue is red with a yellow greasy coating, and his pulse is rapid and slippery. What is the pattern identification for him?

   a. Food stagnation
   b. Damp-heat encumbering the Spleen
   c. Stomach yin deficiency
   d. Stomach fire

94. A 65-year-old male has been suffering from chronic bronchitis for 20 years. He experiences shortness of breath, slight wheezing with a low sound, and more difficulty breathing in than out. The symptoms are induced or aggravated by exertion. He also has arthritis in both knees and has a diagnosis of early Alzheimer's syndrome. He has a pale tongue and a deep weak pulse. What is the pattern identification for him?

   a. Lung qi deficiency
   b. Kidney failing to grasp qi
   c. Heart and Lung qi deficiency
   d. Spleen qi deficiency

95. Jian, a 45-year-old female, has been having frequent dull pain in the epigastrium for over 20 years. Two years ago, she was diagnosed as having a peptic ulcer in the duodenal bulb with chronic superficial gastritis. She took cimetidine and various kinds of Chinese herbs, but experienced little relief; the epigastric pain recurred frequently. Two weeks prior to her visit to your clinic the condition worsened. The pain radiated to the back and was accompanied by nausea and regurgitation of clear fluids. Other symptoms included reduced appetite, a dulling of her sense of taste, and a preference for hot beverages. The epigastric pain was alleviated with local pressure and aggravated by cold weather. The stool was sticky and loose. She has a pale tongue with a thin white coating and a deficient pulse. Which of the following patterns matches her condition?

   a. Stomach yin deficiency
   b. Cold invading the Stomach
   c. Stomach and Spleen yang deficiency with cold
   d. Cold-dampness accumulation in the Spleen and Stomach

96. A 63-year-old woman complains of lower back pain for many years. At age 13 she had polio, which made her left leg significantly shorter, and has had backaches ever since. Her knees ache and she suffers from frequent urination especially at night. She also feels cold, tires easily, and sometimes experiences dizziness and tinnitus. Her tongue is pale and flabby, and her pulse is deep, slow, and weak. The diagnosis for her is lower back pain due to which of the following patterns?

a. Kidney yang deficiency
   b. Kidney qi deficiency
   c. Kidney essence deficiency
   d. Kidney yin deficiency

97. A mother of a nine-year-old boy, Alvin, consults you about the fact that her son has always suffered from nocturnal enuresis, wetting the bed every night. The boy's pediatrician can find no cause. She says he urinates frequently during the day, having trouble remaining continent in the day as well as at night. She states that his urine is clear and that he urinates a lot. Upon questioning, she says he often has cold hands and feet. He has a pale complexion, a pale tongue with slippery coating, a weak and slight rapid pulse. Which of the following patterns may cause this condition?

   a. Kidney qi deficiency
   b. Kidney yang deficiency
   c. Kidney essence deficiency
   d. Kidney yin deficiency

98. Sherman is 47 years old and has been diagnosed with carcinoma of the bladder for four years. He had an operation three years ago and was asymptomatic until now. His current signs and symptoms include burning urination, blood in the urine, frequent and difficult urination, dark urine, backache, slight dizziness, and chilliness. What is the pattern identification for him?

   a. Urinary Bladder damp-heat, Kidney yang deficiency
   b. Urinary Bladder deficiency cold, Kidney yang deficiency
   c. Large Intestine damp-heat, Spleen yang deficiency
   d. Heart fire transmitting to Small Intestine, Spleen yang deficiency

99. Brenda, a 57-year-old female, raised nine children. She looks aged and was diagnosed with early Alzheimer's syndrome and osteoporosis four years ago. Yesterday she came in to your office complaining of aches and weakness of the knees and legs, pain and soreness of the lower back, poor memory, and hair loss. You find that her teeth are loose, her tongue is pale and cracked and peeled, and her pulse is weak. What is the pattern identification for her?

   a. Kidney qi deficiency
   b. Kidney yin deficiency
   c. Kidney yang deficiency
   d. Kidney essence deficiency

100. A 50-year-old man suffered from a severe pain in the left loin with very dark and scanty urine, dry mouth, and night sweats. This pain came in bouts and was caused by a kidney stone lodged in the urethra. The tongue was deep red and very dry, almost completely without coating; the tip was even redder. There was an extremely deep crack in the midline of the tongue with smaller cracks spreading out from it. The pulse at the time of examination was deep and wiry. The diagnosis for him is Kidney stone related to which of the following patterns?

a. Urinary Bladder damp-heat
b. Small Intestine excess fire
c. Large Intestine damp-heat
d. Kidney yin deficiency

101. The patient is a 60-year-old man and his chief complaint is blood in the stools for two months. He has no abdominal pain and his frequent bowel movements are loose. The blood is fresh red, but he does not have hemorrhoids. He feels very tired and cold most of the time, and wears extra clothes even in hot weather. His tongue is pale and flabby with a sticky white coating, and his pulse is weak, especially in the middle position on the right side. The diagnosis for him is hematochezia related to which of the following patterns?

a. Spleen yang deficiency
b. Large Intestine damp-heat
c. Excess heat in the blood
d. Kidney yang deficiency

102. Liza, a 23-year-old college student, complains of discomfort in her chest, palpitations, and shortness of breath upon exertion. She was diagnosed with anemia and hypotension two years ago and has been taking multivitamins and iron since then. She has been on a vegetarian diet for over eight years. Other complaints include cold hands and feet, very light and scanty menstruation, lower backache, loose stools during her period, depression, dizziness, and sometimes dull headaches. She has a blood pressure of 96/60 mmHg, a pale tongue, and a weak pulse. She may suffer from all of the following patterns, EXCEPT:

a. Heart and Kidney yang deficiency
b. Liver qi and blood stagnation
c. Liver blood deficiency
d. Spleen qi deficiency

103. A female patient has a history of acute nephritis and duodenal ulcer. For five years she has been symptom-free, except for some weakness in the limbs, a pale and yellowish complexion, abdominal bloating, poor appetite, shortness of breath, loose stools, and sweating after slight physical exertion. Which of the following patterns matches her condition?

a. Kidney yang deficiency
b. Kidney qi deficiency
c. Spleen qi deficiency
d. Spleen yang deficiency

104. A 47-year-old female patient has had frequent loose stools for over 10 months, both day and night, and the condition is worse after eating cold or oily foods. She is sometimes incontinent when sneezing or coughing. She is always tired and feels cold, has lower backaches, and often feels dizzy. Her tongue is pale, and her pulse is weak and deep. Which of the following patterns relate to her condition?

a. Spleen qi sinking
   b. Kidney yang deficiency
   c. Spleen yang deficiency
   d. All of the above

105. Annie, 27, complains of indigestion. She has been diagnosed with a peptic ulcer, but the medication hasn't helped. She has a very good appetite and always feels hungry, but once she starts to eat, she gets easily full and bloated. She also has a dry mouth and throat, and is constantly sipping water. She gets tired very easily and always has a slight temperature, especially in the afternoon. She complains of night sweats and wakes up easily. You see that her cheeks are slightly flushed and the skin around her lips is very dry. Her pulse is thin. What is the pattern identification for her?

   a. Liver yin deficiency
   b. Kidney yin deficiency
   c. Stomach yin deficiency
   d. Lung yin deficiency

106. A 52-year-old patient was diagnosed with hypertension over 15 years ago and has been taking antenolol 25mg daily for the last 10 years. His job has been extremely stressful in the last couple of months because of a mass layoff in his company. Two weeks ago, he started experiencing headaches, which felt like distention pain in the temple and eye areas. He also felt dizziness with a feeling of being unstable and easily falling. Other symptoms include insomnia, dream-disturbed sleep, irritability, and anger. Yesterday, during a bitter quarrel with his boss, he suddenly felt numbness on the left side of his body, had trouble speaking, dizziness, a loss of balance and coordination, a severe headache, and his face became red with bloodshot eyes. His tongue was red and stiff, and his pulse was wiry and forceful. What would be the current pattern identification for this case?

   a. Heart fire blazing
   b. Phlegm-fire harassing the Heart
   c. Extreme heat generating Liver wind
   d. Liver yang transforming into wind

107. A 34-year-old woman complains of severe anxiety, insomnia, worrying, brooding, palpitations, and mental restlessness. She has headaches affecting the right eye and the right side of the head, and they are severe and throbbing in character. Her periods come irregularly, sometimes later and sometimes earlier; the flow has been heavy and the blood has been dark with clots. She also experiences premenstrual irritability. Her pulse is wiry but thin. She has a thick yellow tongue coating and the tongue body is deep red with red spots along the sides and at the tip, where it is red and swollen. Her condition includes all of the following patterns, EXCEPT:

   a. Liver yang rising
   b. Heart fire blazing
   c. Liver qi and blood stagnation
   d. Heart blood deficiency

108. A 64-year-old woman is seeking treatment for hypertension. Her systolic blood pressure oscillates between 150 and 200 mmHg, and is more of a problem than her diastolic blood pressure, which has always been around 95 mmHg. Her main physical signs and symptoms include a stiff neck, a feeling of pressure in the head, throbbing headaches over the vertex, dizziness, tinnitus, blurred vision, dry eyes, waking up frequently during the night, and a feeling of heat in the evening. Her complexion is dull with red patches on both cheek bones, and her eyes are rather dull and without glimmer. Her tongue is red, redder on the sides, and the coating is very thin. Her pulse is deep, thin, and wiry. The diagnosis for her headache is due to which of the following patterns?

    a. Liver yang rising and Liver yin deficiency
    b. Liver yang transforming into wind
    c. Heart fire blazing with Liver yang rising
    d. Lung qi and Heart qi deficiency

109. A 30-year-old woman comes to your office with a chief complaint of dizziness. When she stands up from her chair, she feels dizzy and sometimes blacks out. She also has numbness of the limbs and muscle twitching. Her menstrual cycle is delayed and her sleep is very light. Sunlight makes her eyes hurt. Her face is pale, tongue is pale, and pulse is weak. Which of the following signs and symptoms would be consistent with her condition?

    a. Poor appetite
    b. Lumbar and knee pain
    c. Brittle and pale nails
    d. Laughing and crying without reason

110. A 43-year-old male patient has been suffering from tension headaches for over five days. The pain is around the eyes and side of the head, and is usually aggravated by stress. He complains of dizziness, irritability, difficulty falling asleep, and dream-disturbed sleep. He also noticed ringing in the ears and a bitter taste in the mouth. He has a red face, red eyes, dry stools, and yellow urine. His tongue is red with a yellow coating, and his pulse is wiry and rapid. His headache is due to which of the following patterns?

    a. Heart fire blazing
    b. Phlegm-fire harassing the Heart
    c. Liver fire blazing
    d. Liver yang rising

111. Two weeks ago a patient woke up in the morning and felt his whole body aching. He was dizzy and having difficulty getting out of bed. Movements of his left upper and lower limbs were limited. Tactile sensation on the left side of the body was also impaired. His speech was affected and it was hard to understand his words, as he could not move his tongue freely. When his family members assisted him out of bed, they found his eyes and mouth twitching towards the right side of the face. At your clinic you noticed that his tongue was deviated to the right and he had a thick

yellow tongue coating. His pulse was wiry and slippery. He was 65 years old and had a history of high blood pressure. He was diagnosed with apoplexy. Which of the following patterns is the best diagnosis for him?

a. Kidney yin deficiency with Liver yang rising
b. Liver wind due to phlegm obstruction
c. Liver qi stagnation with blood stagnation
d. Wind-cold attack with phlegm obstruction

112. A patient likes to drink wine. Recently, he started having frequent urination with less volume than before, and a burning pain during urination. His mouth is dry with a bitter taste, his stools are dry, and he has lower abdominal and hypochondriac distention and pain. He has no desire to drink water, sometimes has fever, and his red tongue has a yellow greasy coating. What is the pattern identification for him?

a. Damp-heat in the Urinary Bladder
b. Heart fire transmitting to the Small Intestine
c. Kidney yin deficiency with damp-heat
d. Liver and Gallbladder damp-heat

113. A 54-year-old male patient complains of discomfort and pain that feels like a tight ache, pressure, fullness, or squeezing in the center of his chest. He also experiences shortness of breath. Physical exam finds that he has profuse cold sweating on the forehead, cold limbs, severe palpitations, and feeble breath. His pulse is faint and irregular. What is the pattern identification for him?

a. Heart qi deficiency
b. Blood obstructing the Heart vessels with Heart blood deficiency
c. Heart yang deficiency
d. Cold obstructing the Heart vessels with Heart yang collapse

114. A 32-year-old male patient presents with the following symptoms after consuming 120g of red ginseng: irritability, red face, restlessness, agitation, fidgeting, vexation, fever, shouting and laughing, unable to sleep, yellow urination, no bowel movements for over three days, thirst, a red tongue with a yellow greasy coating, and a rapid slippery pulse. What is the pattern identification for him?

a. Heart fire blazing
b. Phlegm-fire harassing the Heart
c. Phlegm misting the Heart
d. Heart yin deficiency with heat

115. A 45-year-old female tells you that her sleep quality has been bad in the last two months. Her sleep is restless with tossing and turning and unpleasant dreams. She feels dizziness and experiences a sense of heaviness and oppression of the chest. She also has nausea, palpitations,

and mental restlessness. Upon examination you find her blood pressure to be at 175/96 mmHg. She has a red face, a red tongue with a yellow greasy coating, and her pulse is slippery and rapid. What would be the current pattern identification for her case?

   a. Heart fire blazing with phlegm-fire harassing
   b. Blood stasis obstructing the Heart vessels
   c. Heart yin deficiency
   d. Liver yang rising with Liver and Kidney yin deficiency

116. A 72-year-old woman has been suffering from a persistent cough for five years and has been diagnosed with chronic bronchitis. The cough is productive with sticky yellow sputum and there is a sensation of oppression in the chest. Her body is thin and her skin is dry. Her pulse is slightly slippery on the left distal position. Her tongue is red and dry without coating in the front. Which of the following patterns matches her current condition?

   a. Heat-phlegm in the Lungs with Lung yin deficiency
   b. Phlegm-dampness in the Lungs with Lung qi deficiency
   c. Dryness invading the Lungs
   d. Lung yin and Lung qi deficiency

117. Ming, a 32-year-old male, complains of insomnia for three weeks, waking up during the night, having nightmares, and always dreaming of flying. He also experiences a bitter taste in the mouth, thirst, mental restlessness, and palpitations. He has acne on his face and upper back, canker sores in his mouth, and constipation. He has a red tongue with a thin yellow coating, and a rapid pulse. What is the pattern identification in this case?

   a. Heart yin deficiency
   b. Liver fire blazing
   c. Heart fire blazing
   d. Phlegm-fire harassing the Heart

118. A 45-year-old man has just been diagnosed with essential hypertension. He has a long history of bronchial asthma and has also been recently diagnosed with chronic obstructive pulmonary disease (COPD). He suffers from cough with profuse clear sputum, wheezing, shortness of breath, and palpitations. He feels tired all the time and sweats a lot even without any physical exertion. You find that his voice is very weak when he talks to you. His tongue is pale with a thin white coating and his pulse is weak. Which of the following patterns is the best diagnosis for him?

   a. Liver qi stagnation with Lung qi deficiency
   b. Lung qi and Heart qi deficiency
   c. Cold-phlegm obstructing the Lung
   d. Cold-water shooting into the Lung

119. A 64-year-old female patient has a history of bronchial asthma for over 15 years. A week ago, she contracted the common cold and developed a sensation of oppression and fullness in the chest, dyspnea, rumbling sounds in the throat, and cough with profuse thin white sputum. Other signs and symptoms include shortness of breath, tiredness, and sweating without any physical activity. Her tongue is pale with a white greasy coating, and her pulse is weak and slippery. What would be the outcome of your pattern identification in this case?

    a. Wind-cold invading the Lung
    b. Lung qi and Lung yin deficiency
    c. Lung qi deficiency with cold-phlegm accumulation
    d. Wind-cold invasion with Lung qi deficiency

120. A 32-year-old female patient is diagnosed with a urinary tract infection (UTI) by her primary doctor. Symptoms include frequent urination with urgency and a painful burning sensation. The urine is a scanty amount and dark yellow in color. She has a history of anxiety that has been under control with Xanax for over a year. She complains of thirst and likes to drink cold water. She has a very red tongue, a thin yellow tongue coating, and a rapid pulse. The diagnosis for her painful urinary dribbling disorder syndrome is due to which of the following patterns?

    a. Damp-heat in the Urinary Bladder
    b. Damp-heat in Liver and Gallbladder
    c. Small Intestine excess fire
    d. Heart fire transmits to the Small Intestine

121. James, a 34-year-old male, has been diagnosed with Crohn's disease for over 10 years. His current symptoms include loose stools, borborygmus, and dull abdominal pain that feels better with warmth and pressure. He has cold limbs and clear urine. His tongue is pale with a white coating, and his pulse is deep, slow, and weak. What is the pattern identification for him?

    a. Large Intestine cold-dampness
    b. Large Intestine deficiency cold
    c. Spleen qi deficiency
    d. Kidney yang deficiency

122. Calvin, a 10-year-old boy, had a pool party to celebrate his birthday yesterday. This morning he started complaining of abdominal pain with rumbling sounds. He had watery diarrhea with pain around the umbilicus area. A heat pad helps. He feels chills and his body temperature is 100.4° F. He also has cough with clear thin sputum. His tongue coating is white and thick, while his pulse is superficial and tight. What is the pattern identification for him?

    a. Wind-cold invading the Lung with Large Intestine cold-dampness
    b. Wind-heat invading the Lung with Large Intestine damp-heat
    c. Wind-cold invading the Lung with Large Intestine damp-heat
    d. Wind-heat invading the Lung with Large Intestine cold-dampness

123. A 23-year-old male student has been admitted to the hospital because of acute appendicitis. He has a body temperature of 100.6° F, a pulse rate of 99 bpm, profuse perspiration, and shallow respiration. The pain is in the lower right quadrant. On palpation of the abdomen, marked localized tenderness and some rigidity in the right iliac fossa are noted. Pressure with the fingertip shows the area of greatest tenderness is located near McBurney's point. He hasn't had any bowel movements for over three days, and he drinks a lot of cold water. His tongue is red with a thick, dry, and dark brown coating. His pulse is deep and forceful. What is the pattern identification for him?

   a. Excess heat in the Large Intestine and Stomach
   b. Food stagnation
   c. Large Intestine dryness
   d. Large Intestine damp-heat

124. A 65-year-old patient has been suffering from chronic cough for over 10 months. She complains of persistent cough that is worse in the evenings and has very little phlegm, which is sticky, slightly yellow, and difficult to expectorate. Her cough is usually induced or worsens when she is tired or after exercise. Other symptoms include anxiety, insomnia, fatigue, and sometimes palpitations. She has a red cracked tongue with a very red tip and a scanty tongue coating that is slightly yellow. Her pulse is thin and deep. What is her pattern identification?

   a. Lung qi deficiency
   b. Lung yin deficiency
   c. Heart fire blazing
   d. All of the above

125. A 55-year-old female reports a two-year history of worsening insomnia, coinciding with an increase in menopausal symptoms, including hot flashes, and night sweats. She states that she has had intermittent insomnia since the births of her children 20 years ago, while she also had mild postpartum depression. She is taking flurazepam for her insomnia. She has difficulty falling asleep and wakes up very frequently. The arousals last anywhere from a few minutes to a few hours. She has also noticed having nightmares more frequently than in the past. She never feels rested upon awakening and describes feeling fatigued during the day with low energy. Her other daytime symptoms include low motivation, poor concentration, and her mood is "not great," but she denies feeling particularly depressed. She has had to cut back her time at work to 10-15 hours per week because of her insomnia. Another recent problem she reports is gastroesophageal reflux disease (GERD). Her worst symptoms occur during the night, describing the pain at times as "like having a heart attack." She has a red tongue with a thin yellow coating, and a thin rapid pulse. What is the pattern identification for this patient?

   a. Liver blood deficiency
   b. Heart and Stomach yin deficiency with heat
   c. Heart and Kidney disharmony
   d. All of the above

126. Clint, a 46-year-old male, has been suffering from recurrent asthmatic attacks and cough for the past 10 years. It is usually induced by weather changes. He recently suffered a relapse for two weeks after a cold. He is short of breath and is unable to breathe while lying down. There is slight sweating, chills, and white, foamy, and watery sputum. His appetite is poor and his stools are unformed. His tongue is light red with a white greasy coating, and his pulse is deep, slippery, and weak. What is the pattern identification for this patient?

   a. Lung qi deficiency
   b. Spleen yang deficiency
   c. Cold-phlegm obstructing the Lung
   d. All of the above

127. A 28-year-old female patient has had no menstrual periods for over three months. Before that, she states, her menstruation was scanty and light, usually lasting only two to three days with an average cycle being 35-40 days. She has a dull and sallow complexion with pale lips and nails. She also suffers from dizziness, poor vision, dry eyes, numb and cold hands and feet, poor sleep, easy sweating, and low energy. She has a pale and tender tongue, and a thin weak pulse. What is the pattern identification for her?

   a. Spleen qi deficiency
   b. Liver blood deficiency
   c. Heart and Spleen deficiency
   d. Spleen qi deficiency with Liver blood stagnation

128. A 35-year-old female has been suffering from dysmenorrhea for over 20 years. The cramping usually starts one or two days before her menstrual period and stops on the third or fourth day. The pain is severe, located in the lower abdomen, worse with pressure, and relieved by warmth. She also suffers from severe PMS, distending pain in the breasts, irritability, anger, mood swings, and constipation. Her menstrual cycle is very irregular, from 21-35 days. The color of the blood is very dark with clots. Her tongue is dusky with a thin yellow coating, and her pulse is wiry. The diagnosis for her is dysmenorrhea due to which of the following patterns?

   a. Liver qi stagnation
   b. Liver blood stagnation
   c. Liver qi and blood stagnation
   d. Liver blood stagnation with Liver fire

129. A 54-year-old male patient was diagnosed with Crohn's disease three years ago and is using prednisone. Three weeks ago his symptoms flared up; he started having persistent diarrhea six to ten times per day that contained undigested food. He has also been suffering from fatigue, dizziness, and shortness of breath that is worse with exertion, poor appetite, and a lot of sweating. He lost six pounds in the last three weeks. His tongue is pale with a thin white coating and his pulse is deep and weak. His diarrhea is related to which of the following patterns?

a. Kidney qi deficiency
b. Spleen qi sinking
c. Small Intestine deficiency cold
d. Large Intestine deficiency cold

130. A 56-year-old male patient was diagnosed with acute kidney failure and is on the waiting list for a kidney transplant. Symptoms include pitting edema that is worse in the feet and ankles, scanty urine, a heavy sensation, abdominal distention, decreased appetite, nausea, and vomiting. His BP is 160/100 mmHg, serum creatinine is 6.4mg/dL, BUN is 65mg/dL. He has a dark facial complexion, a white greasy tongue coating, and a deep slippery pulse. Which of the following patterns is related to his condition?

a. Cold-dampness encumbering the Spleen
b. Wind-water invading the Lung
c. Kidney yang deficiency with water retention
d. Kidney water upward invading the Spleen

131. A 23-year-old female patient has been suffering from metrostaxis, a continual dripping and slight loss of blood from the uterus, for over four months. It sometimes stops for two to four days, but then starts right back up again. In the last couple of weeks she also started experiencing dizziness, blurred vision, and a numbness and tingling sensation in her hands. Her menses are dark-colored with blood clots accompanied by pain in the lower abdomen, a dark purple tongue, and a thin hesitant pulse. What is the pattern identification for her condition?

a. Liver qi and blood stagnation
b. Spleen not controlling blood
c. Liver blood deficiency and stagnation
d. Heart qi and blood deficiency

132. A 36-year-old female patient has been diagnosed with chronic fatigue syndrome (CFS) for over 12 months. Clinical manifestations include fatigue, loss of memory, poor concentration, extreme exhaustion lasting more than 24 hours after physical or mental exercise, blurred vision with sensitivity to light, and a tingling sensation in the hands and feet. She might have all of the following signs and symptoms, EXCEPT:

a. Pale and tender tongue
b. Thin and weak pulse
c. Irritability and agitation
d. Shortness of breath

133. Susan, 36 years old, was diagnosed with celiac disease since she was 12. Last month she was tested for small intestinal bacterial overgrowth (SIBO) and it turned out positive. She has been on a gluten-free, diary-free, and vegan diet, but complains of "indigestion" issues. She felt

bloating, gas, abdominal pain, nausea, and vomiting when she eats cold or raw foods. She also complains of fatigue, difficulty maintaining her weight, cold numbness and tingling in her hands and feet, and aching pain in her joints. She noticed that she loses her balance sometimes and has mild cognitive impairment issues such as trouble remembering, difficulty learning new things, poor concentration, and difficulty making decisions. Her menstrual cycle is 32-35 days with light bleeding for three days. She has no abdominal cramps, but does have some lower backache and loose stools. Her blood test indicates anemia and vitamin D and B_{12} insufficiency. She has a pale complexion, a pale small tender tongue with a thin white coating, and a weak pulse. Which of the following patterns does Susan have?

    a. Heart and Liver blood deficiency
    b. Spleen and Kidney yang deficiency
    c. Liver qi and blood stagnation
    d. Both A and B

134. A 12-year-old boy was admitted to the hospital yesterday because of acute nephritis. He suffered from chills, fever, sore throat, and cough with sputum for two days, and then noticed that his face looked puffy and his eyelids were swollen. His urine has been very scanty and a smoky rust color. His BP is 140/90 mmHg, temperature is 100.4° F, and WBC is 15,000/mcL. His tongue is red with a thick yellow coating, and his pulse is superficial, slippery, and rapid. What is the pattern identification?

    a. Dampness encumbering the Spleen
    b. Wind-heat invading the Lung
    c. Yang edema: wind-water invading the Lung
    d. Yin edema: Kidney yang deficiency

135. A patient comes to you complaining of dizziness. His complexion is pale yellowish and lusterless. In a soft voice he tells you that his energy has been especially low lately because of trouble sleeping and feeling anxious. After two weeks of taking an herbal formula for his condition, he now experiences dryness, thirst, and constipation. His pulse feels thin and doesn't have much strength. His tongue is a little pale with teeth marks on the edges. Which of the following patterns is the most appropriate for his condition?

    a. Spleen qi deficiency
    b. Heart blood deficiency
    c. Body fluids deficiency
    d. All of the above

136. A 35-year-old female was diagnosed with endometriosis 12 years ago. She has been taking birth control pills to manage her menstrual cramps. Four months ago she planned to have a baby and stopped the birth control pills. Since then, her menstrual cycle has always been delayed and accompanied by severe cramping and profuse bleeding with clots. Her OBGYN also told her that she has uterine fibroids. Her weight is 182 pounds, her tongue is slightly pale with a thick

greasy coating, and her pulse is wiry and slippery. Which of the following patterns matches her condition?

   a. Blood and phlegm stagnation in the uterus
   b. Kidney essence deficiency with blood deficiency
   c. Liver qi stagnation and blood stagnation in the uterus
   d. Liver blood and Spleen qi deficiency

137. A 14-year-old boy complains of having a cough for a week accompanied by chills, fever, sore throat, and thirst. Since he was little, he catches colds frequently. His body is thin and he is not active. His appetite is normal, but he is very picky and prefers cold and sweet foods and drinks. He continues to cough, producing yellowish sputum. His tongue is red with a thin and slightly yellow coating. His pulse is superficial and slightly rapid. The diagnosis for him is cough due to which of the following patterns?

   a. Wind-cold invading the Lung with cold-phlegm accumulation, Lung qi deficiency
   b. Wind-heat invading the Lung with heat-phlegm accumulation, Lung qi deficiency
   c. Heat-phlegm obstructing the Lung, Lung qi and Lung yin deficiency
   d. Dryness invading the Lung, Lung qi deficiency

138. A 74-year-old woman has been diagnosed with chronic bronchitis for over ten years. Recently, she was diagnosed as having acute pneumonia. She currently has a cough that is easily triggered by cold weather, chest distress and tightness, shortness of breath, and, since yesterday, her face, especially around her eyes, seems swollen. She also complains that her chest feels cold and always wears more layers around her chest. Her face looks very pale and she has noticeably lost weight over the past ten years. Her tongue is pale and purplish with a thin white coating, and her pulse is deep and weak. What is the most appropriate pattern identification for her?

   a. Cold-phlegm obstructing the Lung with Lung qi deficiency
   b. Lung and Kidney yang deficiency with water retention
   c. Lung qi and Lung yang deficiency with water retention
   d. Cold-water shooting into the Lung

139. A 38-year-old male has been suffering from a chronic sore throat for many years. He is a teacher and was a singer at a club. His constitution is good. However, he likes to eat greasy and spicy foods. He drinks a lot of water, but always feels thirsty. He has a feeling of phlegm. His tongue is reddish with some cracks, and his pulse is slippery and thin. What is the most appropriate pattern identification for him?

   a. Excess heat in the Lung channel with damp-heat in the middle burner
   b. Wind-heat invading the Lung, with heat-phlegm accumulation
   c. Lung yin deficiency with phlegm accumulation
   d. Kidney yin deficiency with deficiency heat flaring up

140. A 53-year-old female was referred to the office for evaluation of a chronic cough, productive of large volumes of grossly purulent sputum. She has a history of recurrent respiratory infections that have resulted in five hospitalizations in the past year. In the months preceding her visit to the clinic, she reported producing 1-1.5 cups of sputum daily, requiring 2.5 liters of supplemental oxygen per minute for 12 hours each night. Shortness of breath limited her daily activity considerably. Medical history includes asthma, diagnosed 20 years earlier, an episode of pneumothorax, and suspected chronic obstructive pulmonary disease (COPD). She had quit smoking eleven years previously. Upon pulmonary examination, bilateral breath sounds are audible with a few expiratory wheezes at the lung bases; there are no rales. Chest x-rays reveal very prominent bronchial markings consistent with chronic bronchitis and possibly bronchiectasis; no acute infiltrates have been identified. Her tongue is slightly pale with a greasy coating, and her pulse is weak and slippery. The diagnosis for her is cough due to which of the following patterns?

    a. Kidney yang deficiency with cold-phlegm obstructing the Lung
    b. Liver fire invading the Lung
    c. Lung qi deficiency with phlegm-dampness obstructing the Lung
    d. Spleen qi deficiency with phlegm-dampness obstructing the Lung

141. A 66-year-old man with a smoking history of one pack per day for the past 47 years presents with progressive shortness of breath and chronic cough, productive of yellowish sputum, for the past two years. On examination he appears cachectic and in moderate respiratory distress, especially after walking to the examination room, and has pursed-lip breathing. His neck veins are mildly distended. Lung examination reveals a barrel chest and poor air entry bilaterally with moderate inspiratory and expiratory wheezing. Heart and abdominal examination are within normal limits. Lower extremities exhibit scant pitting edema. He has a red cracked tongue with little coating, and a deep, slippery, and thin pulse. What is the most appropriate pattern identification for him?

    a. Heat-phlegm obstructing the Lung
    b. Kidney qi deficiency, Lung qi and yin deficiency, with phlegm accumulation
    c. Dryness invading the Lung with phlegm accumulation
    d. Lung qi deficiency with heat-phlegm accumulation

142. A 42-year-old female was diagnosed with trigeminal neuralgia a year ago. Her symptoms flare up a couple times a year and are usually triggered by emotional stress or occur after eating spicy foods or drinking alcohol. The latest episode started yesterday after she attended a family party. There is severe, burning, and shooting pain that feels like electric shocks in her left cheek and jaw area, and is triggered by touching her face. Other symptoms include thirst with a preference for cold water, and constipation with dry stools. She has a red tongue with a yellow coating, and a rapid wiry pulse. What is the pattern identification for her current condition?

    a. Liver fire blazing
    b. Heart fire blazing
    c. Stomach fire
    d. Gallbladder heat

143. Othello, 25, complains of having a cough for the past four days. He said he had to walk a quarter of a mile in a winter storm without any rain gear. That same evening, his body temperature increased to 102° F, and he had a headache that felt like being tightly wrapped, severe chills, and nasal congestion. In the last two days he had a productive cough, especially at night. The sputum is white colored. He also has a scratchy throat and poor appetite, but no pain. He has a slightly superficial and rapid pulse, and a thin white tongue coating. What is the correct pattern identification?

    a. Wind-heat invading the Lung
    b. Wind-cold invading the Lung
    c. Wind-cold-dampness invading the Lung
    d. Phlegm-dampness obstructing the Lung

144. A 65-year-old patient has been suffering from chronic cough since her husband died suddenly by heart attack 10 months ago. She was diagnosed with "bronchitis" and had been put on antibiotics three times. She complains of persistent cough that is worse in the evenings, cough with scanty phlegm that is sticky, slightly yellow, and difficult to expectorate. Her cough is usually induced or made worse when she is stressed or tired. Other symptoms include depression, anxiety, insomnia, fatigue, and sometimes palpitations. She has a red cracked tongue with a very red tip and a slightly yellow scanty coating. Her pulse is thin, deep, and wiry. What is her pattern identification?

    a. Heart and Kidney disharmony
    b. Lung yin deficiency with phlegm accumulation, Spleen qi deficiency, Liver qi stagnation, Heart fire blazing
    c. Lung qi and yin deficiency with phlegm accumulation, Liver qi stagnation, Heart fire blazing
    d. Lung and Kidney yin deficiency, Heart and Kidney disharmony

145. A 34-year-old female patient has been having diarrhea and fever for the past two days. She had "fresh" green salad for lunch two days ago in a restaurant and started to feel discomfort hours later. The symptoms include chills, abdominal pain, headache, tenesmus, blood and mucus in the stools, and a burning sensation in the anus. She also has thirst, a sore throat, and scanty, dark yellow urine. Upon physical examination, her body temperature is 102.2° F, and salmonella typhimurium has been found in her stool culture. She has a yellow sticky tongue coating and a slippery rapid pulse. What is the pattern identification for this patient?

    a. Wind-heat invading the Lung with Large Intestine damp-heat
    b. Wind-cold invading the Lung with Large Intestine cold-dampness
    c. Damp-heat accumulation in the middle burner
    d. Liver fire invading the Spleen with Large Intestine damp-heat

146. The patient is a 47-year-old female who has had frequent urination for over 10 years, day and night. She is sometimes incontinent when sneezing or coughing. She is always tired and easily

cold, has lower backaches, and often feels dizzy. Her tongue is pale, and her pulse is weak and deep. Which of the following patterns matches her condition?

   a. Spleen qi deficiency and sinking
   b. Urinary Bladder deficiency cold
   c. Spleen and Kidney yang deficiency
   d. Kidney yang deficiency, Kidney qi failing to consolidate

147. A patient comes to you with a diagnosis of cardiac edema but wants to try Chinese medicine before he tries Western drugs. His primary symptoms are cough with profuse white foamy sputum, dyspnea, shortness of breath that is worse with exercise, chest tightness, low urinary output, body-wide edema that makes it difficult for him to sleep lying down at night, a feeling of general heaviness in his head and body, coldness in his extremities, and no thirst. His pulse is deep and his face is pale and slightly cyanotic, as are his fingers. What is the pattern identification for this patient?

   a. Cold-water shooting into the Lung
   b. Heart and Kidney yang deficiency
   c. Spleen and Kidney yang deficiency
   d. Heart and Spleen deficiency

148. A 52-year-old female patient has type 2 diabetes and takes metformin 500mg daily. Current signs and symptoms include obesity, fatigue, frequent urination, and cold legs and feet. She also has chronic candida vulvovaginitis. She has a pale tongue with a yellow greasy coating, and a slippery and weak pulse. What is the pattern identification?

   a. Spleen and Kidney yang deficiency
   b. Kidney yang deficiency with damp-heat in the lower burner
   c. Dampness accumulation in the middle burner and lower burner
   d. Kidney yin and yang deficiency

149. Elisa, a 32-year-old female, broke up with her boyfriend six months ago and has been living in fear ever since. She always thinks that her ex-boyfriend will harm and kill her. She has called the police more than 10 times, but the police found no evidence. She also complains that her neighbors and some of her friends are on her ex-boyfriend's side, watching her and acting against her, so she is scared to leave her apartment. She also believes that people are unfair, lying, or actively trying to harm her. Other symptoms include timidity, startling easily, irritability, palpitations, trouble sleeping, and always having nightmares. She has lost a lot of weight as she does not dare to eat due to having a bitter taste in her mouth and fearing that someone is trying to poison her. She has a red tongue with a thick, yellow, greasy coating, and a slippery and wiry pulse. What is her pattern identification?

   a. Liver qi stagnation with Liver fire blazing
   b. Gallbladder qi deficiency with Liver qi stagnation
   c. Liver and Gallbladder damp heat
   d. Gallbladder stagnation with phlegm disturbance

150. A 72-year-old male has a history of chronic bronchitis for over 30 years. He suffers from asthmatic breathing and shortness of breath, which are worse on exertion. He has a low voice, cold limbs, pale bluish complexion, spontaneous sweating, and urinary incontinence with cough. He has also been diagnosed with benign prostatic hyperplasia (BPH) with frequent nocturia. He has a pale tongue with a thin coating, and a weak and deep pulse. What is the correct pattern identification for him?

    a. Lung and Kidney yang deficiency
    b. Spleen and Kidney yang deficiency
    c. Lung qi and yang deficiency
    d. Heart and Lung qi deficiency

151. A 40-year-old female has had no menstruation since divorcing her husband three years ago. She is an actress with a very busy schedule and a stressful job. She complains of mood swings, irritability, anger, anxiety, and dream-disturbed sleep. She is on a dairy-free, gluten-free, and sugar-free diet, but still feels bloated, has abdominal distention, and soft stools. Other symptoms include neck and shoulder tension, lower backache, breast distention, and sometimes abdominal cramping. She tested positive for small intestinal bacterial overgrowth (SIBO), and her hormone levels are all in normal range except testosterone being slightly low. She has a red tongue with a thick, yellow, greasy coating, and a thin, wiry and slippery pulse. She is 5'9" tall, weighs 105 pounds, and has a body temperature of 99.1° F. She states that her body temperature is always slightly high. Her condition may be related to which of the following patterns?

    a. Liver qi and blood stagnation
    b. Spleen qi deficiency with dampness
    c. Heart and Kidney disharmony
    d. All of the above

152. A female, who is 38 years old, has been diagnosed with irritable bowel syndrome (IBS) for about five years. Her condition flares up and is aggravated by emotional stress. She has a sallow complexion and tires quickly and frequently. She used to experience more constipation, but now her stools are loose with occasional constipation. She feels bloated in her abdomen, but favors warmth and pressure. She has no nausea or vomiting, but occasionally experiences regurgitation. Her tongue is pale and dusky with a thin coating, and her pulse is weak. What is the pattern identification for her?

    a. Spleen and Stomach disharmony
    b. Liver qi stagnation with Spleen qi deficiency
    c. Spleen qi deficiency and qi stagnation in the middle burner
    d. Dampness in the middle burner

153. A 20-year-old female said she lost over 10 pounds in the last two months even though she has been eating more than before. She states that she has a very good appetite, eats a lot of food, and always feels hungry. She noticed that she has an increased sensitivity to heat, sweats a lot, and drink a lot of cold water. She also complains of nervousness, anxiety and irritability, palpi-

tations, and difficulty sleeping. Other symptoms include frequent urination, three to four bowel movements a day, and a short menstrual cycle with heavy bleeding. During the exam you find that her hands have a slight tremor and there is some swelling at the base of the her neck. She has a red tongue with a thin yellow coating, and a rapid surging pulse. What is her pattern?

   a. Liver yang rising due to Liver and Kidney yin deficiency
   b. Stomach and Heart fire
   c. Liver wind due to excess heat
   d. Spleen and Stomach yin deficiency

154. Robert has had abdominal distention and stuffiness for two days. Other symptoms include poor digestion, bad breath, thirst with a preference for cold drinks, belching with a sour taste, and only one bowel movement in two days with undigested food in the stool. His tongue is red with a thick, yellow, greasy coating, and his pulse is slippery and rapid. What is the pattern identification?

   a. Spleen qi deficiency with damp-heat in the middle burner
   b. Food stagnation with Stomach fire
   c. Stomach qi rebellion due to Stomach yin deficiency
   d. Stomach qi and yin deficiency

155. A 39-year-old man has been enduring a fever for the past five days along with painful blisters on the left side of his waist for the past three days. The pain is severe, burning, continuous, and radiating in nature. The blisters were initially small and few in number, but they later multiplied and wrapped around the left side of his waist. The skin surrounding the vesicles is erythematous and very tender on palpation. Other symptoms include a bitter taste in the mouth, thirst without desire to drink, and red eyes and face. He is an ER nurse and has been under great pressure for the last two months because of a large number of COVID-19 patients flooding the emergency room. He has a red tongue with a thick, yellow, greasy coating, and a wiry and slippery pulse. He has been diagnosed with shingles, also known as herpes zoster. The TCM diagnosis for him is shingles due to which of the following patterns?

   a. Wind rash caused by heat toxicity invading the Lung
   b. Liver and Gallbladder damp-heat
   c. Liver and Gallbladder blood stagnation
   d. Wind-heat invading the Lung with heat-phlegm obstruction

156. A 28-year-old woman complains of edema in her feet for one month. There is no past or current related disease history. She works six days a week in a coffee shop. Beginning several years ago, she has eaten a vegetarian diet off and on. Her body is very thin and pale, and she experiences occasional dizziness, poor energy, and soft stools. Her tongue body is thin, pale, and scalloped on the sides, and her pulse is deep and thin. What is the pattern identification?

   a. Lung and Kidney yang deficiency
   b. Water retention due to Kidney qi deficiency

c. Water retention due to Spleen qi deficiency
d. Dampness accumulation in the lower burner

157. A 35-year-old female patient was diagnosed with a peptic ulcer three months ago. She has upper abdominal discomfort and pain that is worse at night and wakes her up. She also has a feeling of fullness, hunger, or emptiness in the stomach, often 1-2 hours after a meal, but no desire to eat. She has to force herself to eat because of having no appetite, and has lost 20 pounds in the last four months. Other symptoms include chapped lips, nausea, belching, sometimes vomiting, and constipation with dry stools. Her tongue is red with a scanty coating, and her pulse is rapid and thin. What is the pattern identification?

a. Food stagnation
b. Spleen and Stomach yin deficiency
c. Dampness accumulation in the middle burner
d. Spleen and Stomach disharmony

158. A 53-year-old male patient has been diagnosed with Crohn's disease for over five years. He is taking 5mg prednisone per day. His symptoms flare up a couple times a year and is usually triggered by emotional stress. In general, he always feels lassitude, abdominal fullness and bloating, no appetite, depression, and loose stools. Four days ago he started having severe abdominal pain that was resistant to pressure, nausea, diarrhea with bloody stools, tenesmus, and a body temperature of 100.4° F. Other signs and symptoms include thirst, a red tongue with teeth marks, a yellow greasy tongue coating, and a deep, rapid, and slippery pulse. What is the most appropriate pattern identification for his current condition?

a. Liver qi stagnation overacting on the Spleen
b. Spleen qi deficiency, Large Intestine damp-heat
c. Spleen and Stomach disharmony
d. Spleen and Kidney yang deficiency with Liver qi stagnation

159. Two weeks ago, a 20-year-old New York college student started feeling chills, sometimes with shaking, a non-productive cough, headache, stuffy nose, sore throat, and body aches. His illness has gotten worse and become severe in the last two days. Now he complains of shortness of breath that limits his activities along with tightness and pressure in his chest. Other symptoms include having no appetite due to a loss of taste and smell, nausea and occasionally vomiting, going to the toilet 5-6 times a day with watery stools, and a sensation of body heaviness and fatigue. Vital signs are as follows: T: 102.6° F, P: 92 bpm, RR: 24 pm, BP: 118/78 mmHg. His COVID-19 viral test is positive. He has a red tongue with a thick, white, greasy coating, and a superficial, rapid, and slippery pulse. What is his pattern identification?

a. Wind-heat-dampness invading the Lung
b. Cold-dampness encumbering the Spleen
c. Lung qi deficiency
d. All of the above

160. A 21-year-old female vegan primarily eats cold and raw foods with a preference for fruit. Two days ago she noticed fullness and distention with accompanying diarrhea. Inquiry reveals anorexia, no taste, no thirst, and a heavy sensation in her head. Observation shows a dull face and a pale flawbby tongue with a white greasy coating. Palpation demonstrates epigastric and abdominal fullness and a soft and slow pulse. What is the pattern identification for her condition?

    a. Cold-dampness encumbering the Spleen
    b. Damp-heat encumbering the Spleen
    c. Spleen and Stomach disharmony
    d. Spleen yang deficiency with Stomach deficiency cold

161. Mary, a 30-year-old female, complains of indigestion. She has been diagnosed with a peptic ulcer, has dull epigastric burning pain, and medication hasn't helped. Her appetite is normal, but once she starts to eat, she easily gets full and bloated. She also has a dry mouth and throat, and is constantly sipping water. Her menstrual cycle is short with a scanty light-colored flow. She gets tired very easily and always has a slight temperature, especially in the afternoons. She complains of night sweats and wakes up easily. You see that her cheeks are slightly flushed and the skin around her lips are very dry. Her pulse is thin. What is her most probable pattern?

    a. Liver and Spleen disharmony
    b. Spleen qi and Stomach yin deficiency
    c. Liver and Kidney yin deficiency
    d. Spleen and Stomach disharmony

162. Dry stools first and then loose watery stools indicate which of the following patterns?

    a. Large Intestine deficiency cold
    b. Small Intestine deficiency cold
    c. Spleen qi deficiency
    d. Kidney yang deficiency

163. Richard has been sick for one year. He has hepatomegaly below the hypochondria that is 2-3 cm. There are no palpable findings for the spleen. Chief complaint: fixed pain in bilateral hypochondria region that is worse on the right side. His abdomen is distended, and he has lassitude and no appetite. He has taken more than 80 herbal prescriptions to soothe the Liver and regulate the flow of qi, dispel phlegm, and resolve dampness, but symptoms have not improved. He is losing weight, has a bitter taste in the mouth, a dry throat, dizziness, difficulty sleeping, and constipation. He has a red tongue with a crack in the middle and a thin coating. The pulse is wiry, hesitant, and thin. What is the pattern identification for this case?

    a. Liver qi and blood stagnation with phlegm accumulation
    b. Liver yin deficiency with blood stagnation and Spleen qi deficiency
    c. Liver and Kidney yin deficiency
    d. Liver and Gallbladder damp-heat

164. A 30-year-old female comes in to see you, complaining of paroxysmal headaches at the temples and on both sides of the head. She also complains of hypochondrial pain, a bitter taste in the mouth, a poor appetite, and nausea. She does not like eating greasy foods. She is thirsty but does not want to drink. She also has vaginal itching due to candidiasis. Her tongue is slightly red with a thick yellow coating, and her pulse is wiry and slippery. What is the pattern identification for her?

   a. Liver and Gallbladder damp-heat
   b. Liver yang rising
   c. Liver qi and blood stagnation
   d. Liver fire blazing

165. A 34-year-old female is diagnosed with acute hepatitis B. Her chief complaints are fullness of the epigastrium, nausea, no appetite, fatigue, low-grade fever. Other symptoms include sweating, muscle and joint aches, hypochondrial pain, and a bitter taste in the mouth. She is thirsty but can only drink small quantities of water and has dark urine. She has a thick, sticky, yellow tongue coating, and a slippery and wiry pulse. Her skin and sclera are bright yellow. What is her pattern identification?

   a. Liver and Gallbladder damp-heat
   b. Damp-heat encumbering the Spleen with Liver Fire
   c. Damp-heat accumulation in the Spleen
   d. Liver yin deficiency with dampness in the Spleen

166. A 45-year-old woman was diagnosed with a urinary tract infection (UTI) two months ago. After taking 10 days of Macrobid, her UTI symptoms went away, but now she complains of an itchy and burning sensation in her vaginal area with yellow foul-smelling discharge that has lasted a month. She has had this problem several times over the past few years. She is slightly overweight and has lassitude, lethargy, a sensation of heaviness, and feels very sleepy all the time. She has some thirst but doesn't drink much, and she has a bowel movement every other day. Her tongue is red with a greasy yellow coating, and the sides are redder and have teeth marks. Her pulse is wiry and slippery. Her gynecologist diagnosed her with candida infection. What is her pattern identification?

   a. Liver and Gallbladder damp-heat
   b. Spleen qi deficiency with dampness
   c. Heart and Spleen qi deficiency
   d. Damp-heat accumulation in the Spleen

167. Joan, age 32, presents with a chronic distending headache on the right side. She has been consuming a large amount of alcohol for about a year because she has been depressed. The headache usually starts when she goes out into the bright sun, and the pain originates in her right eye, goes over the head, and ends at the occiput. She also complains about occasional right intercostal pain, trouble sleeping, and a bitter taste in the mouth. She has a red complexion and a red tongue with a yellow coating. Her pulse is wiry and rapid. What is the best pattern identification?

a. Liver yang rising
b. Kidney yin deficiency with heat
c. Heart fire blazing
d. Liver fire blazing

168. Which pattern is indicated by the following signs and symptoms: dull pain in the lower abdomen that is relieved by pressure and warmth, borborygmus, soft stools, frequent or clear copious urination, a pale tongue with a thin white coating, and a deep, weak, or slow pulse?

a. Kidney yang deficiency
b. Large Intestine deficiency cold
c. Small Intestine deficiency cold
d. Spleen yang deficiency

169. Kevin, a six-year-old boy, has poor memory and difficulty concentrating in school. He has nightmares that keep him from sleeping and he fights a lot with his sister. His favorite food is ice cream. He has a slightly enlarged red tongue body with a red tip and a thin white coating. Which of the following patterns is the diagnosis for him?

a. Heart fire blazing
b. Liver fire blazing
c. Phlegm misting the Heart
d. Heart blood deficiency

170. A 56-year-old male patient was diagnosed with congestive heart failure (CHF) over three years ago. He complains of palpitations and shortness of breath that becomes worse on exertion. He also has spontaneous sweating, cold limbs, cyanosis of the lips, and a pale, flabby, and tender tongue with a thin white coating. His pulse is thin, weak, and knotted. What is the correct pattern for him?

a. Heart qi deficiency
b. Cold-phlegm obstructing the Heart vessels
c. Heart yang deficiency
d. Heart and Kidney yang deficiency

171. A 54-year-old female complains of having ADHD since age 10. She has poor sleep, anxiety, nervousness, and severe stabbing headaches in the forehead. She is also prone to vaginal candida infections. Her pulse is wiry, rapid, and hesitant. Her tongue is reddish purple and flabby with a crack and a thick yellow coating. What is the pattern identification for her?

a. Liver qi and blood stagnation with damp-heat
b. Heart yin deficiency, blood stasis, damp-heat in the lower burner
c. Heart blood deficiency, Liver blood stagnation with damp-heat
d. Damp-heat in the Liver channel

172. Jane, 48, has been suffering from insomnia and dream-disturbed sleep for over three years. She also has poor memory, palpitations, dizziness, and vertigo. She has had no menstrual period since last year. Laboratory examination shows: FSH 124 mIU/ml, estradiol 20 pg/mL, and LH 48.3 IU/L. Her physician has diagnosed her with menopause syndrome. She has a pale face and tongue, and a weak pulse. What is the pattern identification for her?

   a. Kidney yin deficiency
   b. Spleen qi deficiency
   c. Heart fire blazing
   d. Heart blood deficiency

173. Valerie, a 58-year-old female, has cardiac pain that is stabbing or stuffy in nature at the precordial region or behind the sternum. The pain started 10 minutes ago and refers to the shoulder and arm. She also feels palpitations and has dark purplish tongue and lips. Her pulse is thin and hesitant. What is the pattern identification for her?

   a. Chest blockage due to Heart vessels obstruction by blood stasis
   b. Chest blockage due to Heart vessels obstruction by phlegm
   c. Palpitations due to Heart blood and qi deficiency
   d. Lung abscess due to heat-phlegm accumulation in the Lung

174. A 34-year-old woman seeks treatment from you because she has premature atrial contraction (PVC) and supraventricular tachycardia (SVT). Symptoms include palpitations and a feeling of oppression in her chest. From your interview and examination, you discover that she has mental restlessness, insomnia, dream-disturbed sleep, poor memory, anxiety, uneasiness, malar flush, night sweats, and a dry mouth and throat. Blood tests show that her hormone levels are all in normal range. Her tongue is red with almost no coating and has a crack. Her pulse is thin and rapid. What is the best TCM diagnosis for her?

   a. Insomnia due to Heart and Kidney disharmony
   b. Palpitations due to Heart yin deficiency
   c. Restless organ disorder due to Heart blood deficiency
   d. Menopause syndrome due to Kidney yin deficiency

175. A 52-year-old male has been suffering from hypertension for over 10 years. Recently, he has been experiencing oppression in the chest along with pain in the chest that is sharp and extends to the left shoulder or arm. He also complains of palpitations, breathlessness, dizziness and expectoration of white sputum. He has a flabby tongue with purple spots on the sides, and a slippery and hesitant pulse. What is the most appropriate pattern identification for him?

   a. Heart vessels obstruction by blood stasis
   b. Phlegm misting the Heart
   c. Heart vessels obstruction by blood stasis and cold-phlegm
   d. Water qi encroaching on the Heart

176. A 65-year-old male has had minor heart attacks twice in the past five years. He felt severe left chest pain with a very hot and tight sensation before going to the emergency room. He generally prefers a cooler temperature. His face is reddish and his hands are warm, but his feet are slightly cold. He has frequent palpitations at night, night sweats, constipation, and yellow urine. His tongue is red with purple spots and a yellow coating, while his pulse is wiry and thin. What is the TCM diagnosis for him?

   a. Chest blockage due to Heart vessels obstruction by heat-phlegm
   b. Chest blockage due to Heart vessels obstruction by blood stasis with Heart yin deficiency
   c. Palpitations due to Heart yin deficiency with heat misting the Heart
   d. Palpitations due to Heart fire blazing with Kidney yin deficiency

177. All of following signs or symptoms can appear in Urinary Bladder deficiency cold, EXCEPT:

   a. Urgent and painful urination
   b. Bedwetting
   c. Frequent copious urination
   d. Incontinence

178. Logan, a 64-year-old male patient, has been having acute and severe hiccups ever since he had stomach cancer removal surgery (partial gastrectomy) three days ago. The hiccups are consistent, loud, dry, and accompanied by burning pain. His doctor has put him on medication, but it only helps to stop the hiccups for 30 minutes. The hiccups make it difficult to eat and sleep. He is very tired, thirsty, and stressed. He has a thin red tongue with a lot of cracks and a peeled coating. His pulse is slightly rapid, thin and hesitant. Which of the following patterns is associated with his hiccups?

   a. Liver overacting on the Stomach
   b. Stomach and Spleen disharmony
   c. Kidney and Stomach yin deficiency
   d. Stomach yin deficiency with blood stagnation

179. A 42-year-old female patient complains of vertigo and dizziness. She said it started five weeks ago, occurring suddenly. The vertigo and dizziness were so severe that she had to lie down. She also experienced headache, tinnitus, nausea, and vomiting. The symptoms disappeared after two hours. Since then, she has had a couple of episodes. Her BP is 118/70 mmHg, her tongue is slightly red with a thick yellow coating, and her pulse is wiry and slippery. The diagnosis is vertigo and dizziness due to which of the following patterns?

   a. Liver yang rising
   b. Liver wind with phlegm
   c. Liver blood deficiency
   d. Spleen qi deficiency with phlegm-dampness accumulation

180. Barbara, a 61-year-old female, was diagnosed with Sjögren's syndrome, complains of dry eyes and mouth. Other symptoms include a dry throat, a nonproductive cough that is worse in the evenings, and dry skin with some red rashes on her face. She also has stiffness and aching in her knees and little finger. She is very emotional and cries a lot, feeling depressed and frustrated. She has a red cracked tongue with little coating, and a thin, rapid, and wiry pulse. What is the pattern identification for her?

   a. Liver and Lung yin deficiency
   b. Liver fire attacking the Lung
   c. Kidney and Liver yin deficiency
   d. Dryness invading the Lung

181. A 19-year-old female patient says that she began menstruating at the age of 14, and her period has been irregular since then. Two to three days before her menstrual period she gets breast distention and abdominal cramps. The abdominal cramps become milder in day three and four, and will continue another two days after menses. Her menstrual flow is scanty, thin, and light red in color. Her tongue appears pale on the sides with a thin coating, and her pulse is thin and wiry. What is the pattern identification for this patient's syndrome?

   a. Liver qi and blood stagnation
   b. Liver qi and blood deficiency
   c. Spleen qi deficiency with Liver blood stagnation
   d. Liver qi stagnation with blood deficiency

182. A 16-year-old girl comes in because of abnormal menstruation. She said that she started her period when she was 14 and it has always been on an 18-day cycle. The blood is very fresh red and in large quantity with clots. She also complains of skin breakouts and abdominal cramps for the first two days. She drinks a lot of ice water and often eats salads. Which of the following patterns relates to her condition?

   a. Liver qi and blood stagnation
   b. Spleen qi deficiency not controlling blood
   c. Liver blood stagnation, with heat in the blood
   d. Spleen qi and blood deficiency

183. A 39-year-old female patient is referred by her naturopathic doctor for Addison's disease. She complains of extreme fatigue and lassitude, weight loss due to a decrease in appetite, muscle aches and pain in her lower back and legs, preference for warmth, mental fatigue, brain fog, dizziness or fainting when standing up, loose stools, dull skin color, loss of body hair, no sex drive, and a short menstrual cycle with a scanty flow. Her blood pressure is 75/50 mmHg. She is also very irritable and depressed. Her tongue is pale with teeth marks and a thin glossy coating, and her pulse is faint. What is the pattern identification for her chief complaint?

a. Liver qi stagnation with Spleen qi deficiency
b. Kidney and Spleen yang deficiency
c. Heart blood and Spleen qi deficiency
d. Heart and Kidney disharmony

184. Barbara, age 34, complains of infertility. She has had three unexpected miscarriages during the last eight years. Since her first miscarriage, she has had an irregular menstrual cycle and lower abdominal pain during menstruation. The pain is aggravated by pressure and relieved by warmth. She has a slightly purple tongue with a thin white coating, and a deep wiry pulse. What is the best pattern identification for her?

a. Spleen and Kidney qi deficiency
b. Liver qi and blood stagnation
c. Heart and Kidney disharmony
d. Kidney essence deficiency

185. A 64-year-old female patient complains of swelling of her feet and ankles. It started three years ago and gradually got worse. She was diagnosed with coronary heart disease and hypertension over 10 years ago. Other symptoms include shortness of breath with activity, palpitations, difficulty sleeping, fatigue, weakness, and lower back pain. Her body always feels cold, especially below her waist. Her tongue is pale and tender with a slippery white coating, and her pulse is deep and weak. What is her pattern identification?

a. Yang edema due to dampness accumulating in the Spleen
b. Yin edema due to Heart and Kidney yang deficiency
c. Spleen and Kidney yang deficiency
d. Heart and Kidney disharmony

186. Roger, a 42-year-old Iraq veteran, was diagnosed with post-traumatic stress disorder (PTSD) three years ago. Now his symptoms include mental depression, dullness, muttering, crying and laughing without reason, paraphrenia, muteness, paraphasia, and incoherent speech. He has a thick, white, greasy tongue coating and a slippery pulse. What is the pattern identification for him?

a. Phlegm misting the Heart
b. Heart fire blazing
c. Phlegm-fire harassing the Heart
d. Heart vessels obstruction by phlegm

187. A 64-year-old female patient was diagnosed with chronic bronchitis over three months ago. Symptoms include cough that is worse in the evenings, and viscous white blood-streaked sputum that is difficult to expectorate. Other symptoms include shortness of breath that is worse with

exertion, wheezing, and distress in the chest. Her tongue has cracks in the front along with a thick white coating, and her pulse is deep, thin, and slippery. What is her pattern identification?

    a. Dryness invading the Lung with Lung qi deficiency
    b. Heat-phlegm obstructing the Lung with Lung qi deficiency
    c. Cold-phlegm obstructing the Lung with Lung qi and yin deficiency
    d. Phlegm-dryness obstructing the Lung with Lung qi and yin deficiency

188. A 34-year-old female patient told you that she is very sensitive to all kinds of dairy foods. They always cause her abdominal bloating and distention, borborygmus, even vomiting with clear sticky fluids, loose stools, and dull abdominal pain that is relieved by warmth and pressure. She has a white tongue coating and a weak pulse. What is the pattern identification for her?

    a. Spleen qi deficiency with dampness
    b. Stomach and Large Intestine deficiency cold
    c. Food stagnation
    d. Spleen and Stomach qi deficiency

189. A 45-year-old male patient told you that four years ago his blood test showed HIV positive. At the time, he didn't have any symptoms and so did not receive any treatments. Three months ago he started having diarrhea, going to the bathroom about three to four times per day. His stools were watery and contained undigested food. He has also been suffering from fatigue, dizziness, and shortness of breath that is worse with exertion, poor appetite, and profuse sweating. He has lost 20 pounds in the last three months and cannot tolerate cold. He also urinates more frequently both during the day and night. His tongue is pale with a thin white coating, and his pulse is deep and weak. What is the pattern identification for him?

    a. Spleen qi sinking with Kidney yang deficiency
    b. Spleen qi deficiency with Heart blood deficiency
    c. Dampness accumulation in the Spleen
    d. Kidney qi deficiency

190. A 43-year-old female patient has been diagnosed with hypothyroidism. Her symptoms include fatigue, weakness, spontaneous sweating, coarse and dry hair, dry and rough pale skin, hair loss, muscle cramps with frequent muscle aches, constipation, memory loss, palpitations, and insomnia. Her menstrual cycle is usually 35-42 days or even every other month, with very light scanty bleeding. She has a pale and tender tongue with teeth marks and a thin white coating. Her pulse is thin and weak. What is the most appropriate pattern for her condition?

    a. Kidney yin deficiency with Heart fire blazing
    b. Spleen and Kidney yang deficiency
    c. Liver and Kidney yin deficiency
    d. Heart qi and Liver blood deficiency

191. A 12-year-old boy presents with intense, sharp, stabbing pain in the right lower quadrant that is worse with pressure. He has profuse sweating, thirst, no bowel movements for three days, drinks a lot of water, and a body temperature of 103.2° F. What is the pattern identification for him?

   a. Small Intestine qi stagnation
   b. Large Intestine heat accumulation
   c. Large Intestine damp-heat
   d. Cold invading the Large Intestine

192. A 56-year-old male patient was diagnosed with coronary artery disease. This morning during his routine physical exercise, he suddenly felt a squeezing pain and discomfort in his chest area, and the pain radiated to his left arm and shoulder. He also felt heaviness, tightness, and a sensation of pressure in his chest. Meanwhile, he had shortness of breath, profuse sweating, lightheadedness, dizziness, extreme weakness, and anxiety. His pulse is rapid and irregular. The diagnosis for him is chest blockage due to which of the following patterns?

   a. Heart fire blazing
   b. Liver qi and blood stagnation
   c. Heart qi deficiency and blood stagnation
   d. Heart vessels obstructed by phlegm

193. A 43-year-old female was diagnosed with chronic idiopathic thrombocytopenic purpura (ITP) over three years ago. She says that she gets bruised a lot and has very heavy menstrual bleeding. Other symptoms include fatigue, shortness of breath, and spontaneous sweating. She has a pale complexion, a pale tongue, and a thin weak pulse. Which of the following is the best diagnosis for her?

   a. Bleeding due to Liver blood stagnation
   b. Bleeding due to Lung heat
   c. Bleeding due to Spleen qi deficiency
   d. Bleeding due to Liver fire injuring blood vessels

194. A 40-year-old male patient has been diagnosed with Buerger's disease, also known as thromboangiitis obliterans. Signs and symptoms include coldness and pain in the arch area of the feet. The condition is usually induced or aggravated by exposure to cold and walking, and relieved by warmth and rest. His feet look very pale and turn bluish when exposed to the cold. His tongue is pale purple with a thin white coating, and his pulse is deep, slow, and hesitant. What is the pattern identification?

   a. Blood stagnation due to Liver blood deficiency
   b. Blood stagnation due to Liver qi stagnation
   c. Liver and Gallbladder damp-heat
   d. Kidney yang deficiency with blood stagnation

195. A 23-year-old female has been suffering from abdominal pain for over six months. The pain usually starts one hour after a meal and takes 2-3 hours to stop. It is a dull and twisted kind of pain in the lower left quadrant of her abdomen. She has been on a vegan and gluten-free diet, and has a history of anorexia. Other symptoms include bloating, poor appetite, low energy, depression, anxiety, 2-3 bowel movements a day with soft stools, and bruising easily. Her menstruation cycle is 21 days with light-colored bleeding for seven days and no cramps. Ultrasound, x-ray, gastroscopy, colonoscopy, and blood test results are all negative. Physical exam shows a weight of 110 lbs, height of 5'6", a pale face and lips, a pale tongue with teeth marks, and a weak wiry pulse. What is the pattern identification?

    a. Stomach blood stagnation with Spleen qi deficiency
    b. Liver and Stomach disharmony
    c. Spleen and Stomach disharmony
    d. Liver qi stagnation with Spleen qi deficiency

196. A 35-year-old female was diagnosed with Crohn's disease last year. She complains of abdominal cramps that are consistent and worse after eating seafood. The pain is also aggravated during her menstrual cycle. She has 3-5 bowel movements a day with watery stools that do not contain blood. Other symptoms include bloating and distention, poor appetite, low energy, depression, anxiety, cold limbs, and nocturnal urination averaging three times a night. She weighs only 105 lbs and is 5'6" tall. She has a pale tongue with a slightly thick coating and a weak pulse. What is the pattern identification for her?

    a. Spleen yang deficiency with dampness
    b. Spleen and Kidney yang deficiency
    c. Large Intestine cold-dampness
    d. Large Intestine damp-heat

197. Jane, a 48-year-old female diagnosed with post-traumatic stress disorder (PTSD), has been suffering from insomnia and dream-disturbed sleep for over three years. She also experiences poor memory, palpitations, dizziness, vertigo, nervousness, timidity, startling easily, paranoia, and shortness of breath. She has had no menstrual period since last year, and denies having hot flashes and night sweats. Her face and tongue are both pale, and her pulse is weak. What is the correct diagnosis?

    a. Heart blood and Gallbladder qi deficiency
    b. Heart and Spleen deficiency
    c. Spleen and Kidney yang deficiency
    d. Heart and Kidney disharmony

198. A 38-year-old female has been suffering from nightmares for over 20 years, dreaming every night and always woken up by her dreams. She also suffers from anxiety, depression, insecurity, lack of confidence, frequent panic attacks, and a bitter taste in the mouth. She was abused in her childhood and has been treated by psychotherapists for many years. Additionally, she has been

diagnosed with chronic interstitial cystitis, causing frequent and urgent urination, but no burning pain. Her tongue is red, redder at the tip, and has a slightly thick yellow coating. Her pulse is wiry and slippery. Which of the following patterns relates to her condition?

   a. Gallbladder stagnation with phlegm disturbance
   b. Liver qi stagnation with heat
   c. Heart fire transmitting to the Small Intestine
   d. All of the above

199. Esther, 27, is 70 days pregnant and complains of increasing episodes of severe vomiting of clear saliva for the last two weeks. It has been so bad that she has not been able to eat. Recently, she began feeling nausea, poor appetite, dizziness, shortness of breath, and an aversion to speaking. She has become so debilitated that she can hardly get out of bed. Her tongue is pale with a thin white coating and her pulse is slippery and weak. What is the pattern identification?

   a. Liver and Stomach disharmony
   b. Liver qi stagnation with Spleen qi deficiency
   c. Stomach yin deficiency
   d. Spleen and Stomach disharmony with qi deficiency

200. Clint, 46, has been suffering from recurrent asthmatic attacks and coughing for the past 10 years. It is usually induced by weather changes. He recently suffered a relapse for two weeks after a cold. He is short of breath and unable to breathe while lying down. He has slight sweating, chills, and white foamy watery sputum. His appetite is poor and his stools are unformed. His tongue is light red with a white greasy coating, and his pulse is deep, slippery, and weak. What is the diagnosis for this patient?

   a. Cold-water shooting into the Lung with Spleen yang deficiency
   b. Cold-water shooting into the Heart with Kidney yang deficiency
   c. Cold-phlegm obstructing the Lung
   d. Lung qi deficiency with phlegm-dampness accumulation

201. A 35-year-old female complains of amenorrhea for more than six months. She tells you she always has scanty and light menstrual flow and a long menstrual cycle of 30-35 days. Other signs and symptoms include tiredness, dizziness, loose stools, poor appetite, blurred vision, and numbness and tingling of the limbs. Upon examination, you find that she has a sallow complexion and a pale tongue that is paler on the sides. Her pulse is hesitant. What is the pattern identification for her?

   a. Liver and Heart blood deficiency
   b. Kidney essence deficiency
   c. Liver qi and blood stagnation
   d. Liver blood deficiency with Spleen qi deficiency

202. Your patient is a 25-year-old male with nocturnal emissions, and his condition has been getting worse over the last couple months. During the day, he experiences mental fatigue, poor focus, brain fog, and weakness in his legs and back. Even when he does get to sleep, it is usually very restless and he frequently has night sweats. He is prone to tongue sores, although he does not have them now. His tongue is red with little coating and his pulse is thin and rapid. What is the pattern identification?

   a. Heart blood and Spleen qi deficiency
   b. Heart and Kidney disharmony
   c. Heart fire blazing
   d. Liver blood deficiency

203. Malcolm, a 56-year-old school teacher, complains of brain fog and mental fatigue. He has just finished writing his book. He has been having insomnia for the past four years, as he dreams frequently and wakes very easily. He also has palpitations, dizziness, lassitude, loose stools, and poor memory. He was diagnosed with hypothyroidism and has been taking synthroid. He looks pale. His tongue is pale with little coating, and his pulse feels thin and weak. What is his pattern identification?

   a. Liver blood and Gallbladder qi deficiency
   b. Heart and Kidney disharmony
   c. Heart blood and Spleen qi deficiency
   d. Heart fire blazing

204. A 45-year-old female lost her job two months ago. She complains of depression, anger, frustration, difficulty falling sleep, oppression in the chest, and frequent sighing. Other symptoms include poor appetite, abdominal bloating, loose stools, fatigue, and shortness of breath. She also notices that her menstruation was very scanty and short in the last two months. She has a pale tongue and a weak pulse. What is the pattern identification?

   a. Liver and Stomach disharmony with qi and blood deficiency
   b. Liver qi stagnation and blood deficiency with Spleen qi deficiency
   c. Phlegm misting the Heart
   d. Spleen and Stomach disharmony

205. A middle-aged man has had a productive cough for a month. His voice is weak and the cough is worse after exercise. He experiences some sensation of fullness in his abdomen just after eating as well as feeling somewhat sleepy. He also feels some sensation of phlegm. He doesn't smoke and only drinks moderate amounts of beer or wine in the evenings. His urination is fine but he has sluggish bowel movements. His pulse is thin and very weak in both front positions. His tongue is flabby with a thin white coating. What is the pattern identification?

   a. Cold-phlegm obstructing the Lung
   b. Lung and Kidney qi deficiency with phlegm

c. Wind-cold invading the Lung
d. Lung and Spleen qi deficiency with phlegm

206. A 28-year-old female student complains of insomnia and feeling stressed from final examinations. She is the nervous type and wakes up frequently during the night, has very low energy, and feels slightly dizzy. Her concentration and memory are getting worse. She has occasional palpitations and feels overwhelmed from her relationships. Her complexion is slightly sallow. She tires easily and sometimes falls asleep in class. Her appetite has decreased. Her tongue is pink with a thin white coating. Her pulse is thin and deep. What is her pattern identification?

   a. Heart blood and Spleen qi deficiency
   b. Heart and Kidney disharmony
   c. Spleen and Kidney yang deficiency
   d. Liver qi stagnation with Heart fire blazing

207. The chief complaint for a 36-year-old male patient is stress related to his job and relationships with coworkers. He feels upper abdominal tightness and irritable bowel movements. His appetite varies depending on his emotional changes. He is slightly depressed with occasional insomnia, involving difficulty falling asleep because of his busy mind. Overall, his body is healthy, he consistently exercises, and he has no other complaints. He has a red tongue with a slightly thick coating, and a deep, wiry, and slightly slippery pulse. What is the pattern identification for him?

   a. Heart and Spleen deficiency
   b. Liver and Stomach disharmony with Heart blood deficiency
   c. Liver and Spleen disharmony with Heart fire blazing
   d. Heart and Kidney disharmony with Spleen qi deficiency

208. A 50-year-old female complains of having irregular menses for about half a year and reports that recently she started feeling hot in her upper body, especially her chest and neck. She has also been experiencing slight night sweats. She feels better in the morning and worse later in the day and at night. She is very irritable, and feels shoulder and neck tension when she experiences stress. She has dry skin, eyes, and mouth, and doesn't drink enough water. Her urination is yellow and she is slightly constipated. Her tongue is red, but pale on the sides, with a very thin coating. Her pulse is slippery and rapid. What is the pattern identification?

   a. Heart and Kidney disharmony
   b. Liver and Kidney yin deficiency with Liver blood deficiency
   c. Liver qi stagnation with Kidney yin deficiency
   d. Liver blood deficiency

209. An 84-year-old man has had pitting edema of the lower legs for over 10 years. He is able to walk, but very sluggishly. His lower back has no pain, but feels stiff. He complains that his feet feel cold all the time so he wears something on his feet during all seasons. He has frequent urination,

especially at night, when he has to urinate 2-3 times. He likes drinking wine at dinner, but he does not smoke. He feels some gas and bloating after his meals, and feels a heavy sensation in his body and limbs. His tongue is deep purple with a very thick gray coating. His pulse is wiry, slippery, and deeper in the rear positions. What is the diagnosis?

   a. Damp-heat encumbering the Spleen
   b. Edema due to dampness encumbering the Spleen
   c. Edema due to Heart and Kidney yang deficiency
   d. Edema due to Spleen and Kidney yang deficiency

210. Beatrice, 78, has been suffering from hiccups for five days. She states that five days ago she had a big argument with her son and the hiccups developed immediately afterward. Her hiccups are continuous, clear, and forceful. She has a feeling of an uncontrollable upsurge of gas with fullness in the epigastrium and hypochondrium. Her appetite has decreased and she has occasional acid regurgitation. She also has a bitter taste in her mouth and suffers from restlessness and insomnia. Her tongue is cracked and slightly red with little coating, and her pulse is thin and wiry. What is the pattern identification?

   a. Liver fire with excess heat in the Stomach
   b. Liver and Stomach disharmony with Heart and Kidney disharmony
   c. Stomach yin deficiency with excess cold invading the Stomach
   d. Spleen and Stomach disharmony with Liver and Stomach disharmony

211. A 56-year-old male has been suffering from chronic obstructive pulmonary disease (COPD), due to emphysema for over 15 years. He complains of cough with profuse white sputum, wheezing, and shortness of breath. He feels tired all the time. He also complains of no appetite, loose stools, and sweating a lot even without any exertion. You find that his voice is very weak when he talks to you. His tongue is pale with a thick white coating, and his pulse is weak and slippery. What is the pattern identification?

   a. Lung and Spleen yang deficiency with cold-phlegm
   b. Lung and Kidney qi deficiency with cold-phlegm
   c. Lung and Spleen qi deficiency with cold-phlegm
   d. Lung and Kidney yin deficiency with cold-phlegm

212. A 31-year-old woman has been suffering from periodic severe abdominal pain for six months. During an attack, she would feel slightly feverish and weak, and her stools would become loose. The abdominal pain would be aggravated by physical exertion and has been most prominent in the left illiac fossa. She has also been diagnosed with diverticulitis. Two months ago, she developed a foul-smelling yellowish-green vaginal discharge, her appetite decreased significantly, and she felt more tired and weak in general. She had also experienced some bleeding in between her menstrual periods, and swelling of the ankles. Her tongue is peeled except for some thin yellow coating in the center, and her tongue body is thin. Her pulse is thin, rapid, slippery, and wiry at both proximal positions. All of the following patterns are related to her condition, EXCEPT:

a. Spleen qi deficiency
b. Large Intestine qi and blood stagnation
c. Liver and Gallbladder damp-heat
d. Liver qi stagnation

213. A 27-year-old female complains of having hoarseness for over six months. At onset, she had a sore throat, a "thickened" voice, cough, and thirst. Spraying the throat with a tincture of benzoin provided no relief, nor did warm acrid herbs or cool bitter herbs. She also complains of restlessness, disturbed sleep, tinnitus, a dry throat, and weakness and soreness in the lower back and knees. The hoarseness has made speaking very difficult. She has a red tongue with a scanty coating, and a thin and rapid pulse. What is the pattern identification for her at this time?

a. Heat congesting the Lung, Heart fire blazing
b. Lung yin deficiency, Heart and Kidney disharmony
c. Lung qi deficiency, phlegm-fire harassing the Heart
d. Lung qi and yin deficiency, Liver qi stagnation with heat

214. George is a 20-year-old student at a local community college with a history of schizophrenia. On several recent occasions, he experienced sudden absolute panic. During these episodes, his heart would pound, he would tremble, his mouth would get dry, and he would feel as if the walls were caving in. The feelings only last a few minutes, but when they occur the only thing that seems to relieve his fear is walking around his apartment and reminding himself that he is in control. He has also experienced irritability and trouble sleeping, having nightmares all the time. His face looks red and his skin breaks out. His tongue is red with a thick, yellow, greasy coating and his pulse is rapid, slippery, and wiry. What is the pattern identification for him?

a. Phlegm-fire harassing the Heart
b. Phlegm misting the Heart
c. Heart fire blazing
d. Liver qi stagnation

215. *Yáng míng* organ [*fǔ*] pattern from the six-channel pattern identification system matches which of the following *zàng fǔ* patterns?

a. Stomach fire
b. Damp-heat in Liver and Gallbladder
c. Heat congested in the Lung
d. Large Intestine heat accumulation

216. Martha, a 74-year-old woman with a history of rheumatic fever while in her twenties, presented to her practitioner with complaints of increasing shortness of breath and palpitations upon exertion. She also noted that the typical swelling she has had in her ankles for years has started to get worse over the past two months, making it especially difficult to get her shoes on toward the end of the day. In the past week, she has had a decreased appetite, some nausea and vomiting, and tenderness in the right upper quadrant of the abdomen. On physical examination,

Martha's jugular veins are noticeably distended. Auscultation of the heart reveals a low-pitched rumbling systolic murmur, heard best over the left upper sternal border. She looks pale and her hands and feet are cold. She has a pale flabby tongue with a white slippery coating, and a deep weak pulse. What is the pattern identification for her?

   a. Heart and Kidney disharmony
   b. Spleen and Kidney yang deficiency
   c. Lung and Heart qi deficiency
   d. Heart, Spleen, and Kidney yang deficiency

217. All of the following symptoms can appear in both Gallbladder stagnation with phlegm disturbance and phlegm-fire harassing the Heart, EXCEPT:

   a. Dizziness and nausea
   b. Bitter taste in the mouth
   c. Greasy tongue coating, slippery pulse
   d. Insomnia, palpitation

218. A 54-year-old female computer programmer complains of "heart pounding." She describes the episodes as a feeling of fullness in her neck and a racing heart. The events do not seem to be triggered by stress or physical exertion, and have occurred at all times during the day and night. She estimates that they occur about 10 times a day. The palpitations last about five minutes and then subside. They are not associated with chest pain or shortness of breath. In addition, she complains of increasing irritability and difficulty concentrating at work, both of which have become noticeable over the past 12 months. She describes herself as having always been the nervous type, but over the past year, a tremor in both hands has made it difficult for her to use a keyboard. She also reports having lost weight over the past three months, as she feels hunger but no desire to eat. She complains of mild insomnia and notices that she has recently started feeling uncomfortable at night when there are lots of covers over her. She denies any history of depression or anxiety disorders, does not drink coffee or alcohol, and does not take any medication. Her tongue is red with a thin yellow coating, and her pulse is thin and rapid. Which of the following patterns matches her condition?

   a. Heart and Kidney disharmony
   b. Wind due to Liver yin deficiency
   c. Stomach yin deficiency
   d. All of the above

219. Richard, 50, had a Colles fracture of his right arm two years ago. The injury healed after orthopedic treatment. However, the patient complains of having weakness in his right arm ever since and has become depressed from worrying about not being able to continue his work as a driver. During the past year, he developed insomnia and started having poor memory. Neurological and EEG examinations revealed no abnormalities. There was no history of hypertension. Patient is taking Prozac 300mg, but it has not been helpful enough. During consultation, you find that the patient has a dull pale complexion, appears gloomy, responds slowly, and laughs and

cries for no apparent reason, but exhibits no manic behavior. His appetite is poor and he complains of feeling fullness in the chest. He has difficulty falling asleep and often has nightmares. The tongue is pale with a greasy white coating and his pulse is wiry and thin. What is the pattern identification for him?

    a. Blood stagnation in the Small Intestine channel, Liver qi stagnation
    b. Phlegm misting the Heart, Liver qi stagnation, Heart and Spleen deficiency
    c. Phlegm obstructing the Heart vessels, Heart and Kidney disharmony, Spleen qi deficiency
    d. Phlegm-fire harassing the Heart, blood stagnation in the Small Intestine channel, Spleen qi deficiency

220. A 32-year-old woman has been suffering from painful periods for two years. The pain occurs in the hypogastrium, lateral abdomen, and sacrum. It is dull in character and associated with a bearing down sensation. Her periods are regular and the menstrual blood is slightly dark with a few clots. She also suffers from premenstrual tension with irritability and pronounced distention of the breasts and abdomen. She has been taking contraceptive pills for 10 years and the periods became painful when she stopped taking them. She has been given a progesterone pill but this has not helped the dysmenorrhea at all. Apart from the menstrual issues, she also suffers from irritable bowel syndrome, which causes her spastic pain in the abdomen with alternating constipation and diarrhea—a problem she has had for 10 years. Further inquiry revealed that she sometimes has blurry vision, occasionally feels dizzy, and experiences a tingling sensation in her limbs. Her tongue is slightly pale on the sides, and her pulse is thin and wiry. What is the current pattern identification for her?

    a. Liver qi and blood stagnation, Liver blood deficiency, Liver and Spleen disharmony
    b. Spleen qi deficiency, Liver qi and blood deficiency, Kidney yin deficiency
    c. Spleen and Stomach disharmony, Liver qi stagnation
    d. Liver qi stagnation due to Liver and Kidney yin deficiency, food stagnation with heat

221. Joy, a 50-year-old female, has been suffering from cough for six weeks. She received treatment at an urgent care clinic for bronchitis when it started and took a course of PCE 500 and a cough suppressant/expectorant. The fever, malaise, and colored-sputum resolved within seven days, but she still completed her 10-day course of medication. Overall, she is feeling better except for her cough, which comes "in spasms" and makes her feel like she can't get enough air. She has also noticed that if she walks up two flights of stairs at work or across the parking lot when it is cold, she will start coughing. Occasionally at night, she will cough a lot and hear wheezing. The over-the-counter cough preparations she has tried are not helping. She has been able to work at her secretarial job, but finds that if she talks too much or sits by someone with strong perfume, she will also start coughing. Her tongue is red with a scanty coating, and her pulse is thin and slightly wiry. What is the pattern identification for her?

    a. Wind-cold invading the Lung with heat-phlegm accumulation
    b. Cold dryness invading Lung, Lung qi deficiency
    c. Lung and Kidney yin deficiency, Liver qi stagnation
    d. Lung qi and yin deficiency with wind

222. Diane is a 54-year-old postmenopausal woman who has come to your office with the chief complaint of a cough that has increased over the past six months, accompanied by sputum and a sense of breathlessness. The sputum is thin and slightly yellow, and is more noticeable in the mornings. This has been an ongoing problem for several years. Over the past two years, she has been treated three times in the ER for a "respiratory infection" by being prescribed an "inhaler" as well as antibiotics. She has also been suffering from seasonal "hay fever" since childhood and takes HCTZ 25mg once daily for her hypertension. Her bowel movements tend to be dry. She has a slightly red tongue with a crack towards the back and a thick, slightly yellow coating. Her pulse is thin, deep, and slightly slippery. What is the pattern identification for her?

   a. Phlegm-dampness obstructing the Lung, Spleen and Kidney qi deficiency
   b. Lung qi deficiency with phlegm-dampness obstruction, Kidney yin deficiency
   c. Wind-cold invading the Lung, Lung and Kidney yin deficiency
   d. Liver fire invading the Lung

223. Mr. Lee is a 73-year-old retired construction worker who presents with complaints of fatigue and shortness of breath. The symptoms have appeared gradually over the past 5-10 years. He admits to frequent episodes of bronchitis, about 3-4 times a year, and currently smokes about two packs of cigarettes per day. He started smoking at age 20. He also admits to a gradual weight loss of 30 pounds in the past five years. He has a productive cough "most all of the time" that is worse in the mornings. His sputum is mostly clear to white, at times copious and tenacious. His shortness of breath is worse with any activity, such as climbing 10 steps on the stairs, walking half a block, or carrying a bag of groceries from the car. These activities cause him to sit a while and wait for his breathing to "settle down" before proceeding with other activities. He also has palpitations with lightheadedness several times a week, plus edema of the feet over the last year. His appetite has decreased and he feels bloated at times. He was diagnosed with benign prostatic hyperplasia (BPH) a couple years ago and has frequent urination at night. His tongue is flabby and pale with teethmarks and a thick white coating. His pulse is deep and weak. Which of the following patterns matches his condition?

   a. Kidney yang deficiency with water retention
   b. Spleen yang deficiency with dampness accumulation
   c. Lung qi deficiency with cold-phlegm obstruction
   d. All of the above

224. Which of the following signs and symptoms are common in Kidney yang deficiency with water effusion, cold-water shooting into the Lung, and water qi encroaching on the Heart?

   a. Edema, cold limbs, pale face, pale flabby tongue with slippery coating, weak and slippery pulse
   b. Cough with profuse white foamy sputum, facial edema, dyspnea, inability to lie down flat
   c. Palpitations, oppression or pain in the chest, shortness of breath, facial edema, inability to lie down flat
   d. Pitting edema worse below the waist, epigastric and abdominal distention and oppression, poor appetite, loose stools

225. A patient started violently vomiting this morning. Which of the following patterns may be the cause?

   a. Exopathogens invading the Stomach
   b. Food stagnation
   c. Liver overacting on the Stomach
   d. All of the above

226. All of the following patterns may be related to yang-type jaundice, EXCEPT:

   a. Damp-heat encumbering the Spleen
   b. Liver and Gallbladder damp-heat
   c. Liver fire blazing
   d. Gallbladder heat

227. With improper or delayed treatment, Kidney qi deficiency pattern may develop into which of the following patterns?

   a. Kidney yang deficiency
   b. Kidney yin deficiency
   c. Kidney failing to grasp qi
   d. All of the above

228. A 67-year-old male patient presents to the emergency department with acute onset shortness of breath and dyspnea. Symptoms started two days ago and have progressively gotten worse. He reports difficulty breathing when he lies down, pain and tightness in his chest, forgetfulness, fatigue, feeling cold and requiring blankets, increased urinary frequency, incontinence, and swelling in his lower extremities. He was diagnosed with chronic obstructive pulmonary disease (COPD) one year ago. He has a pale flabby tongue with a white greasy coating, and a deep, weak, and slippery pulse. What is the pattern identification for him?

   a. Wind-cold invading the Lung
   b. Kidney and Lung qi deficiency
   c. Cold-phlegm obstructing the Lung
   d. Cold-water shooting into the Lung

229. A 65-year-old female patient has been suffering from a cough for over six years. She was diagnosed with chronic obstructive pulmonary disease (COPD). She has a non-productive cough, shallow breathing, low energy, dry mouth and throat, and a hoarse voice. She was smoking two packs of cigarettes a day for 40 years and stopped six years ago. She also complains of lower backache and arthritis pain in her left knee. Other symptoms include constipation and poor sleep. She has a red cracked tongue with a scanty coating, and a thin slippery pulse. What is the pattern identification for her?

   a. Heat-phlegm obstructing the Lung
   b. Heat congesting the Lung
   c. Dryness invading the Lung
   d. Lung and Kidney yin deficiency

230. A two-year-old boy was admitted to the hospital due to pneumonia with symptoms of respiratory distress, dyspnea, chills, and fever. He was treated with antibiotics, but two days later, his mother found that he looked puffy and swollen in the face, worse around the eyelids, and that he hadn't urinated since the night before. A diagnosis of acute glomerulonephritis was determined after a series of blood and urine tests. What is the pattern identification for this boy?

    a. Wind-cold invading the Lung
    b. Wind-heat invading the Lung
    c. Wind-water invading the Lung
    d. Cold-water shooting into the Lung

231. A 35-year-old male veteran was diagnosed with post-traumatic stress disorder (PTSD). He spent nine months on the battlefield six years ago. Since then, he has been having nightmares almost daily. Other symptoms include fright, being easy startled, timidity, and susceptibility. He is very angry about the war, irritable, and depressed. He is under the care of a therapist and has been taking antidepressants for over six years. He has a red tongue with a thick, yellow, greasy coating, and a slippery and wiry pulse. What is the pattern identification for him?

    a. Gallbladder stagnation with phlegm disturbance
    b. Liver qi stagnation with heat
    c. Gallbladder heat
    d. Liver and Gallbladder damp-heat

232. A 34-year-old male patient suffers from periodontitis and wants to use Chinese herbs to help his condition. His gums are swollen and have been bleeding for four days, especially after he eats very spicy food. In general, he loves to drink ice water, has a very good appetite, and is prone to constipation. He has a red tongue with a yellow coating, and a slippery and rapid pulse. What is the pattern identification for him?

    a. Food stagnation
    b. Stomach fire
    c. Heart fire
    d. Liver fire

233. A 42-year-old female was diagnosed with Lyme disease four years ago. She suffers from mental fogginess, poor concentration, fatigue, difficulty sleeping, dizziness, vertigo, numbness and tingling in the hands and feet, palpitations, shortness of breath, blurry vision, dull headache, chest pain, and rib soreness. She also complains of droopy eyelids, heaviness of the body, neck and back stiffness, feeling cold all the time, and daily bowel movements with loose stools. She has been on a vegan and gluten-free diet for over three years and has lost 30 pounds during that time, now weighing 105 pounds. Her menses have been absent for over two years. She has a pale complexion, a pale and small tongue with a thick, white, greasy coating, and a weak pulse. Which of the following patterns matches her condition?

a. Heart and Kidney yang deficiency
b. Liver qi stagnation due to blood deficiency
c. Spleen qi deficiency with dampness
d. All of the above

234. A 37-year-old male patient was diagnosed with Crohn's disease 15 years ago. He has been symptom-free for the last 12 years. Two days ago, he started having diarrhea after he had a seafood salad. He has watery stools three to five times a day. Meanwhile, he feels fullness, distention, and abdominal cramping that is relieved by bowel movements or after applying heat. He has no desire to eat and feels slimy in the mouth. Other symptoms include feeling heavy and tired, no thirst, and no fever. He has a slightly pale tongue with a white glossy coating, and a slippery pulse. What is his current condition?

a. Spleen and Kidney yang deficiency
b. Cold-dampness encumbering the Spleen
c. Large Intestine cold-dampness
d. Spleen qi deficiency with dampness

235. A 32-year-old female patient is admitted to the hospital with the complaint of severe epigastric pain. The pain is located in her upper abdominal area, radiates to the back, and is worse with eating or pressure. It began two hours ago after she attended a BBQ party, where she had three cans of beer, BBQ beef, and potato salad. She felt nauseous and vomited three times. She also has abdominal bloating, distention, and diarrhea with sticky stools. She was diagnosed with a gallbladder stone a few years ago. Physical exam shows: BBT: 100.4° F, HR: 94, and BP: 128/82mmH. Her skin and sclera are a yellowish color, her tongue is red with a thick, yellow, greasy coating, and her pulse is rapid and slippery. Blood tests show her amylase level is 320 U/L, lipase level is 290 U/L, and serum bilirubin level is 3.5mg per dL. What is her pattern identification?

a. Large Intestine damp-heat
b. Damp-heat encumbering the Spleen
c. Liver and Gallbladder damp-heat
d. Food stagnation

236. A 48-year-old woman with a history of chronic alcoholism is admitted to the hospital because of abdominal pain, fever, and jaundice. She had been drinking more than one pint of liquor per day before she developed anorexia and nausea about one week ago. Soon thereafter, she began having continuous epigastric and right upper quadrant pain, along with postprandial vomiting. There was no evidence of "coffee grounds" vomitus, hematemesis, or melena. She has been feeling feverish but denies shaking chills. She has been working as a secretary for over 25 years and the job has been very stressful, which is why she started drinking and gradually increased the volume. One month ago she became increasingly tired and weak. Her appetite has been poor for the past few months and she has lost about 20 pounds. Physical examination shows BBT 101.2° F, pulse 96/min, and respiration 18/min. Her face is sunken with temporal wasting, her sclera are

icteric, and her nail beds are pale without clubbing. There is a blotchy redness over the hypothenar regions that blanches with pressure. Spider angiomas are seen on the upper back. The liver is 18 cm in span, firm, and tender. Abdominal palpation shows that there is shifting dullness and bulging flanks. There is a vague tenderness over the entire abdomen, most marked in the right upper quadrant. She has a pale purple tongue with a yellow greasy coating, and a deep, thin, and choppy pulse. Laboratory tests include WBC 18,200/mcL, RBC 3.2/mcL, platelets 112,000/mcL, creatinin 1.9mg/100 ml, Liver panel SGOT 260 IU, SGPT 86 IU, ALP 470 IU, and bilirubin 4.7mg/100 ml. PT is 15. A liver biopsy was done: fatty infiltration, some focal hepatonecrosis, and alcoholic hyaline (Mallory bodies) were seen. The diagnosis for her is alcoholic liver disease. What is the pattern identification for her?

   a. Liver and Gallbladder damp-heat
   b. Liver qi and blood deficiency
   c. Liver qi and blood stagnation
   d. All of the above

237. The patient, 36, reported to a gynecological clinic in the 6th week of pregnancy with vaginal bleeding. All previous six pregnancies ended in miscarriage between the 7th and 9th weeks of pregnancy. The patient has not been treated for other chronic diseases, her BMI is 17.5, and she does not smoke or drink. The patient has been menstruating regularly every 28 days but has spotting 3-5 days before her menstrual periods, which are painful and abundant. A hematoma of 1.5×2 cm was reported in the internal mouth of the uterus. Other symptoms include fatigue, sleepiness, no appetite due to morning sickness, and lower back pain that has worsened since pregnancy. She has a pale complexion, a slightly pale tongue with a thin white coating, and a weak pulse. What is her pattern identification?

   a. Kidney qi failing to consolidate
   b. Spleen qi sinking
   c. Kidney essence deficiency
   d. Kidney yang deficiency

238. A 54-year-old male patient was diagnosed with ulcerative colitis over five years ago. He has been treated by specialists with antibiotics or corticosteroids when his symptoms are bad. He has constipation between episodes. Two weeks ago he had a business trip for four days and started having loose stools again. Now his bowel movements are 4-6 times a day with soft loose stools and borborygmus. Meanwhile, he has dull pain in his lower abdomen that is relieved by warmth. He has noticed that his diarrhea gets worse when he eats salads or seafood, making his stools watery and muddy like duck droppings. His urination is normal. He is six feet tall, weighs 155 pounds, and goes to the gym three times a week. He has a slightly pale flabby tongue with a thin white coating, and a deep slow pulse. What is the pattern for his current condition?

   a. Small Intestine deficiency cold
   b. Large Intestine deficiency cold
   c. Kidney yang deficiency
   d. Large Intestine cold-dampness

239. John, a 74-year-old male patient, has been suffering from constipation for over 15 years. He has been taking laxatives to relieve his symptoms, but increased his dosage in the last couple of weeks when his symptoms got worse. He has dry stools that are difficult to evacuate and he feels very tired after he defecates. He has also been diagnosed with benign prostatic hyperplasia (BPH), having symptoms of dysuria, dripping, and nocturnal polyuria. Other symptoms include chilliness, lower backache, dry mouth, thirst, and dry skin. He has a slightly pale tongue with a dry white coating, and a weak pulse. Which of the following patterns matches with his condition?

   a. Large Intestine heat with Kidney yin deficiency
   b. Large Intestine dryness with Kidney yang deficiency
   c. Small Intestine deficiency cold and Kidney yang deficiency
   d. Liver qi stagnation with Kidney yin deficiency

240. Ted, a 65-year-old male patient diagnosed with chronic renal failure (stage IV), has symptoms of pitting edema in his lower extremities, epigastric and abdominal distention and oppression, loose stools, and scanty white foaming urine. He also complains of nausea, decreased appetite, high blood pressure, drowsiness, lethargy, cold body and limbs, and lower back pain. He has a dull complexion, a pale and flabby tongue with a slippery white coating, and a weak pulse. Which pattern is the most appropriate for his condition?

   a. Kidney yang deficiency
   b. Spleen yang deficiency
   c. Kidney water upward invading the Spleen
   d. Cold-dampness encumbering the Spleen

241. Linda, a 28-year-old female, complains of chest pain, insomnia, palpitations, migraine headache, lower abdominal pain and distention before and during periods, excessive menstrual bleeding that is dark red and has clots, and a mass on her neck. Her tongue is purplish red with prickles on the tip and has a thin yellow coating. Her pulse is slippery and wiry. The Western medical diagnosis for her is thyroiditis. What is the pattern identification for her?

   a. Heart fire with Liver qi and blood stagnation
   b. Heart and Kidney disharmony
   c. Liver qi stagnation with Liver yang rising
   d. Heart and Kidney yang deficiency

242. A 54-year-old female complains of having recurrent urinary tract infections over the last two years, with a new infection that started yesterday. Symptoms include a frequent urge to urinate, cloudy strong-smelling urine sometimes with blood, a feeling of pressure in her lower abdomen, lethargy, and lower backache. Meanwhile, she also suffers from hot flashes, night sweats, and trouble sleeping. Urinalysis suggests bacterial infection. Physical exam shows that her temperature is 99.2° F, respiratory rate is 21 breaths per minute, and heart rate is 85 bpm. She has a red tongue with a thick yellow coating, and a thin slippery pulse. What is the pattern identification for her?

a. Urinary Bladder damp-heat with Kidney yin deficiency
b. Liver and Gallbladder damp-heat
c. Heart fire transmits to the Small Intestine
d. Wind-heat invasion with Urinary Bladder damp-heat

243. A 58-year-old African-American male patient had a cerebrovascular accident (CVA) two weeks ago. He now suffers from hemiplegia on his right side. During the physical examination you find that there are big scars on his chest and right inner leg, the results of bypass surgery three years ago. His right hand and ankle are swollen. Blood pressure is 180/90 mmHg. His tongue is flabby with a purplish color and has a thick, yellow, greasy coating, and his sublingual veins are purple and extended. His pulse is wiry, slippery, and choppy. Which of the following patterns best matches his condition?

a. Liver yang rising due to Liver and Kidney yin deficiency
b. Liver wind attack with phlegm and blood stagnation
c. Liver wind due to yin deficiency
d. Heart and Kidney disharmony

244. Amber, a 26-year-old patient, presents to the clinic complaining of lower belly pain and increased urinary frequency for seven months. Her daytime urinary frequency ranges from 20-35 times with nocturia about 6-8 times. The patient's suprapubic pain is 6/10 in intensity and fluctuates quite markedly. She experiences no associated symptoms such as fever; weight, appetite, or bowel changes; or any antecedent infection. She has been in a relationship with her boyfriend for four years, and she experiences mild pelvic pain during sexual intercourse. Her urinalysis and urine culture are insignificant. Laboratory investigations, including complete blood count, fasting blood glucose, hemoglobin A1c, erythrocyte sedimentation rate (ESR), thyroid function tests, and liver function tests were all within normal limits. Pelvic ultrasound and cystoscopy are insignificant. The diagnosis for her condition is interstitial cystitis. She also complains of having trouble sleeping, nervousness, restlessness, and feeling tense. She often feels her heart beat and has difficulty breathing when stressed. She has a red tongue with a redder tip, a thin yellow tongue coating, and a slippery and wiry pulse. Which of the following patterns matches her condition?

a. Urinary Bladder damp-heat
b. Damp-heat in the Liver and Gallbladder channel
c. Heart fire transmits to the Small Intestine
d. Kidney yin deficiency with damp-heat accumulation

245. Joseph, a 45-year-old male, complains of headache and neck stiffness that is worse in the occipital area, and aggravated by turning his head. He also experiences dizziness, brain fog, difficulty concentrating, and hand tremor. He noticed that his headache gets worse every time he eats salty food. He is a professional chef, doesn't take any medications, does not smoke, and only drinks socially. His BP is 200/110 mmHg. He has a red tongue, with a thin yellow coating, and a wiry and slippery pulse. What is his pattern identification?

a. Wind-phlegm disturbing upward
b. Liver and Kidney yin deficiency
c. Liver yang rising
d. Heart fire with Kidney yin deficiency

246. Meredith, a 34-year-old female, was diagnosed with polycystic ovarian syndrome (PCOS), and placed on birth control pills since age 16 to help regulate her periods and reduce her acne breakouts. Since she stopped the pill two years ago, she has had a few periods, but they are not completely regular as they sometimes skip a month or two. Physical exam shows that her blood pressure is 130/90 mmHg, BMI is 29, and skin breakouts on her chin and back as well as excess facial and body hair. Other symptoms include low energy, depression, anxiety, lower backache, and loose stools during her menstruation. Her blood test shows LH 12 mlU/ml, FSH 3.8 mlU/ml, testosterone 0.49ng/ml, DHEA-S 249 ug/dl, TSH 4.2 uIU/ml, and fasting blood sugar 6.2 mmol/l. She has a slightly pale tongue with teeth marks and a thick, white, greasy tongue coating. Her pulse is deep, thin, and slippery. Which of the following patterns matches her condition?

a. Spleen qi deficiency
b. Kidney qi deficiency
c. Phlegm stagnation
d. All of the above

247. Jean, a 39-year-old female patient, has a history of H. pylori infection. For the last couple of weeks she traveled a lot and did not eat regularly. Now she complains of epigastric pain that happens after missing meals and is relieved by a heat pack or warm drink. She also has mild nausea, regurgitation, poor appetite, loose stools (2-3 times a day), and cold hands and feet. She has a deep thin pulse, and a pale tongue with a white greasy tongue coating. What is the correct pattern?

a. Spleen and Kidney yang deficiency and dampness accumulation
b. Liver and Spleen disharmony with Kidney yang deficiency
c. Spleen and Stomach Yang deficiency with dampness accumulation
d. Stomach fire

248. A 30-year-old female has had migraines that occur twice a month for the last 15 years. The pain is located behind the eyes and occasionally at the vertex. There is nausea with vomiting of bile when the condition is severe. She has a tendency towards constipation, a bitter taste in the mouth, occasional gastric reflux, irritability, and difficulty falling asleep. While taking her history, she criticized her previous healthcare practitioners. Her pulse is wiry and rapid, and her tongue is red with a thin yellow coating. What is the pattern identification?

a. Phlegm-heat in the Gallbladder
b. Liver blood deficiency and Liver qi stagnation
c. Liver fire blazing and overacting on the Stomach
d. Spleen and Stomach disharmony

249. A 35-year-old female tests positive for small intestinal bacterial overgrowth (SIBO). She has abdominal bloating and distention, belching, nausea, and an aversion to food. She also complains of frequent pain in her epigastric area. Eating food doesn't help, and cold food or drink makes it worse. Other symptoms include loose stools and sometimes constipation. She has taken antibiotics, which make her symptoms much better, but then they recur a month after she stops taking the antibiotics. She has a thick greasy tongue coating, and a slippery pulse. Which of the following patterns matches her condition?

   a. Liver and Stomach disharmony
   b. Spleen and Stomach disharmony
   c. Liver and Spleen disharmony
   d. Food stagnation

250. Eric, a 79-year-old male patient, has been having chronic non-productive cough for over six months. Coughing is worse in the evenings or when talking, and there is scanty whitish sputum. He has also been suffering from constipation for many years with dry stools that are difficult to evacuate and bowel movements every 2-3 days. He has been taking blood pressure medication (beta-blockers) for over 20 years. He has a red cracked tongue with a slightly yellow scanty coating, and a thin and slow pulse. Which of the following patterns matches his condition?

   a. Lung yin deficiency with Large Intestine dryness
   b. Phlegm-dryness obstructing the Lung with Large Intestine yin deficiency
   c. Kidney and Lung yin deficiency
   d. Lung yin deficiency with Kidney yang deficiency

Answer Key

1.	c	26.	a	51.	c	76.	b
2.	a	27.	b	52.	d	77.	c
3.	b	28.	c	53.	c	78.	b
4.	b	29.	c	54.	d	79.	c
5.	b	30.	c	55.	c	80.	c
6.	d	31.	a	56.	b	81.	d
7.	a	32.	b	57.	b	82.	b
8.	b	33.	a	58.	b	83.	b
9.	c	34.	b	59.	c	84.	a
10.	d	35.	b	60.	d	85.	a
11.	d	36.	c	61.	a	86.	b
12.	b	37.	a	62.	a	87.	a
13.	a	38.	c	63.	c	88.	d
14.	d	39.	d	64.	d	89.	b
15.	d	40.	b	65.	b	90.	b
16.	b	41.	d	66.	c	91.	a
17.	c	42.	b	67.	d	92.	c
18.	c	43.	c	68.	c	93.	a
19.	c	44.	d	69.	a	94.	b
20.	d	45.	a	70.	c	95.	c
21.	d	46.	b	71.	d	96.	a
22.	a	47.	a	72.	c	97.	b
23.	c	48.	c	73.	d	98.	a
24.	b	49.	d	74.	b	99.	d
25.	d	50.	a	75.	c	100.	d

101. a	126. d	151. d	176. b
102. b	127. b	152. b	177. a
103. c	128. c	153. b	178. d
104. d	129. b	154. b	179. b
105. c	130. a	155. b	180. a
106. d	131. c	156. c	181. d
107. d	132. c	157. b	182. c
108. a	133. d	158. b	183. b
109. c	134. c	159. d	184. b
110. c	135. d	160. a	185. b
111. b	136. a	161. b	186. a
112. d	137. b	162. d	187. d
113. d	138. c	163. b	188. b
114. b	139. c	164. a	189. a
115. a	140. c	165. b	190. d
116. a	141. b	166. a	191. b
117. c	142. c	167. d	192. c
118. b	143. c	168. c	193. c
119. c	144. c	169. a	194. d
120. c	145. a	170. c	195. d
121. b	146. d	171. b	196. b
122. a	147. a	172. d	197. a
123. a	148. b	173. a	198. d
124. d	149. d	174. b	199. d
125. d	150. a	175. c	200. a

201.	d	226.	c
202.	b	227.	d
203.	c	228.	d
204.	b	229.	d
205.	d	230.	c
206.	a	231.	a
207.	c	232.	b
208.	b	233.	d
209.	d	234.	b
210.	b	235.	b
211.	c	236.	d
212.	d	237.	a
213.	b	238.	b
214.	a	239.	b
215.	d	240.	c
216.	d	241.	a
217.	a	242.	a
218.	d	243.	b
219.	b	244.	c
220.	a	245.	c
221.	d	246.	d
222.	b	247.	c
223.	d	248.	c
224.	a	249.	b
225.	d	250.	b

Bibliography

PREMODERN TEXTS

Appendices to the Classified Classic (類經附翼 *lèi jīng fù yì*): Zhang Jing-Yue, 1624

Case Records as a Guide to Clinical Practice (臨證指南醫案 *Lín zhèng zhǐ nán yī àn*): Ye Tian-Shi, 1746.

Basic Questions: Discourse on Mechanisms for Preserving Life (素問病機氣宜保命集 *sù wèn bìng jī qì yí bǎo mìng jí*): Liu Wan-Su, 12th century

Classic of Difficulties (難經 *Nàn Jīng*): Anonymous, 1st century CE.

Craft of Medicines and Patterns for Children (小兒藥証直訣 *xiǎo ér yào zhèng zhí jué*): Qian Yi, 1119

Discussion of Blood Patterns (血證論 *Xuè zhèng lùn*): Tang Rong-Chuan, 1884

Discussion of Cold Damage (傷寒論 *Shāng hán lùn*): Zhang Zhong-Jing, c. 220

Discussion of the Origins of the Symptoms of Disease (諸病源侯論 *Zhū bìng yuán hòu lùn*): Chao Yuan-Fang, 610

Emergency Formulas Worth a Thousand Gold Pieces (備急千金要方 *bèi jí qiān jīn yào fang*): Sun Si-Miao, 652

Essentials from the Golden Cabinet (金匱要略 *Jīn guì yào lùe*): Zhang Zhong-Jing, c. 220

Essential Pivot of Diagnosis (診家樞要 *Zhěn jiā shū yào*): Hua Shou, 1359

Golden Mirror of the Medical Tradition (醫宗金鑑 *Yī zōng jīn jiàn*): Wu Qian, 1742

Origins of Medicine (醫學啟源 *yī xué qí yuán*), Zhang Yuan-Su, 1186

Pulse Classic (脈經 *Mài jīng*): Wang Shu-He, c. 3rd century

Thorough Understanding of Cold Damage (傷寒指掌 *Shāng hán zhǐ zhǎng)*: Wu Kun-An, 1796

Treasury Classic (中藏經 *Zhōng càng jīng*): Attributed to Hua Tuo, c. 200

Treatise on Causes and Symptoms of Diseases (諸病源侯論 *zhū bìng yuán hòu lùn*): Chao Yu-an-Fang, 610

Treatise on the Spleen and Stomach (脾胃論 *Pí wèi lùn*): Li Dong-Yuan, c. 13th century

Yellow Emperor's Inner Classic: Basic Questions (黃帝內經素問 *Huáng dì nèi jīng sù wèn*): Anonymous, c. 200

Yellow Emperor's Inner Classic: Divine Pivot (黃帝內經靈樞 *Huáng dì nèi jīng líng shū*): Anonymous, c. 200

CONTEMPORARY TEXTS

Chen Jia-Xu. *Diagnostics of Traditional Chinese Medicine, 9th Edition* (中醫診斷學 *Zhōng yī zhén duàn xué*). Beijing: Academy Press, 2018

Cheng Xin-Nong. *Chinese Acupuncture and Moxibustion. 3rd Edition.* Beijing: Foreign Languages Press, 2018

Dan Bensky, Volker Scheid, Andrew Ellis, Randall Barolet. *Chinese Herbal Medicine: Formulas & Strategies, 2nd Edition. Seattle:* Eastland Press, 2009.

Deng Tie-Tao. *A Study of Diagnosis in Chinese Medicine, 9th Edition* (中醫診斷學 *Zhōng yī zhén duàn xué*). Beijing: People's Medical Publishing House, 1987

Fei Zhao-Fu. *Traditional Chinese Medicine Diagnosis Lecture Handout (*中醫診斷學講稿 *zhōng yī zhěn duàn xué jiǎng gǎo).* Beijing: People's Medical Publishing House, 2008

Kaptchuk, Ted J. *The Web That Has No Weaver.* New York: Congdon & Weed, 1983

Sun Guang-Ren. *Basic Theories of Traditional Chinese Medicine, Key Points of Analysis* (中醫基礎理論難點解析 *zhōng yī jī chǔ lǐ lùn nán diǎn jiě xī*). Beijing: Chinese Medicine Publishing House, 2005

Sun Guang-Ren, Zheng Hong-Xin. *Basic Theories of Traditional Chinese Medicine, 9th Edition* (中醫基礎理論 *Zhōng yī jī chǔ lǐ lùn*). Beijing: Academy Press, 2018

Maciocia, Giovanni. *Diagnosis in Chinese Medicine: A Comprehensive Guide, 2nd Edition.* Edinburgh: Churchill Livingstone, 2018

Maciocia, Giovanni. *The Foundations of Chinese Medicine, 3rd Edition.* Edinburgh: Churchill Livingstone, 2015

Qi Nan and Yang Fu Gou. *Zang Fu and Clinical Practice in Chinese Medicine* (中醫藏象与临床 *zhōng yī zàng xiàng yǔ Lín chuáng*). Beijing: Chinese Medicine Ancient Book Publishing House, 2001

Wiseman, Nigel and Feng Ye. *A Practical Dictionary of Chinese Medicine.* Brookline, MA.: Paradigm Publications, 1998

Yi Qiao, Al Stone. *Traditional Chinese Medicine Formula Study Guide. Santa Rosa, CA*: Snow Lotus Press, 2000

Yi Qiao, Al Stone. *Traditional Chinese Medicine Diagnosis Study Guide. Seattle*: Eastland Press, 2008

Zhao Jin-Ze. *A Study of Pattern Identification in Chinese Medicine Diagnosis* (中醫證狀鑒別診斷學 *zhōng yī zhèn zhuàng jiàn bié zhěn duàn xué*). Beijing: People's Medical Publishing House, 1984

Zhao Jin-Ze. *A Study of Symptom Identification in Chinese Medicine Diagnosis* (中醫症狀鑒別診斷學 *zhōng yī zhèng zhuàng jiàn bié zhěn duàn xué*). Beijing: People's Medical Publishing Hourse, 1984

Zhu Wen-Feng. *A Study of Diagnosis in Chinese Medicine* (中醫診斷學 *zhōng yī zhén duàn xué*). Beijing: People's Medical Publishing House, 1999

General Index

A

abdominal cold pain, pattern differentiation, 305
abnormal respiration
    definition, 30
    etiology and pathomechanisms, 30
    in Lung disease, 30
acid regurgitation
    etiology and pathomechanisms, 137–138
    as Stomach manifestation, 137–138
acupuncture
    blood deficiency generating wind, 100
    blood stagnation in Stomach, 154
    cold invading Lung, 48
    cold invading Stomach, 150
    cold stagnation in Liver channel, 105
    cold-dampness encumbering Spleen, 73
    cold-water shooting into Lung, 54
    damp-heat encumbering Spleen, 75
    extreme heat generating wind, 99
    food stagnation pattern, 153
    Gallbladder heat, 189
    Gallbladder qi deficiency, 188
    Gallbladder stagnation with phlegm disturbance, 192
    Heart and Kidney disharmony, 223
    Heart and Kidney yang deficiency, 221
    Heart and Lung qi deficiency, 212
    Heart and Spleen deficiency, 215
    Heart blood deficiency, 15
    Heart fire blazing, 18
    Heart fire transmits to Small Intestine, 226
    Heart qi deficiency, 11
    Heart vessels obstruction, 24
    Heart yang collapse, 13
    Heart yang deficiency, 12
    Heart yin defiiency, 16
    Heat congesting Lung, 52
    Kidney essence deficiency, 132
    Kidney failing to grasp qi, 121
    Kidney qi deficiency, 118
    Kidney qi failing to secure, 119
    Kidney water invading Spleen, 276
    Kidney yang deficiency, 124
    Kidney yang deficiency with water effusion, 127
    Kidney yin deficiency, 130
    Large Intestine cold-dampness, 174
    Large Intestine damp-heat, 176
    Large Intestine deficiency cold, 170
    Large Intestine dryness, 173
    Large Intestine Heat accumulation, 179
    Liver and Gallbladder damp-heat, 255
    Liver and Kidney yin deficiency, 243
    Liver and Spleen disharmony, 246
    Liver and Stomach disharmony, 247
    Liver blood deficiency, 88
    Liver blood stagnation, 106
    Liver fire blazing, 93
    Liver fire invading Lung, 251
    Liver qi deficiency, 294
    Liver qi stagnation, 92
    Liver yang deficiency, 298
    Liver yang rising, 95
    Liver yang transforming wind, 98
    Liver yin deficiency, 89
    Lung and Kidney yin deficiency, 239
    Lung blood deficiency, 282
    Lung qi deficiency, 35
    Lung yang deficiency, 278
    phlegm misting Heart, 21
    phlegm-fire harassing Heart, 19
    Small Intestine deficiency cold, 161

Small Intestine excess fire, 163
Small Intestine qi stagnation, 164
Spleen and Kidney yang deficiency, 233
Spleen and Lung deficiency, 230
Spleen and Stomach disharmony, 236
Spleen not controlling blood, 67
Spleen qi deficiency, 64
Spleen qi sinking, 65
Spleen yang deficiency, 68
Spleen yin deficiency, 71
Stomach deficiency cold, 146
Stomach excess with Spleen deficiency, 317
Stomach fire, 148
Stomach qi deficiency, 311
Stomach yin deficiency, 143
turbid phlegm obstructing Lung, 50
Urinary Bladder damp-heat, 203
Urinary Bladder deficiency cold, 200
wind-cold invading Lung, 37
wind-cold-dampness invading body surface, 261
wind-heat invading Lung, 39
wind-water invading Lung, 47
yin deficiency generating wind, 102
aging
Kidney disease and, 112
in Large Intestine disease, 166
in Small Intestine patterns, 157
in Spleen patterns, 58
in Stomach patterns, 137
in Urinary Bladder patterns, 197
amenorrhea, Kidney yin deficiency in, 327–328
Appendices to the Classified Classic (類經附翼 *lèi jīng fù yì*), 323
appetite, poor in Spleen disease, 59
ascending and descending movements, 329
Liver and Lung functions, 249
Spleen and Stomach coordination of, 234
attributive channels (歸經 *guī jīng*), 331

B

Basic Questions (素問 *sù wèn*), 315
Kidney yin deficiency in, 327–328
Liver qi deficiency in, 290
Lung skin and hair links, 279
Lung yang deficiency in, 277
Spleen yin deficiency in, 313
Basic Questions: Discourse on Mechanisms for Preserving Life (素問病機氣宜保命集 *sù wèn bìng jī qì yí bǎo mìng jí*), 331
belching
etiology and pathomechanisms, 138
as Stomach manifestation, 137–138
big qi (大氣 *dà qì*), 227
bile storage and secretion, by Gallbladder, 183
bitter taste, in Gallbladder patterns, 184–185
bleeding, in Spleen disease, 61
bloating and distention, 60–61
as Stomach manifestation, 139–140
blood
control by Spleen, 58
Liver storage and regulation functions, 79–80
blood circulation
Heart and Liver roles, 215–216
Heart and Spleen roles, 213
Liver and Spleen/Stomach roles, 244–245
blood deficiency generating wind, 100
blood production, Heart and Spleen roles, 212–213
blood stagnation in Kidney (淤血阻腎 *yū xuě zú shèn*), 327
blood stagnation in Stomach, 154
bow (引 *yǐn*), from Liver wind, 289

C

canker sores, 8
channel connections, Liver and Lung, 249
channel pattern identification (經絡辯證 *jīng luò biàn zhèng*), 336–337
Chao Yuan-Fang, 330
Chen Wu-Ze, 322
Chen Xiu-Yan, 322
Chen Ziming, 280
chest distress/pain, 7
definition, 7
etiology and pathomechanisms, 7–8

chills and fever
    definition, 29
    etiology and pathomechanism, 29
    in Lung disease, 29

Chinese Internal Medicine (中醫內科學 *zhōng yī nèi kē xué*), 324

chronic illness
    in Gallbladder patterns, 184
    in Heart patterns, 4
    in Large Intestine disease, 166
    in Liver patterns, 80
    and Lung disease, 29
    in Small Intestine patterns, 157
    in Spleen patterns, 58
    in Stomach patterns, 137
    in Urinary Bladder patterns, 197

Classic of Difficulties (難經 *nán jīng*)
    Liver deficiency in, 292
    mìng mén concept in, 321, 322

clear orifices (清竅 *qīng qiào*), 301

cold extremities, Kidney yang deficiency and, 304

cold invading Lung
    clinical manifestations, 47
    vs. cold-phlegm obstructing Lung, 50–51
    definition, 47
    diseases and treatments, 48
    etiology and pathogenesis, 47
    vs. wind-cold invading Lung, 50–51

cold invading Stomach
    acupuncture, 150
    clinical manifestations, 149
    vs. cold-dampness encumbering Spleen, 152
    definition, 149–150
    diseases and treatments, 150
    etiology and pathogenesis, 150
    herbal formulas, 150
    vs. Stomach deficiency cold, 151

cold stagnation in Liver channel
    acupuncture, 105
    clinical manifestations, 104
    definition, 105
    diseases and treatments, 105
    etiology and pathogenesis, 104–105
    herbal formulas, 105

cold-dampness encumbering Spleen
    clinical manifestations, 71
    vs. cold invading Stomach, 152
    vs. damp-heat encumbering Spleen, 76
    definition, 71
    diseases and treatments, 72
    etiology and pathogenesis, 71–72
    vs. water-dampness immersion, 73–74

cold-phlegm obstructing Lung
    vs. cold invading Lung, 50–51
    vs. cold-water shooting into Lung, 55
    vs. wind-cold invading Lung, 50–51

cold-water shooting into Lung
    acupunctue, 54
    clinical manifestations, 53
    vs. cold-phlegm obstructing Lung, 55
    definition, 52
    diseases and treatments, 54
    etiology and pathogenesis, 53–54
    herbal formulas, 54
    vs. Kidney water invading Spleen, 276–277
    vs. Kidney yang deficiency, 128, 276–277
    vs. Kidney yang deficiency with water effusion, 276–277
    vs. water qi encroaching on Heart, 273–274
    vs. water qi encroaching on Heart, 128

Collected Treatises of Jing-Yue (景岳全書 *jǐng yuè quán shū*), 325

compound patterns, 207
    common, 209
    Heart and Kidney compound patterns, 218–224
    Heart and Liver compound patterns, 215–218
    Heart and Lung patterns, 210–212
    Heart and Small Intestine compound patterns, 224–227
    Heart and Spleen compound patterns, 212–215
    identifying, 208–209

Liver and Gallbladder compound patterns, 252–256
Liver and Kidney compound patterns, 240–243
Liver and Kidney yin deficiency, 241–242
Liver and Lung compound patterns, 249–252
Liver and Spleen/Stomach compound patterns, 244–248
Lung and Kidney compound patterns, 236–239
Spleen and Kidney compound patterns, 230–233
Spleen and Lung compound patterns, 227–230
Spleen and Stomach compound patterns, 233–236

Comprehensive Outline of the Materia Medica (本草綱目 *běn cǎo gāng mù*), 280

Comprehensive Recording of Sage-like Benefit from the Zheng He Era (聖濟總錄 *shèng jí zǒng lù*), 325–326

congenital weakness
　in Gallbladder patterns, 184
　in Heart patterns, 4
　in Liver patterns, 80

constipation, in Large Intestine disease patterns, 167

constitution
　and Large Intestine disease, 166
　and Small Intestine patterns, 157
　and Spleen patterns, 58
　and Stomach patterns, 137
　in Urinary Bladder patterns, 197
　weak, and Kidney disease, 112

constrained Spleen, *vs.* Stomach excess with Spleen deficiency, 317–318

constraint (郁 *yù*), 301

continuous palpitations (怔忡 *zhēng chōng*), 5

coolness-dryness (涼燥 *liáng zào*), 41
　invading Lung, 42

corporeal soul (魄 *pò*), 26

cough
　definition, 31
　etiology and pathomechanism, 31
　in Lung disease, 31

coursing and discharging (疏泄 *shū xiè*), 79

coursing and storage, 240

Craft of Medicines and Patterns for Children (小兒藥証直訣 *xiǎo ér yào zhèng zhí jué*), 324, 325, 331

Criterion of Syndrome and Treatment (證治準繩 *zhèng zhì zhǔn shéng*), 292

D

Damp-heat accumulating in Kidney (濕熱蘊腎 *shī rè yùn shèn*), 327

Damp-heat encumbering Spleen
　acupuncture, 75
　vs. cold-dampness encumbering Spleen, 76
　definition, 74
　diseases and treatment, 75
　etiology and pathogenesis, 75–76
　herbal formulas, 75
　vs. Large Intestine damp-heat, 177–178
　vs. Liver and Gallbladder damp-heat, 302–303

damp-heat in middle burner, *vs.* damp-heat in Spleen and Stomach, 319–320

damp-heat in Spleen and Stomach, *vs.* damp-heat in middle burner, 319–320

dampness (濕 *shī*), 262–268
　vs. yin, 313

dampness invasion, 58

decision-making, Gallbladder and, 183–184

deficiency patterns
　compound patterns, 209
　in Heart disease, 9
　in Kidney disease, 116
　in Large Intestine disease, 168
　in Liver disease, 86
　in Lung disease, 33
　in Small Intestine disease, 160
　in Spleen disease, 63
　in Urinary Bladder disease, 199

descending functions, Stomach and, 137

developmental abnormalities, 113

diarrhea, in Large Intestine disease patterns, 166–167
diet
    in Gallbladder patterns, 184
    and Heart patterns, 4
    in Spleen patterns, 58
    in Kidney patterns, 112
    in Large Intestine disease, 166
    in Liver patterns, 80
    in Lung disease, 29
    in Small Intestine patterns, 157
    in Stomach patterns, 137
    in Urinary Bladder patterns, 197
digestion
    Liver and Gallbladder functions, 252–253
    Liver and Spleen/Stomach roles, 244
Discussion of Cold Damage and Miscellaneous Diseases (傷寒雜病論 *shāng hán zá bìng lùn*), 330, 337
diseases and treatments
    blood deficiency generating wind, 100
    blood stagnation in Stomach, 154
    cold invading Lung, 48
    cold invading Stomach, 150
    cold stagnation in Liver channel, 105
    cold-dampness encumbering Spleen, 72
    damp-heat encumbering Spleen, 75
    dryness invading Lung, 42
    extreme heat generating wind, 99
    food stagnation, 153
    Gallbladder heat, 189
    Gallbladder qi deficiency, 188
    Gallbladder stagnation with phlegm disturbance, 192
    Heart and Kidney disharmony, 223
    Heart and Kidney yang deficiency, 221
    Heart and Lung qi deficiency, 212
    Heart and Spleen deficiency, 215
    Heart blood deficiency, 15
    Heart fire blazing, 18
    Heart fire transmits to Small Intestine, 226
    Heart qi deficiency, 11
    Heart vessels obstruction, 24
    Heart yang collapse, 13
    Heart yang deficiency, 12
    Kidney essence deficiency, 132
    Kidney failing to grasp qi, 121
    Kidney qi deficiency, 118
    Kidney qi failing to secure, 119
    Kidney water invading Spleen, 276
    Kidney yang deficiency, 124
    Kidney yang deficiency with water effusion, 127
    Kidney yin deficiency, 130
    Large Intestine cold-dampness, 174
    Large Intestine damp-heat, 176
    Large Intestine deficiency cold, 170
    Large Intestine dryness, 173
    Large Intestine heat accumulation, 179
    Liver and Gallbladder damp-heat, 255
    Liver and Kidney yin deficiency, 243
    Liver and Spleen disharmony, 246
    Liver and Stomach disharmony, 247
    Liver blood deficiency, 88
    Liver fire blazing, 93
    Liver fire invading Lung, 251
    Liver qi deficiency, 294
    Liver yang deficiency, 298
    Liver yang rising, 95
    Liver yang transforming wind, 98
    Liver yin deficiency, 89
    Lung and Kidney yin deficiency, 239
    Lung blood deficiency, 282
    Lung qi deficiency, 35
    Lung yang deficiency, 278
    Lung yin deficiency, 36
    phlegm misting Heart, 21
    phlegm-fire harassing Heart, 19
    Small Intestine deficiency cold, 161
    Small Intestine excess fire, 163
    Small Intestine qi stagnation, 164
    Spleen and Kidney yang deficiency, 233
    Spleen and Lung deficiency, 230
    Spleen and Stomach disharmony, 236
    Spleen not controlling blood, 67
    Spleen qi deficiency, 64

Spleen qi sinking, 65
Spleen yang deficiency, 68
Spleen yin deficiency, 71
Stomach deficiency cold, 146
Stomach excess with Spleen deficiency, 317
Stomach fire, 148
Stomach qi deficiency, 311
Stomach yin deficiency, 143
turbid phlegm obstructing Lung, 50
Urinary Bladder damp-heat, 203
Urinary Bladder deficiency cold, 200
wind-cold-dampness invading body surface (風寒濕襲表 *fēng hán shī xí biǎo*), 261
wind-water invading Lung, 47
yin deficiency generating wind, 102
dispersing and descending, Lung and, 28
Divine Pivot (靈樞 *líng shū*), 321
Kidney excess concept in, 325
dizziness (暈 *yūn*), 289
dryness and dampness, Spleen/Stomach regulation, 234
dryness invading Lung
clinical manifestations, 41
definition, 41
diseases and treatments, 42
etiology and pathogenesis, 41–42
vs. exterior dryness, 43
vs. Liver fire invading Lung, 282–283
vs. Lung yin deficiency, 43–44, 282–283
dryness, Lung patterns caused by, 42

E

edema, yang *vs.* yin, 264
eight principles pattern identification (八網辯證 *bā gāng biàn zhèng*), xv, 37, 335
Emergency Formulas Worth a Thousand Gold Pieces (備急千金要方 *bèi jí qiān jīn yào fang*), 331
emotional activities
Heart and Liver roles, 216
Liver and Gallbladder functions, 253
emotional disorders, Liver patterns and, 81

emotional regulation, Heart and Kidney roles, 220
emotional stress
in Gallbladder patterns, 184
in Heart patterns, 4
in Liver patterns, 80
in Lung disease, 29
in Small Intestine patterns, 157
in Spleen patterns, 58
in Stomach patterns, 137
epigastric bloating/distention, as Stomach manifestation, 139–140
epilepsy (癇 *xián*), 6
erectile dysfunction, Kidney/Liver yang deficiency in, 304–305
essence (精 *jīng*), 320
acquired/postnatal, 320
congenital/prenatal, 320
Spleen and Kidney roles, 230–231
storage by Kidney, 109–110
varieties of, 320–321
essence and blood storage, Liver and Kidney roles, 240
Essence of Chinese Medicine (醫經精義 *yī jīng jīng yì*), 280
essence qi (精氣 *jīng qì*), 108
Essentials from the Golden Cabinet (金匱要略 *jīn guì yào luè*), 330
Lung yang deficiency in, 277
etiology and pathogenesis
abnormal respiration, 30
abnormal urination, 158
bitter taste, 184–185
bleeding, 61
bloating and distention, 60–61
blood deficiency generating wind, 100
blood stagnation in Stomach, 154
chest distress/pain, 7–8
chills and fever, 29
cold invading Lung, 47
cold invading Stomach, 150
cold stagnation in Liver channel, 105
cold-dampness encumbering Spleen, 71–72

cold-water shooting into Lung, 53–54
cough, 31
damp-heat encumbering Spleen, 75–76
dampness patterns, 264
diarrhea/loose stools, 166–167
difficult urination, 197
dryness invading Lung, 41–42
emotional disorders, 81
epigastric bloating/distention, 139–140
extreme heat generating wind, 99
food stagnation pattern, 153
frequent urination, 198
Gallbladder disease patterns, 184
Gallbladder heat, 188–189
Gallbladder qi deficiency, 187–188
Gallbladder stagnation with phlegm disturbance, 191
growth and development abnormalities, 113
Heart and Kidney disharmony, 222
Heart and Kidney yang deficiency, 221
Heart and Liver blood deficiency, 217
Heart and Lung qi deficiency, 211
Heart and Spleen deficiency, 214
Heart blood deficiency, 14–15
Heart fire blazing, 17–18
Heart fire transmits to Small Intestine, 225–226
Heart qi deficiency, 10
Heart vessels obstruction, 23–24
Heart yang collapse, 12–13
Heart yang deficiency, 11–12
Heart yin deficiency, 16
heat congesting Lung, 51–52
insomnia, 6
Kidney disease, general, 112
Kidney essence deficiency, 131
Kidney failing to grasp qi, 121
Kidney qi deficiency, 117
Kidney qi failing to secure, 118–119
Kidney water invading Spleen, 275
Kidney yang deficiency, 123
Kidney yang deficiency with water effusion, 127

Kidney yin deficiency, 129–130
Large Intestine cold-dampness, 173–174
Large Intestine damp-heat, 175–176
Large Intestine deficiency cold, 169–170
Large Intestine dryness, 173
Large Intestine heat accumulation, 179
Liver and Gallbladder damp-heat, 254
Liver and Kidney yin deficiency, 241–242
Liver and Spleen disharmony, 245–246
Liver and Stomach disharmony, 247
Liver blood deficiency, 87
Liver blood stagnation, 105
Liver disease patterns, 80
Liver fire, 285, 287
Liver fire blazing, 92–93
Liver fire invading Lung, 250
Liver heat, 287
Liver qi deficiency, 293–294
Liver qi stagnation, 91
Liver yang deficiency, 297–298
Liver yang rising, 94–95
Liver yang transforming wind, 98
Liver yin deficiency, 88–89
loose stools, 59–60, 158
lumbar and knee pain and weakness, 112
Lung and Kidney yin deficiency, 238–239
Lung blood deficiency, 281–282
Lung qi deficiency, 34
Lung yang deficiency, 278
Lung yin deficiency, 35–36
menstrual disorder, 84
palpitations, 5
phlegm misting Heart, 21
phlegm-fire harassing Heart, 19
poor appetite, 59
reproductive and sexual function disorders, 113
shén disturbance, 7
Small Intestine deficiency cold, 161
Small Intestine excess fire, 162
Small Intestine qi stagnation, 163–164
Spleen and Kidney yang deficiency, 232
Spleen and Lung deficiency, 229–230

Spleen and Stomach disharmony, 235
Spleen not controlling blood, 66
Spleen patterns, 58
Spleen qi deficiency, 63, 65
Spleen yang deficiency, 67
Spleen yin deficiency, 70
Stomach clinical manifestations, 137–138
Stomach deficiency cold, 145–146
Stomach excess with Spleen deficiency, 316
Stomach fire, 147–148
Stomach patterns, general, 137
Stomach qi deficiency, 310–311
Stomach yin deficiency, 142
timidity and paranoia, 185–186
turbid phlegm obstructing Lung, 48–49
Urinary Bladder damp-heat, 202–203
Urinary Bladder deficiency cold, 199–200
urinary incontinence, 198
water metabolism disorders, 114
water qi encroaching on Heart (水氣凌心 shuǐ qì líng xīn), 268–269
wind syndrome, 82–83
wind-cold invading Lung, 36–37
wind-cold-dampness invading body surface (風寒濕襲表 fēng hán shī xí biǎo), 260
wind-water invading Lung, 46
yin deficiency generating wind, 101
etiology pattern identification (病因辨證 bìng yīn biàn zhèng), xv
excess above (上亢 shàng kàng), with deficiency below, 301
excess patterns
    compound patterns, 209
    in Heart disease, 9
    in Kidney disease, 116
    in Large Intestine disease, 168
    in Liver disease, 86
    in Lung disease, 33
    in Small Intestine disease, 160
    in Spleen disease, 63
    in Urinary Bladder disease, 199
excess/deficiency patterns, in Liver disease, 86
exogenous febrile diseases, pattern identification methods, 339

exopathogenic factors
    in Gallbladder patterns, 184
    in Large Intestine disease, 166
    in Liver disease, 80
    in Small Intestine disease, 157
    Spleen patterns from, 58
    Stomach patterns from, 137
    in Urinary Bladder patterns, 197
exterior dryness, vs. dryness invading Lung, 43
exterior patterns, 261
    in Lung disease, 33
exterior wind-cold, vs. wind-cold invading Lung, 37–38
exterior wind-heat, vs. wind-heat invading Lung, 40–41
extreme heat generating wind, 99

F

facial complexion, pale or dark, in Heart patterns, 8
Fang Yu, 324
febrile diseases, pattern identification methods, 339
fever
    alternating with chills (寒熱往來 hán rè wǎng lái), 306–307, 309
    with chills (惡寒發熱 wù hán fā rè), 306, 309
    comparative patterns and treatments, 309
    due to qi deficiency, 313
    high (高燒 gāo shāo), 307
    low-grade (低燒 dī shāo), 307–308, 309
    pattern differentiation, 306–308
    tidal (潮熱 cháo rè), 307, 309
    unsurfaced (身熱不揚 shēn rè bù yáng), 307, 309
Fine Formulas for Women (婦人良方大全 fù rén liáng fāng dà quán), 280
five types of developmental delay (五遲 wǔ chí), 113, 291
five types of flaccidity (五軟 wǔ ruǎn), 113, 291
fixed Kidney disorder (腎著 shèn zhuó), 326

food and drink
    decomposition of, 136
    diseases and treatments, 153
    Stomach reception of, 136
food aversion, as Stomach manifestation, 138–139
food stagnation
    acupuncture, 153
    clinical manifestations, 153
    definition, 153
    etiology and pathogenesis, 153
    herbal formulas, 153
Formulas for Succoring the Sick (濟生方 *jǐ shēng fāng*), 322
four levels pattern identification (衛氣營血辯證 *wèi qì yíng xuě biàn zhèng*), 337, 339
fright palpitations (驚悸 *jīng jì*), 4
fǔ (腑) organs, 135

G

Gallbladder
    bile storage and secretion functions, 183
    decision-making and judgment functions, 183–184
    digestion functions, 183
    pathological changes and clinical manifestations, 184–186
    physiological characteristics and functions, 183–184
Gallbladder disease patterns, 183
    bitter taste in, 184–185
    common etiological factors, 184
    common patterns, 186–187
    deficiency patterns, 187
    excess patterns, 187
    Gallbladder heat, 188–189
    Gallbladder qi deficiency, 187–188
    Gallbladder stagnation with phlegm disturbance, 191–192
    jaundice in, 185
    pattern summary, 195
    timidity and paranoia in, 185–186

Gallbladder heat
    clinical manifestations, 188
    definition, 188
    diseases and treatments, 189
    etiology and pathogenesis, 188–189
    vs. Gallbladder stagnation with phlegm disturbance, 192–193
    vs. Liver and Gallbladder damp-heat, 255–256
    vs. Liver fire blazing, 189–190
Gallbladder qi deficiency
    acupuncture, 1
    clinical manifestations, 187
    definition, 187
    diseases and treatments, 188
    etiology and pathogenesis, 187–188
    herbal formulas, 188
Gallbladder stagnation with phlegm disturbance
    acupuncture, 192
    clinical manifestations, 191
    definition, 191
    diseases and treatments, 192
    etiology and pathogenesis, 191
    vs. Gallbladder heat, 192–193
    vs. Heart fire blazing, 193–194
    herbal formulas, 192
    vs. phlegm-fire harassing Heart, 194–195
gathering qi (宗氣 *zōng qì*), production by Spleen and Lung, 227–228
guiding channels (引經 *yǐn jīng*), 331–332

H

hand cramp (搦 *nuò*), 289
Heart
    blood vessels and, 3
    excess patterns, 9
    function summary, 4
    housing *shén*, 3
    miscellaneous signs and symptoms, 8
    physiological characteristics and functions, 2–3

Heart and Kidney compound pattern
    emotional regulation roles, 220
    Heart and Kidney disharmony, 222–223
    Heart and Kidney yang deficiency, 220–221
Heart and Kidney compound patterns, 218
    essence and blood generation roles, 219–220
    pathophysiological relationship, 218
    yin and yang harmony roles, 218–219
Heart and Kidney disharmony
    acupuncture, 223
    clinical manifestations, 222
    definition, 22
    diseases and treatments, 223
    etiology and pathogenesis, 222
    vs. Heart fire blazing, 223–224
    herbal formulas, 223
Heart and Kidney yang deficiency
    acupuncture, 221
    clinical manifestations, 220
    definition, 220
    diseases and treatments, 221
    etiology and pathogenesis, 221
    herbal formulas, 221
Heart and Liver blood deficiency
    clinical manifestations, 217
    definition, 217
    etiology and pathogenesis, 217
Heart and Liver compound pattern, Heart and Liver blood deficiency, 217–218
Heart and Liver compound patterns, 215
    blood circulation roles, 215–216
    mental-emotional activities and, 216
    pathophysiological relationship, 215–216
Heart and Lung compound patterns, 210
    Heart and Lung qi deficiency, 210–212
    pathophysiological relationships, 210
Heart and Lung qi deficiency
    acupuncture, 212
    defined, 210
    diseases and treatments, 212
    etiology and pathogenesis, 211
    herbal formulas, 212

Heart and Small Intestine compound patterns, 224
    Heart fire transmits to Small Intestine, 225–226
    pathophysiological relationship, 224–225
Heart and Spleen compound patterns, 212
    blood circulation functions, 213
    blood production functions and, 212–213
    Heart and Spleen deficiency, 213–215
    pathophysiological relationship, 212–213
Heart and Spleen deficiency
    acupuncture, 215
    clinical manifestations, 213
    definition, 213
    diseases and treatments, 215
    etiology and pathogenesis, 214
    herbal formulas, 215
Heart blood deficiency
    clinical manifestations, 14
    definition, 14
    diseases and treatments, 15
    etiology and pathogenesis, 14–15
    vs. Heart yin deficiency, 16–17
Heart disease
    chest distress/pain, 7–8
    clinical manifestations, 4–8
    common patterns, 9
    deficiency patterns, 9
    insomnia in, 5–6
    palpitations in, 4–5
    patterns summary, 25
    shén disturbance, 6–7
Heart fire blazing
    acupuncture, 18
    clinical manifestations, 17
    definition, 17
    diseases and treatments, 18
    etiology and pathogenesis, 17–18
    vs. Gallbladder stagnation with phlegm disturbance, 193–194
    vs. Heart and Kidney disharmony, 223–224
    herbal formulas, 18
    vs. Liver fire blazing, 93–94
    vs. phlegm-fire harassing Heart, 20

Heart fire transmits to Small Intestine
    acupuncture, 226
    clinical manifestations, 225
    definition, 225
    diseases and treatments, 226
    etiology and pathogenesis, 225–226
    herbal formulas, 226
    vs. Small Intestine excess fire, 226–227
Heart patterns, 2
    etiological factors, 4
    Heart blood deficiency, 14–15
    Heart fire blazing, 17–18
    Heart qi deficiency, 10–11
    Heart vessels obstruction, 22–24
    Heart yang collapse, 12–14
    Heart yang deficiency, 11–12
    Heart yin deficiency, 15–16
    phlegm misting Heart, 20–21
    phlegm-fire harassing Heart, 18–19
    summary chart, 25
Heart qi deficiency
    clinical manifestations, 10
    definition, 10
    diseases and treatments, 11
    etiology and pathogenesis, 10
    vs. Heart yang collapse, 13–14
    vs. Heart yang deficiency, 13–14
Heart vessels obstruction
    acupuncture, 22
    clinical manifestations, 22–23
    definition, 22
    diseases and treatments, 24
    etiology and pathogenesis, 23–24
    herbal formulas, 22
Heart yang collapse
    clinical manifestations, 12
    definition, 12
    diseases and treatments, 13
    etiology and pathogenesis, 12–13
    vs. Heart qi deficiency, 13–14
    vs. Heart yang deficiency, 13–14
Heart yang deficiency
    clinical manifestations, 11

definition, 11
    diseases and treatments, 12
    etiology and pathogenesis, 11–12
    vs. Heart qi deficiency, 13–14
    vs. Heart yang deficiency, 13–14
Heart yang deficiency (心陽虛 xīn yáng xū)
    clinical manifestations, 271–272
    vs. water qi encroaching on Heart, 271–273
Heart yin deficiency
    clinical manifestations, 15
    definition, 15
    etiology and pathogenesis, 16
    vs. Heart blood deficiency, 16–17
Heat congesting Lung
    acupuncture, 52
    clinical manifestations, 51
    definition, 51
    diseases and patterns, 52
    etiology and pathogenesis, 51–52
    vs. heat-phlegm obstructing Lung, 52–53
    herbal formulas, 52
    vs. Liver fire invading Lung, 251–252
    vs. wind-heat invading Lung, 52–53
heat pathogen, attacking Heart, 4
heat-phlegm obstructing Lung
    vs. heat congesting Lung, 52–53
    vs. wind-heat invading Lung, 52–53
heavenly dew (天癸 tiān guǐ), 328
herbal formulas
    blood deficiency generating wind, 100
    blood stagnation in Stomach, 154
    cold invading Lung, 48
    cold invading Stomach, 150
    cold stagnation in Liver channel, 105
    cold-dampness encumbering Spleen, 73
    cold-water shooting into Lung, 54
    damp-heat encumbering Spleen, 75
    extreme heat generating wind, 99
    fever differentiated patterns, 309
    food stagnation pattern, 153
    Gallbladder heat, 189
    Gallbladder qi deficiency, 188

Gallbladder stagnation with phlegm disturbance, 192
Heart and Kidney disharmony, 223
Heart and Kidney yang deficiency, 221
Heart and Lung qi deficiency, 212
Heart and Spleen deficiency, 215
Heart blood deficiency, 15
Heart fire blazing, 18
Heart fire transmits to Small Intestine, 226
Heart qi deficiency, 11
Heart yang collapse, 13
Heart yang deficiency, 12
Heart yin deficiency, 16
Heat congesting Lung, 52
Kidney essence deficiency, 132
Kidney failing to grasp qi, 121
Kidney qi deficiency, 118
Kidney qi failing to secure, 119
Kidney water invading Spleen, 276
Kidney yang deficiency, 124, 305
Kidney yang deficiency with water effusion, 127
Kidney yin deficiency, 130
Large Intestine cold-dampness, 174
Large Intestine damp-heat, 176
Large Intestine deficiency cold, 170
Large Intestine dryness, 173
Large Intestine heat accumulation, 179
Liver and Gallbladder damp-heat, 255
Liver and Kidney yin deficiency, 243
Liver and Spleen disharmony, 246
Liver and Stomach disharmony, 247
Liver blood deficiency, 88
Liver blood stagnation, 106
Liver fire, 287
Liver fire blazing, 93
Liver heat, 287
Liver qi deficiency, 294
Liver qi stagnation, 92
Liver yang deficiency, 298, 305
Liver yang rising, 95
Liver yang transforming wind, 98
Liver yin deficiency, 89
Lung and Kidney yin deficiency, 239
Lung blood deficiency, 282
Lung qi deficiency, 35
Lung yang deficiency, 278
phlegm misting Heart, 21
phlegm-fire harassing Heart, 19
Small Intestine deficiency cold, 161
Small Intestine excess fire, 163
Small Intestine qi stagnation, 164
Spleen and Kidney yang deficiency, 233
Spleen and Lung deficiency, 230
Spleen and Stomach disharmony, 236
Spleen not controlling blood, 67
Spleen qi deficiency, 64
Spleen qi sinking, 65
Spleen yang deficiency, 68
Spleen yin deficiency, 71
Stomach deficiency cold, 146
Stomach excess with Spleen deficiency, 317
Stomach fire, 148
Stomach qi deficiency, 311
Stomach yin deficiency, 143
turbid phlegm obstructing Lung, 50
Urinary Bladder damp-heat, 203
Urinary Bladder deficiency cold, 200
wind-cold invading Lung, 37
wind-cold-dampness invading body surface (風寒濕襲表 fēng hán shī xí biǎo), 261
wind-heat invading Lung, 39
wind-water invading Lung, 47
Yin deficiency generating wind, 102
hiccups
    etiology and pathomechanisms, 138
    as Stomach manifestation, 137–138
Hua Tuo, 295
Huang Gong-Xiu, 322
hundred vessels, 27
hypochondriac distention, 82
hysteria (百合病 bǎi hé bìng), 6

Important Formulas Worth a Thousand Gold Pieces (千金要方 qiān jīn yào fāng), 295

impotence. *See* erectile dysfunction
improper treatment
    in Large Intestine disease, 166
    in Liver patterns, 80
    in Small Intestine patterns, 157
    Spleen pattern etiologies, 58
    in Stomach patterns, 137
insomnia
    definition, 5
    etiology and pathomechanism, insomnia, 6
    in Heart disease, 5–6
interior patterns, 261
    in Lung disease, 33
internal wind, clinical manifestations, 289–290
interstitial spaces (腠理 *còu lǐ*), 26
Introduction to Medicine (醫學入門 *yī xué rù mén*), 322
irritability and restlessness (煩躁 *fán zào*), 6
itching (癢 *yǎng*), 290

J

jaundice, in Gallbladder disease patterns, 185
jerk (挚 *zhì*), 289
Judgment and Treatment for Similar Patterns (類証治裁), 322

K

Ke Yun-Bo, 325
Key Link of Medicine (醫貫 *yī guàn*), 322
Kidney
    essence storage function, 109–110
    growth and development functions, 109
    miscellaneous signs and symptoms, 114–115
    pathological changes and clinical manifestations, 112–115
    physiological characteristics and functions, 108–111
    as power organ (作強之官 *zuò qiáng zhī guān*), 108, 304
    qi reception by, 111
    reproductive functions, 109
    role in Liver yang deficiency, 303–305
    as root of yin and yang, 109–110
    water metabolism functions, 110–111
Kidney disease patterns, 108
    common patterns, 115–116
    deficiency patterns, 116, 324–325
    etiological factors, 112
    excess patterns, 116
    growth and developmental abnormalities, 113
    Kidney essence deficiency, 131–132
    Kidney failing to grasp qi, 120–121
    Kidney qi deficiency, 117–118
    Kidney qi failing to secure, 118–119
    Kidney yang deficiency, 122–124
    Kidney yang deficiency with water effusion, 126–127
    Kidney yin deficiency, 129–130
    lumbar and knee soreness/weakness, 112
    pattern summary, 134
    relationship and development, 133
    reproductive disorders, 113
    sexual function disorders, 113
    water metabolism disorders, 114
Kidney essence deficiency
    acupuncture, 132
    clinical manifestations, 131
    definition, 131
    diseases and treatments, 132
    etiology and pathogenesis, 131
    herbal formulas, 132
    vs. Kidney yin deficiency, 132–133
Kidney essence, defined, 320–321
Kidney excess patterns, 325–327
Kidney failing to consolidate, 327
Kidney failing to grasp qi
    acupuncture, 121
    clinical manifestations, 121
    definition, 120
    diseases and treatments, 121
    etiology and pathogenesis, 121
    herbal formulas, 121
    vs. Kidney qi deficiency, 125–126
    vs. Kidney qi failing to secure, 125–126

Kidney qi deficiency *(continued)*
    vs. Kidney yang deficiency, 125–126
    vs. Lung qi deficiency, 122
Kidney qi deficiency
    acupuncture, 118
    definition, 117
    diseases and treatments, 118
    etiology and pathogenesis, 117
    herbal formulas, 118
    vs. Kidney failing to grasp qi, 125–126
    vs. Kidney qi failing to secure, 125–126
    vs. Kidney yang deficiency, 125–126
Kidney qi failing to secure
    acupuncture, 119
    clinical manifestations, 118
    definition, 118
    diseases and treatments, 119
    etiology and pathogenesis, 118–119
    herbal formulas, 119
    vs. Kidney failing to grasp qi, 125–126
    vs. Kidney qi deficiency, 125–126
    vs. Kidney yang deficiency, 124–125, 125–126
    vs. Spleen qi sinking, 120
Kidney water invading Spleen
    acupuncture, 276
    clinical manifestation, 275
    vs. cold-water shooting into Lung, 276–277
    definition, 275
    diseases and treatments, 276
    etiology and pathogenesis, 275
    herbal formulas, 276
    vs. Kidney yang deficiency, 276–277
    vs. water qi encroaching on Heart, 276–277
Kidney yang deficiency
    acupuncture, 124
    clinical manifestations, 122–123
    vs. cold-water shooting into Lung, 276–277
    definition, 122
    diseases and treatments, 124
    etiology and pathogenesis, 123
    herbal formulas, 124
    vs. Kidney failing to grasp qi, 125–126
    vs. Kidney qi deficiency, 125

    vs. Kidney qi failing to secure, 124–125, 125–126
    vs. Kidney water invading Spleen, 276–277
    vs. Kidney yang deficiency with water effusion, 276–277
    vs. Large Intestine deficiency cold, 170–171
    vs. Liver yang deficiency, 303–305
    vs. mìng mén fire decline, 323
    vs. Spleen yang deficiency, 170–171
    vs. Urinary Bladder deficiency cold, 200–201
    vs. water qi encroaching on Heart, 276–277
Kidney yang deficiency with water effusion
    acupuncture, 127
    clinical manifestations, 126
    vs. cold-water shooting into Lung, 128, 276–277
    definition, 126
    diseases and treatments, 127
    etiology and pathogenesis, 127
    herbal formulas, 127
    vs. Kidney water invading Spleen, 276–277
    vs. Kidney yang deficiency, 276–277
    vs. water qi encroaching on Heart, 128, 276–277
Kidney yang, defined, 320–321
Kidney yin
    defined, 320–321
    mìng mén water as, 323
Kidney yin deficiency
    acupuncture, 130
    in amenorrhea and menorrhagia, 327–328
    clinical manifestations, 129
    definition, 129
    diseases and treatments, 130
    etiology and pathogenesis, 129–130
    herbal formulas, 130
    vs. Kidney essence deficiency, 132–133
knee soreness/weakness, 112

L

Lantai Criterion (蘭臺軌範), 324
Large Intestine
    miscellaneous signs and symptoms, 168

physiological characteristics and functions, 165
reabsorption functions, 165
transportation functions, 165
Large Intestine cold-dampness
    acupuncture, 174
    clinical manifestations, 173
    definition, 173
    diseases and treatments, 174
    etiology and pathogenesis, 173–174
    herbal formulas, 174
    vs. Large Intestine damp-heat, 176–177
    vs. Large Intestine deficiency cold, 174–175
Large Intestine damp-heat
    acupuncture, 176
    clinical manifestations, 175
    vs. damp-heat encumbering Spleen, 177–178
    definition, 175
    diseases and treatments, 176
    etiology and pathogenesis, 175–176
    herbal formulas, 176
    vs. Large Intestine cold-dampness, 176–177
    vs. Large Intestine heat accumulation, 181
Large Intestine deficiency cold
    acupuncture, 170
    clinical manifestations, 169
    definition, 169
    diseases and treatments, 170
    etiology and pathogenesis, 169–170
    herbal formulas, 170
    vs. Kidney yang deficiency, 170
    vs. Large Intestine cold-dampness, 174–175
    vs. Small Intestine deficiency cold, 171–172
    vs. Spleen yang deficiency, 170–171
Large Intestine disease patterns, 165
    common etiological factors, 166
    common patterns, 168–169
    constipation in, 167
    deficiency patterns, 168
    diarrhea/loose stools in, 166–167
    excess patterns, 168
    Large Intestine cold-dampness, 173–174
    Large Intestine damp-heat, 175–176
    Large Intestine deficiency cold, 169–170
    Large Intestine dryness, 172–173
    Large Intestine heat accumulation, 178–179
    pathological changes and clinical manifestations, 166–168
    pattern summary, 182
Large Intestine dryness
    acupuncture, 173
    clinical manifestations, 172
    definition, 172
    diseases and treatments, 173
    etiology and pathogenesis, 173
    herbal formulas, 173
    vs. Large Intestine heat accumulation, 180
    vs. Stomach yin deficiency, 144–145
Large Intestine heat accumulation
    acupuncture, 179
    clinical manifestations, 178
    definition, 178
    diseases and treatments, 179
    etiology and pathogenesis, 179
    herbal formulas, 179
    vs. Large Intestine damp-heat, 181
    vs. Large Intestine dryness, 180
leakage conditions, 327
Li Chan, 322
Li Dong-Yuan, 313
Li Shizhen, 280
Li Zhong-Zi, 324
Lin Pei-Qin, 322
Liu Chun, 324
Liu Wan-Su, 331
Liver
    blood storage and regulation functions, 79–80
    coursing and discharging functions, 79
    miscellaneous signs and symptoms, 85–86
    pathological changes and clinical manifestations, 81–85, 288
    physiological characteristics and functions, 78
    as unyielding organ (剛臟 *gāng zàng*), 294

Liver and Gallbladder
    emotional activity functions, 253
    pathophysiological relationship, 252–253
Liver and Gallbladder compound patterns, 252
    Liver and Gallbladder damp-heat, 253–255
Liver and Gallbladder damp-heat
    acupuncture, 255
    clinical manifestations, 253
    vs. damp-heat encumbering Spleen, 302–303
    definition, 253
    diseases and treatments, 255
    etiology and pathogenesis, 254
    vs. Gallbladder heat, 255–256
    herbal formulas, 255
Liver and Kidney
    coursing and storage coordination, 240
    essence and blood storage roles, 240
    pathophysiological relationship, 240–241
    yin and yang mutual control, 240
Liver and Kidney compound patterns, 240
Liver and Kidney yin deficiency
    acupuncture, 242
    clinical manifestations, 241
    definition, 241
    diseases and treatments, 242
    etiology and pathogenesis, 241–242
    herbal formulas, 242
    vs. Liver yang rising, 242–243
Liver and Lung
    channel connection, 249
    pathophysiological relationship, 249
    qi regulation functions, 249
Liver and Lung compound patterns, 249
    Liver fire invading Lung, 250–251
Liver and Spleen disharmony
    acupuncture, 246
    clinical manifestations, 245
    definition, 245
    diseases and treatments, 246
    etiology and pathogenesis, 245–246
    herbal formulas, 246
    vs. Liver and Stomach disharmony, 248

Liver and Spleen/Stomach
    blood circulation roles, 244–245
    digestion roles, 244
    pathophysiological relationship, 244–245
Liver and Spleen/Stomach compound patterns, 244
    Liver and Spleen disharmony, 245–246
    Liver and Stomach disharmony, 246–247
Liver and Stomach disharmony
    acupuncture, 247
    clinical manifestation, 247
    definition, 246
    diseases and treatments, 247
    etiology and pathogenesis, 247
    herbal formulas, 247
    vs. Liver and Spleen disharmony, 248
Liver blood deficiency
    acupuncture, 88
    clinical manifestations, 87
    definition, 87
    diseases and treatments, 88
    etiology and pathogenesis, 87
    herbal formulas, 88
    vs. Liver yin deficiency, 90
Liver blood stagnation
    acupuncture, 106
    clinical manifestations, 105
    definition, 105
    diseases and treatments, 106
    etiology and pathogenesis, 105
    herbal formulas, 106
Liver disease patterns, 78
    blood deficiency generating wind, 100
    cold stagnation in Liver channel, 104–105
    common etiological factors, 80
    common patterns, 85–86
    deficiency patterns, 86
    emotional disorders and, 81
    excess patterns, 86
    excess/deficiency patterns, 86
    extreme heat generating wind, 99
    hypochondriac distention and, 82
    Liver Blood deficiency, 87–88

Liver blood stagnation, 105–106
Liver fire blazing, 92–93
Liver qi stagnation, 90–92
Liver wind stirring internally, 97
Liver yang rising, 94–95
Liver yang transforming wind, 97–98
Liver yin deficiency, 88–89
menstrual disorders and, 83–84
pattern summary, 107
relationship and development, 106
wind syndrome and, 82–83
yin deficiency generating wind, 101–102
Liver downward oppress (下迫 xià pò), 288
Liver fire
vs. Liver heat, 287
pattern differentiation, 285–286
varying manifestations, 285
Liver fire attacking Lung, 286
Liver fire attacking Stomach, 286
Liver fire blazing
acupuncture, 93
clinical manifestations, 92
definition, 92
differentiation from other Liver fire patterns, 286
diseases and treatments, 93
etiology and pathogenesis, 92–93
vs. Gallbladder heat, 189–190
vs. Heart fire blazing, 93–94
herbal formulas, 93
vs. Liver qi stagnation, 301–302
vs. Liver yang rising, 95–96, 301–302
Liver fire impairing yin, 286
Liver fire invading Lung
acupuncture, 251
clinical manifestations, 250
definition, 250
diseases and treatments, 251
vs. dryness invading Lung, 282–283
etiology and pathogenesis, 250
vs. heat congesting Lung, 251
herbal formulas, 251
vs. Lung yin deficiency, 282–283

Liver fire with phlegm, 286
Liver heat, *vs.* Liver fire, 287
Liver qi deficiency, 290–293
acupuncture, 294
affecting lower body, 292
affecting middle body, 291–292
clinical manifestations, 293
definition, 293
diseases and treatments, 294
etiology and pathogenesis, 293–294
herbal formulas, 294
and Liver yang, 293
Spleen energetics and, 299–301
vs. Spleen qi deficiency, 299–301
upper body pathology, 291
Liver qi rebellion, *vs.* Liver qi stagnation, 284–285
Liver qi stagnation
acupuncture, 92
clinical manifestations, 90
definition, 90
diseases and treatments, 92
etiology and pathogenesis, 91
herbal formulas, 92
vs. Liver fire blazing, 301–302
vs. Liver qi rebellion, 284–285
vs. Liver yang rising, 301–302
pathogenesis, 284–285
pathological changes, 288
Liver random movement (竄行 cuàn xíng), 288
Liver syncope (厥脱 jué tuō), 288
Liver transverse rebellion (横逆 héng nì), 288
Liver upward disrupt (上擾 shàng rǎo), 288
Liver wind stirring internally, 97
pattern summary, 102
Liver yang deficiency, 294–296
acupuncture, 298
clinical manifestations, 296–297
definition, 297
diseases and treatments, 298
etiology and pathogenesis, 297–298
herbal formulas, 298
Kidney energetics and, 303–305

vs. Kidney yang deficiency, 303–305
Liver channel signs and symptoms, 296
organ signs and symptoms, 295
Liver yang rising
    acupuncture, 95
    clinical manifestations, 94
    definition, 94
    etiology and pathogenesis, 94–95
    herbal formulas, 95
    vs. Liver and Kidney yin deficiency, 242–243
    vs. Liver fire blazing, 95–96
    vs. Liver yang transforming wind, 102–103
    vs. Liver yin deficiency, 96–97
Liver yang transforming wind
    acupuncture, 98
    clinical manifestations, 98
    definition, 97
    diseases and treatments, 98
    etiology and pathogenesis, 98
    herbal formulas, 98
    vs. Liver yang rising, 102–103
    vs. wind-phlegm disturbing upward, 103–104
Liver yin deficiency
    acupuncture, 89
    clinical manifestations, 88
    definition, 88
    diseases and treatments, 89
    etiology and pathogenesis, 88–89
    herbal formulas, 89
    vs. Liver blood deficiency, 90
    vs. Liver yang rising, 96–97
loose stools, 59–60
    in Small Intestine disease, 158
Lou Ying, 324
lower back soreness/weakness, 112
Lung
    as blood organ (肺為血臟 *fèi wéi xuě zàng*), 279
    and corporeal soul (魄 *pò*), 26
    dispersing and descending function, 28
    dredging and regulating function, 28
    exopathogenic factors invading, 44–45
    as florid canopy (華蓋 *huá gài*), 26
    governing hundred vessels, 27
    as minister organ (相傅之官 *xiāng fù zhī guan*), 26
    miscellaneous signs and symptoms, 32
    physiological characteristics and functions, 26–29
    qi governing and control by, 27
    role in protective qi (衛氣 *wèi qì*), 28
    skin and hair links, 279
    water metabolism and, 28
Lung and Kidney
    mutual nourishment and replenishment, 237–238
    pathophysiological relationship, 236–238
    respiration roles, 237
    water metabolism roles, 236
Lung and Kidney compound patterns, 236
    Lung and Kidney yin deficiency, 238–239
Lung and Kidney yin deficiency
    acupuncture, 239
    clinical manifestations, 238
    definition, 238
    diseases and treatments, 239
    etiology and pathogenesis, 238–239
    herbal formulas, 239
Lung atrophy (肺痿 *fèi wěi*), 277
Lung blood deficiency
    acupuncture, 282
    clinical manifestations, 280–281
    diseases and treatments, 282
    etiology and pathogenesis, 281–282
    herbal formulas, 282
    historical mentions, 279–280
Lung disease
    abnormal respiration in, 39
    chills and fever in, 29
    common patterns, 33
    cough in, 31
    pathological changes and clinical manifestations, 29–32
Lung disease patterns, 26
    cold invading Lung, 47–48
    cold-water shooting into Lung, 53–54

common etiological factors, 28–29
common patterns, 33
coolness-dryness invading Lung, 42
deficiency patterns, 33
dryness invading Lung, 41–42
excess patterns, 33
exterior patterns, 33
heat congesting Lung pattern, 51–52
interior patterns, 33
Lung qi deficiency, 34–35
Lung yin deficiency, 35–36
pattern summary, 56
turbid phlegm obstructing Lung, 48–50
warmth-dryness invading Lung, 42
wind-cold invading Lung, 36–37
wind-heat invading Lung, 38–39
wind-water invading Lung, 46–47
Lung qi deficiency
clinical manifestations, 34
definition, 34
diseases and treatments, 35
etiology and pathogenesis, 34
vs. Kidney failing to grasp qi, 122
Lung yang deficiency
acupuncture, 278
clinical manifestations, 278
definition, 277
diseases and treatments, 278
vs. dryness invading Lung, 282–283
etiology and pathogenesis, 278
herbal formulas, 278
Lung yin deficiency, *vs.* Liver fire invading Lung, 282–283
Lung yin deficiency
clinical manifestation, 35
definition, 35
diseases and treatments, 36
vs. dryness invading Lung, 43–44
etiology and pathogenesis, 35–36

M

main water pattern (正水證 *zhèng shuǐ zhèng*), 275

Medical Checklist (醫學網目 *yī xué gāng mù*), 324
Medical Collected Works (秦伯末醫文集 *qín bó mò yī wén jí*), 296
Medical Notes (醫林繩墨 *yī lín shéng mò*), 324
Medical Origin (醫學啟源 *yī xué qí yuán*), 331
Medical Story (醫學正傳 *yī xué zhèng zhuàn*), 322, 324
Medical Three Character Classic (醫學三字經 *yī xué sān zì jīng*), 322
memory problems, in Heart patterns, 8
menorrhagia, Kidney yin deficiency in, 327–328
menstrual disorders, in Liver disease patterns, 83–84
middle qi insufficiency (中氣不足 *zhōng qì bù zú*), 311–312
middle qi sinking (中氣下陷 *zhōng qì xià xiàn*), 313
mìng mén
as gate of vitality, 321
between Kidneys, 322
as motive force between Kidneys, 322
physiological functions, 323
mìng mén fire (命門之火 *mìng mén zhī huǒ*), 108, 110
defined, 320–321
mìng mén water (命門之水 *mìng mén zhī shuǐ*), defined, 320–321
mìng mén fire decline, 323
moving qi (動氣 *dòng qì*), 227

N

nausea
etiology and pathomechanisms, 138
as Stomach manifestation, 137–138
New Compilation of Materia Medica (本草求真 *běn cǎo qiú zhēn*), 322
numbness and tingling (麻 *má*), 289
nutritive qi (營氣 *yíng qì*), 38

O

organ and tissue relationships, xvii

organ relationships, xvii
Origin of Materia Medica (本經逢原 *běn jīng féng yuán*), 322
Origin of Medicine (醫學啟源 *yī xué qǐ yuán*), 324
original yang (元陽 *yuán yáng*), 110

P

palpitations
    continuous, 5
    definition, 4
    etiology and pathomechanisms, 5
    fright palpitations (驚悸 *jīng jì*), 4
    in Heart disease, 4–5
panting (喘 *chuǎn*), 30
paranoia, in Gallbladder disease patterns, 185–186
paraphasia (錯語 *cuò yǔ*), 7
pathogenesis. *See* etiology and pathogenesis
pathogenic factors, in *shén* disturbance, 7
pattern identification (辯證 *biàn zhèng*), 333
    dynamic approach, 333–334
    holistic approach, 333
pattern identification methods, xv–xvi, 333
    channel pattern identification (經絡辯證 *jīng luò biàn zhèng*), 336–337, 338
    eight principles pattern identification (八綱辨證 *bā gāng biàn zhèng*), xv, 335, 338, 339
    etiology pattern identification (病因辨證 *bìng yīn biàn zhèng*), xv, 335–336, 338
    four levels pattern identification (衛氣營血辯證 *wèi qì yíng xuě biàn zhèng*), 337, 339
    qi, blood and body fluids method, xv, 335, 338
    relationships among, 338–339
    six channels pattern identification (六經辯證 *liù jīng biàn zhèng*), 337, 339
    Triple Burner pattern identification (三焦辯證 *sān jiāo biàn zhèng*), 338, 339
    zàng fǔ pattern identification (臟腑辯證 *zàng fǔ biàn zhèng*), 336
Patterns, Cause, Pulse and Treatment (証因脈治 *zhèng yīn mài zhì*), 313

pectoral qi, 227, 228
Penetrating and Conception vessels, 328
phlegm
    characteristics and indications, 49
    clinical manifestations, 49
phlegm (痰 *tán*), 262, 266–267
phlegm misting Heart
    acupuncture, 21
    clinical manifestations, 18–19
    definition, 20
    diseases and treatments, 21
    etiology and pathogenesis, 21
    herbal formulas, 21
    vs. phlegm-fire harassing Heart, 22
phlegm-fire harassing Heart
    acupuncture, 19
    clinical manifestations, 19
    definition, 18
    diseases and treatments, 19
    etiology and pathogenesis, 19
    vs. Gallbladder stagnation with phlegm disturbance, 194–195
    vs. Heart fire blazing, 20
    herbal formulas, 19
    vs. phlegm misting Heart, 22
phlegm-thin mucus (痰飲 *tán yǐn*), 265
physical overstrain, Kidney disease and, 112
Precious Mirror of Oriental Medicine (東醫寶鑒 *dōng yī bǎo jiàn*), 326
Primary Study Medical Classic (醫經小學 *yī jīng xiǎo xué*), 324
primary yang (原陽 *yuán yáng*), 320–321
    mìng mén fire as, 322
primary yin (原陰 *yuán yīn*), 320–321
    mìng mén water as, 323
propping thin mucus (支飲 *zhī yǐn*), 266
protective qi (衛氣 *wèi qì*), 38, 52
Pulse Classic (脈經 *mài jīng*), 322, 330
pulse, Heart patterns, 8

Q

qi reception, Kidney governance, 111
qi transformation (氣化 *qì huà*), 46, 110

qi, blood, and body fluids pattern identification, xv, 335
qi, Lung as governor and controller, 27
Qian Yi, 324, 331
    on Kidney deficiency, 325
Qin Bo-Mo, 296
Qin Jing-Min, 313
Qin Jing-Ming, 280

R

Re-editing Yan's Formulary for Succoring the Sick (重輯嚴氏濟生方), 295
reabsorption functions, Large Intestine, 165
receiving and transforming, Small Intestine and, 156
Records of Heartfelt Experiences in Medicine with Reference to the West (醫學衷中參西錄 *yī xué zhōng zhōng cān xī lù*), 291
reproductive disorders, Kidney and, 113
reproductive essence (*tiān kúi*), 113
reproductive essence (生殖之精 *shēng zhí zhī jīng*), 321
Required Book for Grandmaster (醫宗必讀), 324
respiration
    abnormal (*See* abnormal respiration)
    Lung and Kidney roles in normal, 237
restless organ disorder (臟躁 *zàng zào*), 6

S

Sacred and Favorite Formulas from Tai Ping Era (太平聖惠方 *tài píng shèng huì fāng*), 325
sending up, Spleen and, 58
separating clear from turbid, Small Intestine and, 156
sexual function disorders, Kidney and, 113
sexual overstrain, Kidney disease and, 112
shaking and swinging (動 *dòng*), 290
shén disturbance, 6–7
    definition, 6
    etiology and pathomechanisms, 7
Shen Jin-Ao, 324

shén, Heart as house of, 3
shortage of qi (少氣 *shǎo qì*), 30
shortness of breath (短氣 *duǎn qì*), 30
sight anomalies, from internal wind, 289
six channels pattern identification (六經辯證 *liù jīng biàn zhèng*), 337
Small Intestine
    miscellaneous signs and symptoms, 159
    physiological characteristics and functions, 156–157
    receiving and transforming functions, 156
    separation of clear and turbid by, 156
Small Intestine deficiency cold
    acupuncture, 161
    clinical manifestations, 160
    definition, 160
    diseases and treatments, 161
    etiology and pathogenesis, 161
    herbal formulas, 161
    vs. Large Intestine deficiency cold, 171–172
    vs. Urinary Bladder deficiency cold, 201–202
Small Intestine disease patterns, 156
    abnormal urination in, 157–158
    common etiological factors, 157
    common patterns, 160
    deficiency patterns, 160
    excess patterns, 160
    loose stools in, 158
    pathological changes and clinical manifestations, 157–159
    pattern summary, 164
    Small Intestine deficiency cold, 160–161
    Small Intestine excess fire, 162–163
    Small Intestine qi stagnation, 163–164
Small Intestine excess fire
    acupuncture, 163
    clinical manifestations, 162
    definition, 162
    diseases and treatments, 163
    etiology and pathogenesis, 162
    vs. Heart fire transmits to Small Intestine, 226–227
    herbal formulas, 163
    vs. Urinary Bladder damp-heat, 203–204

Small Intestine qi stagnation
    acupuncture, 164
    clinical manifestations, 163
    definition, 163
    diseases and treatments, 164
    etiology and pathogenesis, 163–164
    herbal formulas, 164
smoking, and Lung disease, 29
soliloquies (獨語 *dú yǔ*), 7
sovereign fire (君火 *jūn huǒ*), 2
spasm (抽 *chōu*), 289
spillage thin mucus (溢飲 *yì yǐn*), 266
Spiritual Pivot (靈樞 *líng shū*), 279
    Liver qi stagnation/rebellion in, 284
Spleen
    constrained, 317–318
    control of blood, 58
    favoring dryness and disfavoring dampness, 313
    as granary organ (食廩之官 *shí lǐn zhī guān*), 57
    miscellaneous signs and symptoms, 61–62
    physiological characteristics and functions, 57–58
    sending up functions, 58
    transformation and transportation functions, 58
Spleen and Kidney
    essence generation and storage, 230–231
    water metabolism regulation function, 231
Spleen and Kidney compound patterns, 230
    pathophysiological relationship, 230–231
    Spleen and Kidney yang deficiency, 231–233
Spleen and Kidney Yang deficiency
    acupuncture, 233
    clinical manifestations, 232
    definition, 231
    diseases and treatments, 233
    etiology and pathogenesis, 232
    herbal formulas, 233
Spleen and Lung compound pattern, Spleen and Lung deficiency, 229–230

Spleen and Lung compound patterns, 227
    gathering qi production, 227–228
    pathophysiological relationship, 227–229
    water metabolism regulation, 228–229
Spleen and Lung deficiency
    acupuncture, 230
    clinical manifestation, 229
    definition, 229
    diseases and treatments, 230
    etiology and pathogenesis, 229–230
    herbal formulas, 230
Spleen and Stomach
    complementary ascending and descending movements, 234
    dryness and dampness regulation by, 234
    ingestion, transportation, transformation roles, 234
    pathophysiological relationship, 233–234
Spleen and Stomach compound patterns, 233
    Spleen and Stomach disharmony, 235–236
Spleen and Stomach disharmony
    acupuncture, 236
    clinical manifestations, 235
    definition, 235
    diseases and treatments, 236
    etiology and pathogenesis, 235
    herbal formulas, 236
Spleen disease
    bleeding in, 61
    bloating and distention in, 60–61
    loose stools in, 59–60
    pathological changes and clinical manifestations, 59
    poor appetite and, 59
Spleen disease patterns, 57
    cold-dampness encumbering Spleen, 71–72
    common etiological factors, 58
    common patterns, 62–63
    damp-heat encumbering Spleen, 74–76
    deficiency patterns, 63
    excess patterns, 63
    pattern summary, 77
    Spleen not controlling blood, 66–67

Spleen qi deficiency, 63–64
Spleen qi sinking, 64–65
Spleen yang deficiency, 67–68
Spleen yin deficiency, 70–71
Spleen not controlling blood
    acupuncture, 67
    clinical manifestations, 66
    definition, 66
    diseases and treatments, 67
    etiology and pathogenesis, 66
    herbal formulas, 67
    vs. Spleen qi deficiency, 68–69
    vs. Spleen qi sinking, 68–69
    vs. Spleen yang deficiency, 68–69
Spleen qi deficiency
    acupuncture, 64
    clinical manifestations, 63
    definition, 63
    diseases and treatments, 64
    etiology and pathogenesis, 63, 65
    herbal formulas, 64
    vs. Liver qi deficiency, 299–301
    vs. Spleen not controlling blood, 68
    vs. Spleen qi sinking, 68–69
    vs. Spleen yang deficiency, 68–69
    vs. Stomach qi deficiency, 311–312
Spleen qi sinking
    acupuncture, 65
    clinical manifestations, 65
    definition, 64
    etiology and pathogenesis, 65
    herbal formulas, 65
    vs. Kidney qi failing to secure, 120
    vs. Spleen not controlling blood, 68–69
    vs. Spleen qi deficiency, 68–69
    vs. Spleen yang deficiency, 68–69
Spleen yang deficiency
    acupuncture, 68
    clinical manifestations, 67
    definition, 67
    diseases and treatments, 68
    etiology and pathogenesis, 67–68
    herbal formulas, 68
    vs. Kidney yang deficiency, 170–171
    vs. Large Intestine deficiency cold, 170–171
    vs. Spleen not controlling blood, 68–69
    vs. Spleen qi deficiency, 68–69
    vs. Spleen qi sinking, 68–69
    vs. Stomach deficiency cold, 146–147
Spleen yin deficiency, 313–315
    acupuncture, 71
    clinical manifestations, 70
    definition, 70
    diseases and treatments, 71
    etiology and pathogenesis, 70
    herbal formulas, 71, 315
    vs. Stomach yin deficiency, 143–144
Spleen Yin, major physiological functions, 314
Standard for Diagnosis and Treatment (證治準繩 *zhèng zhì zhǔn shéng*), 272
Stomach
    decomposition functions, 136
    descending functions, 137
    epigastric bloating/distention and, 139–140
    food and drink reception functions, 136
    food aversions and, 138–139
    miscellaneous signs and symptoms, 140
    physiological characteristics and functions, 136–137
Stomach deficiency cold
    acupuncture, 146
    clinical manifestations, 145
    vs. cold invading Stomach, 151
    definition, 145
    diseases and treatments, 146
    etiology and pathogenesis, 145–146
    herbal formulas, 146
    vs. Spleen yang deficiency, 146–147
Stomach disease patterns, 136
    acid regurgitation in, 137–138
    belching in, 137–138
    blood stagnation in Stomach, 154
    cold invading Stomach, 149–150
    common etiological factors, 137
    common patterns, 141
    deficiency patterns, 141

excess patterns, 141
food stagnation, 153
hiccups in, 137–138
nausea in, 137–138
pattern summary, 155
Stomach deficiency cold, 145–146
Stomach fire, 147–148
Stomach yin deficiency, 142–143
vomiting in, 137–138

Stomach excess with Spleen deficiency
acupuncture, 317
clinical manifestations, 315
vs. constrained Spleen, 317–318
definition, 315
diseases and treatments, 317
etiology and pathogenesis, 316
herbal formulas, 317

Stomach fire
acupuncture, 148
clinical manifestations, 147
definition, 147
diseases and treatments, 148
etiology and pathogenesis, 147–148
herbal formulas, 148
vs. Stomach yin deficiency, 148–149

Stomach qi deficiency
acupuncture, 311
clinical manifestations, 310
definition, 310
diseases and treatments, 311
etiology and pathogenesis, 310–311
herbal formulas, 311
vs. Spleen qi deficiency, 311–312

Stomach yin deficiency
acupuncture, 143
clinical manifestations, 142
definition, 142
diseases and treatments, 143
etiology and pathogenesis, 142
herbal formulas, 143
vs. Large Intestine dryness, 144–145
vs. Spleen Yin deficiency, 143–144
vs. Stomach fire, 148–149

Sun Simiao, 325, 331
on Liver yang deficiency, 295
suspended thin mucus (懸飲 *xuán yǐn*), 266
sweating, in Heart patterns, 8
Symptoms, Causes, Pulse, and Treatment (症因脈治 *zhèng yīn mài zhì*), 280
syncope (厥脫 *jué tuō*), from internal wind, 290
Systemic Compilation of the Internal Clinic (類經附翼 *lèi jīng fù yì*), 322

T

Taiping Holy Prescriptions for Universal Relief (太平聖惠方 *tài píng shèng huì fāng*), 291
Tang Rong-Chuan, xvi
Tang Zong-Hai, 314
Ten Books of Dong Yuan, Blue Room Secret Treasures (東垣十書, 蘭室密藏 *dōng yuán shí shū, lán shì mì zàng*), 328
Textbook TCM Diagnosis (中醫診斷學 *zhōng yī zhěn duàn xué*), 324
thin mucus (飲 *yǐn*), 262, 265–266
obstructing Heart, 268, 269
thin mucus obstructing Heart, *vs.* water-dampness invading upward, 270
thin mucus patterns, 266, 268
Thousand Ducat Formulas (備急千金要方 *bèi jí qiān jīn yào fāng*), 325
Three Reason Formula (三因方 *sān yīn fāng*), 322
timidity, in Gallbladder disease patterns, 185–186
tongue tip, red in Heart patterns, 8
tongue ulcers, 8
Traditional Chinese Medicine Fundamental Theory (中醫基礎理論 *zhōng yī jī chǔ lǐ lùn*), 279, 326
transformation and transportation
coordination by Spleen and Stomach, 234
Spleen and, 58
transportation functions, Large Intestine, 165
Treasury Classic (中藏經 *zhōng cáng jīng*), 291
early pattern development theory in, 330
Kidney excess in, 325
Liver yang deficiency, 295

Treatise on Blood Syndromes (血証論), 314
Treatise on Causes and Symptoms of Diseases (諸病源候論 zhū bìng yuán hòu lùn), 330
Treatise on Cold Damage and Miscellaneous Diseases (傷寒雜病論 shāng hán zá bìng lùn), 291
    Liver yang deficiency in, 295
tremor (颤 chàn), 289
Triple Burner, no patterns of its own, 135
Triple Burner pattern identification (三焦辯證 sān jiāo biàn zhèng), 338
true fire (真火 zhēn huǒ), 110, 321
True Lineage of Medicine (醫學正傳 yī xué zhèng zhuàn), 328
true water (真水 zhēn shuǐ), 321
true yang (真陽 zhēn yáng), 110, 321
    mìng mén fire as, 323
true yin (真陰 zhēn yīn), 320–321
    mìng mén water as, 323
turbid phlegm obstructing Lung
    clinical manifestations, 48–49
    definition, 48
    diseases and treatments, 50
    etiology and pathogenesis, 48–49
turbid dampness encumbering Kidney (濕濁困腎 shī zhuó kùn shèn), 326

U

upper stifling breath (上氣 shàng qì), 30
upward gaze (竄 cuàn), 289
Urinary Bladder
    difficult urination, 197
    frequent urination, 197–198
    miscellaneous signs and symptoms, 198
    physiological characteristics and functions, 196
    urine excretion function, 196
    urine storage function, 196
Urinary Bladder damp-heat
    acupuncture, 203
    definition, 202
    diseases and treatments, 203
    etiology and pathogenesis, 202–203
    herbal formulas, 203
    vs. Small Intestine excess fire, 203–204
Urinary Bladder deficiency cold
    acupuncture, 200
    clinical manifestations, 199
    definition, 199
    diseases and treatments, 200
    etiology and pathogenesis, 199–200
    herbal formulas, 200
    vs. Kidney yang deficiency, 200–201
    vs. Small Intestine deficiency cold, 201–202
Urinary Bladder patterns, 196
    common etiological factors, 197
    common patterns, 198–199
    deficiency patterns, 199
    excess patterns, 199
    pathological changes and clinical manifestations, 197–198
    pattern summary, 205
    Urinary Bladder damp-heat, 202–203
    Urinary Bladder deficiency cold, 199–200
urinary incontinence, 197–198
urination
    difficult, 197
    frequent, 197–198
urination abnormalities, in Small Intestine disease, 157–158
urine, in Heart patterns, 8

V

vertigo (暈 yūn), 289
vomiting
    etiology and pathogenesis, 138
    as Stomach manifestation, 137–138

W

Wang Shu-He, 322, 330
warmth-dryness (溫燥 wēn zào), 41
warmth-dryness invading Lung, 42
water (水 shuǐ), 262, 264–265
    pattern etiology and pathogenesis, 265

water and food essence (水谷之精 *shuǐ gǔ zhī jīng*), 320
water metabolism
    disorders of, 262–268
    Kidney and, 110–111
    Kidney and disorders of, 114
    Lung and Kidney roles, 236
    regulation by Spleen and Kidney, 231
    Spleen and Lung regulation of, 228–229
Water qi encroaching on Heart (水氣凌心 *shuǐ qì líng xīn*)
    acupuncture, 270
    clinical manifestation, 268
    vs. cold-water shooting into Lung, 128, 273–274, 276–277
    definition, 268
    diseases and treatments, 270
    etiology and pathogenesis, 268–269
    vs. Heart yang deficiency, 271–273
    herbal formulas, 270
    vs. Kidney water invading Spleen, 276–277
    vs. Kidney yang deficiency, 276–277
    vs. Kidney yang deficiency with water effusion, 128, 276–277
water-dampness (水濕 *shuǐ shī*), 267
    invading upward, 268, 269
water-dampness immersion, *vs.* cold-dampness encumbering Spleen, 73–74
water-dampness invading upward (水濕上犯 *shuǐ shī shàng fàn*), 268
    vs. thin mucus obstructing Heart, 270
water-thin mucus (水飲 *shuǐ yǐn*), 268
wheezing (哮 *xiào*), 30
wind syndrome, 82–83
wind-cold invading Lung
    acupuncture, 37
    clinical manifestations, 36
    vs. cold invading Lung, 50–51
    vs. cold-phlegm obstructing Lung, 50–51
    definition, 36
    diseases and treatments, 37
    etiology and pathogenesis, 36–37
    vs. exterior wind-cold, 37–38
    herbal formulas, 37
    vs. wind-heat invading Lung, 39–40
wind-cold-dampness invading body surface (風寒濕襲表 *fēng hán shī xí biǎo*)
    acupuncture, 261
    clinical manifestations, 260
    definition, 260
    diseases and treatments, 261
    etiology and pathogenesis, 260
    herbal formulas, 261
    vs. wind-cold-dampness painful obstruction disorder, 261–262
wind-cold-dampness painful obstruction disorder (風寒濕痺証 *fēng hán shī bì zhèng*), 261–262
wind-heat invading Lung
    acupuncture, 39
    clinical manifestations, 38
    definition, 38
    diseases and treatments, 39
    etiology and pathogenesis, 38–39
    vs. exterior wind-heat, 40–41
    vs. heat congesting Lung, 52–53
    vs. heat-phlegm obstructing Lung, 52–53
    herbal formulas, 39
    vs. wind-cold invading Lung, 39–40
wind-phlegm disturbing upward, *vs.* Liver yang transforming wind, 103–104
wind-water invading Lung
    acupuncture, 47
    clinical manifestations, 46
    definition, 46
    diseases and treatments, 47
    etiology and pathogenesis, 46
    herbal formulas, 47
wind, clinical manifestations of internal, 289–290
Wondrous Lantern for Peering into the Origin and Development of Miscellaneous Disease (雜病源流犀燭), 324

X

Xu Ling-Tai, 324

Y

Yan He, 295
Yan Yong-He, 322
yang edema, 264
yang madness (狂 *kuáng*), 6
Yellow Emperor's Inner Classic (黃帝內經 *huáng dì nèi jīng*), 284, 314, 315
    early *zàng fǔ* pattern identification development in, 329–330
    Kidney excess concept in, 325
    Liver qi deficiency in, 290, 299
Yin deficiency generating wind
    acupuncture, 102
    clinical manifestations, 101
    definition, 101
    diseases and treatments, 102
    etiology and pathogenesis, 101
    herbal formulas, 102
yin edema, 264, 275
yin madness (癲 *diān*), 6
Yu Tuan, 322, 324

Z

zàng (臟) organs, 1
zàng fǔ organs, nature, character, pathological changes, xvi
zàng fǔ pattern identification (臟腑辯證 *zàng fǔ biàn zhèng*)
    defined, xv
    embryonic stage, 329–330
    first systematic organization, 330
    history and development, 329, 332
    as identification method, 326
    method and procedure, xvi–xvii
    promotion and widespread usage, 332
    second systematic organization and improvement, 330–331
    third systematic organization and maturation, 331–332
Zhang Jing-Yue, 322
    on Kidney deficiency, 325
    on Kidney excess, 325
    on *mìng mén* fire, 323
Zhang Lu, 322
Zhang Xichun, 291, 314
Zhang Yuan-Su, 324, 331
Zhang Zhongjing, 330, 337
    on Liver qi deficiency, 291
    on Liver yang deficiency, 295
    on Lung yang, 277
Zhao Xian-Ke, 322, 323
Zhu Danxi, 290, 294
    on Spleen yin deficiency, 313